EMERGING TECHNOLOGIES IN HEALTHCARE

MATTHEW N. O. SADIKU

ROTIMI A. K. JAIYESIMI

JOYCE B. IDEHEN

SARHAN M. MUSA

AuthorHouse™
1663 Liberty Drive
Bloomington, IN 47403
www.authorhouse.com
Phone: 833-262-8899

Because of the dynamic nature of the Internet, any web addresses or links contained in this book may have changed since publication and may no longer be valid. The views expressed in this work are solely those of the author and do not necessarily reflect the views of the publisher, and the publisher hereby disclaims any responsibility for them.

Any people depicted in stock imagery provided by Getty Images are models, and such images are being used for illustrative purposes only. Certain stock imagery © Getty Images.

This book is printed on acid-free paper.

ISBN: 978-1-6655-2843-6 (sc)
ISBN: 978-1-6655-2844-3 (hc)
ISBN: 978-1-6655-2842-9 (e)

Library of Congress Control Number: 2021911656

Print information available on the last page.

Published by AuthorHouse 09/24/2021

authorHOUSE®

Dedicated to our spouses:

Janet, Morenike, Osato, and Lama

BRIEF TABLE OF CONTENTS

1 INTRODUCTION 1

2 WEARABLE HEALTHCARE TECHNOLOGIES 15

3 TELEMEDICINE 25

4 ELECTRONIC AND MOBILE HEALTH 39

5 INTERNET OF THINGS IN HEALTHCARE 48

6 SMART HEALTHCARE 63

7 HEALTHCARE BIG DATA 80

8 ARTIFICIAL INTELLIGENCE IN HEALTHCARE 95

9 MACHINE LEARNING IN HEALTHCARE 111

10 NATURAL LANGUAGE PROCESSING IN HEALTHCARE 123

11 HEALTHCARE CHATBOTS 134

12 HEALTHCARE ROBOTICS 143

13 HEALTHCARE DRONES 155

14 AMBIENT INTELLIGENCE IN HEALTHCARE 166

15 HEALTHCARE BLOCKCHAIN 176

16 NANOMEDICINE 188

17 VIRTUAL AND AUGMENTED REALITY IN HEALTHCARE 201

18 HEALTHCARE BUSINESS INTELLIGENCE 214

19 HEALTHCARE 4.0 225

20 3D PRINTING IN HEALTHCARE 236

21 HEALTHCARE SOCIAL MEDIA 250

22 HEALTHCARE GAMIFICATION 264

23 FUTURE OF HEALTHCARE TECHNOLOGIES 278

24 INDEX 291

PREFACE

Health is regarded as one of the global challenges for mankind. Healthcare is a complex system that covers processes of diagnosis, treatment, and prevention of diseases. It constitutes a fundamental pillar of the modern society. The healthcare industry is one of the largest industries in developed nations in terms of job creation, number of employees, and expenditure. A modern healthcare system typically consists of the service providers (i.e., doctors, nurses), healthcare management (i.e. administrators), information technology, the consumers (i.e., patients), the insurance companies (payers), and pharmaceutical drug provider. Such a modernized healthcare system should provide healthcare services to people at any time and from anywhere. As a service industry, healthcare organization is always challenged with efficiencies, equities, and provision of qualities in delivering services.

Modern healthcare is technological healthcare. Technology is everywhere. Technology surrounds every aspect of 21st century life. It is in the cell phones we use, the cars we drive, and even the food we eat. Although technology and healthcare have gone hand and hand for decades, healthcare is increasingly becoming more prone to technology. The digital revolution seeks to transform healthcare and empower citizens in taking charge of their own health.

The healthcare industry is changing rapidly around the world due to breakthroughs in digital technologies that are being adopted to meet various challenges. Healthcare will become increasingly digitized in the future. Today, technology buzzwords abound— Big Data, Cloud Computing, Artificial Intelligence (AI), Machine Learning (ML), Robots, Chatbots, 3D Printing, Telemedicine, Virtual Reality (VR), Augmented Reality (AR), Blockchain, Health Wearable, and the Internet of Medical Things. These emerging technologies, while not new in other industries, are increasingly being used in healthcare because of their potential and proven value. The management of these technologies and medical devices is critical to the continued success of healthcare systems in both developed and developing nations.

This book focuses on twenty one emerging technologies in the healthcare industry. An emerging technology is one that holds the promise of creating a new economic engine and is trans-industrial. Emerging technological trends are rapidly transforming businesses in general and healthcare in particular in ways that we find hard to imagine. Artificial intelligence (AI), machine learning, robots, blockchain, cloud computing, Internet of things (IoT), and augmented & virtual reality are some of the technologies at the heart of this revolution and are covered in this book. Technologies have turned the traditional healthcare into smart healthcare. The convergence of these technologies is upon us and will have a huge impact on the patient experience.

The book is organized into 23 chapters. The first chapter is an introduction to emerging technologies. Chapter 2 covers applications of wearable technologies in healthcare. Chapter 3 discusses telemedicine, which refers to the remote delivery of clinical care through communication technologies. Chapter 4 discusses the two concepts of ehealth and mhealth. Electronic health (ehealth) refers to the use of information and communication technology to enable health care. Mobile health (or mHealth) refers to the practice of medicine via mobile devices such as mobile phones, tablet computers, personal digital assistants, and wearable devices. Chapter 5 provides an introduction to the use of Internet of things in the healthcare domain. Internet of things (IoT) is the global interconnection of several heterogeneous devices.

Chapter 6 is about smart healthcare, which involves using smart technologies for health purposes. Chapter 7 is on big data analysis in the healthcare sector. Big data refers to massive amount of data generated through digitization of all sorts of information, including health records. In chapter 8, we discuss artificial intelligence, which is the use of computer science to develop machines that can be trained to learn, reason, communicate, and make humanlike decisions Chapter 9 is on machine learning, which is a branch of artificial intelligence that is based on the notion that systems can learn from data, identify patterns, and make decisions with minimal human intervention. In chapter 10, we cover natural language processing, another branch of artificial intelligence, which is used for extracting the elements of concerns from raw plain text information. In chapter 11, we address chatbots, which are artificial intelligence programs designed to simulate human conversation via text or speech. Chapter 12 provides an introduction to healthcare robots and their applications.

In chapter 13 discusses the use of drones in the field of healthcare. Drones are autonomous or remotely controlled multipurpose aerial vehicles driven by aerodynamic forces. Chapter 14 is on the application of ambient intelligence in healthcare. Ambient intelligence refers to electronic environments that are sensitive and responsive to the presence of people (patients, doctors, nurses, and informal caregivers).

Chapter 15 is on the use of blockchain in healthcare. Blockchain consists of a shared or distributed database used to maintain a growing list of transactions. Chapter16 is on nanomedicine, which is essentially the medical application of nanotechnology to the diagnosis, management, and treatment of disease. In chapter 17, we explain their two concepts of concepts of virtual and augmented reality technologies and their uses in healthcare. Virtual reality is a computer simulation system that can create and simulate virtual worlds. Augmented reality refers to technology that overlays information and virtual objects on real-world scenes in real-time. Chapter 18 covers the use of business intelligence in healthcare. Business intelligence refers to the tools and systems that play a major role in the planning process of an organization. Chapter 19 deals with Healthcare 4.0, which is essentially the healthcare extension of Industry 4.0 in healthcare system. In chapter 20, we provide an introduction on how 3DP is used in healthcare industry. 3D printing is the means of producing three dimensional solid objects from a digital model. Chapter 21 provides an introduction on how, where, and why social media are being used in the healthcare sector. Social media can be regarded as the collection of Internet-based tools that help a user to connect, collaborate, and communicate with others in real time. Chapter 22 in on how gamification is used in healthcare. Gamification (or game-based approach) is basically adapting game-design elements (fun, play, transparency, reward, incentive, competition, and challenge) and game-thinking to non-game services and applications. The last chapter focuses on the future of these emerging technologies.

We would like to thank Dr. Kayode Shope and his colleagues for reviewing the manuscript.

DETAILED TABLE OF CONTENTS

CHAPTER 1 INTRODUCTION 1

1.1 INTRODUCTION 1
1.2 CONCEPT OF EMERGING TECHNOLOGY 2
1.3 EMERGING HEALTHCARE TECHNOLOGIES 2
1.4 APPLICATIONS OF EMERGING HEALTHCARE TECHNOLOGIES 8
1.5 BENEFITS 10
1.6 CHALLENGES 11
1.7 CONCLUSION 11
REFERENCES 12

CHAPTER 2 WEARABLE HEALTHCARE TECHNOLOGIES 15

2.1 INTRODUCTION 15
2.2 WEARABLES 15
2.3 WEARABLES IN HEALTHCARE 17
2.4 APPLICATIONS OF WEARIABLES IN HEALTHCARE 18
2.5 BENEFITS 21
2.6 CHALLENGES 22
2.7 CONCLUSION 23
REFERENCES 23

CHAPTER 3 TELEMEDICINE 25

3.1 INTRODUCTION 25
3.2 CONCEPT OF TELEMEDICINE 26
3.3 TYPES OF TELEMEDICINE 27
3.4 APPLICATIONS OF TELEMEDICINE 28
3.5 BENEFITS 34
3.6 CHALLENGES 35
3.7 CONCLUSION 36
REFERENCES 36

CHAPTER 4   ELECTRONIC AND MOBILE HEALTH **39**

4.1 INTRODUCTION 39
4.2 CONCEPT OF ELECTRONIC HEALTH 40
4.3 CONCEPT OF MOBILE HEALTH 40
4.4 APPLICATIONS...43
4.5 BENEFITS... 44
4.6 CHALLENGES 44
4.7 CONCLUSION... 46
REFERENCES.. 46

CHAPTER 5   INTERNET OF THINGS IN HEALTHCARE **48**

5.1 INTRODUCTION 48
5.2 OVERVIEW ON INTERNET OF THINGS...................................49
5.3 WHY HEALTHCARE NEEDS IOT 51
5.4 INTERNET OF MEDICAL THINGS 53
5.5 APPLICATIONS OF IoT IN HEALTHCARE 54
5.6 BENEFITS..56
5.7 CHALLENGES..58
5.8 CONCLUSION 60
REFERENCE 60

CHAPTER 6   SMART HEALTHCARE... **63**

6.1 INTRODUCTION 63
6.2 CONCEPT OF SMART HEALTHCARE 64
6.3 ENABLING TECHNOLOGIES 66
6.4 FEATURES OF SMART HEALTHCARE 68
6.5 APPLICATIONS AND SERVICES 69
6.6 SMART HOSPITALS 70
6.8 SMART MEDICATION...73
6.9 BENEFITS..74
6.10 CHALLENGES...75
6.11 CONCLUSION 76
REFERENCES...77

CHAPTER 7   HEALTHCARE BIG DATA **80**

7.1 INTRODUCTION 80
7.2 WHY BIG DATA IN HEALTHCARE 81
7.3 BIG DATA CHARACTERISTICS 82

7.4 BIG DATA ANALYTICS 83
7.5 BIG DATA ETHICS 84
7.6 APLICATIONS IN HEALTHCARE..85
BENEFITS.. 88
CHALLENGES 89
CONCLUSION 91
REFERENCES..92

CHAPTER 8   ARTIFICIAL INTELLIGENCE IN HEALTHCARE 95

8.1 INTRODUCTION 95
8.2 OVERVIEW ON ARTIFICIAL INTELLIGENCE.............................96
8.3 APPLICATIONS IN HEALTHCARE 100
8.4 INTERNATIONAL TRENDS..103
8.5 BENEFITS..105
8.6 CHALLENGES 105
8.7 CONCLUSION...107
REFERENCES..107

CHAPTER 9   MACHINE LEARNING IN HEALTHCARE 111

9.1 INTRODUCTION 111
9.2 OVERVIEW ON MACHINE LEARNING 112
9.3 EXTREME LEARNING MACHINE 114
9.4 APPLICATIONS OF ML IN HEALTHCARE 115
9.5 BENEFITS..118
9.6 CHALLENGES 118
9.7 CONCLUSION...119
REFERENCES.. 120

CHAPTER 10 NATURAL LANGUAGE PROCESSING IN HEALTHCARE.......... 123

10.1 INTRODUCTION 123
10.2 NLP BASICS 124
10.3 DIFFERENT ASPECTS OF NLP 125
10.4 APPLICATIONS IN HEALHCARE...126
10.5 GLOBAL HEALTHCARE NLP 129
10.6 BENEFITS...130
10.7 CHALLENGES..131
10.8 CONCLUSION..131
REFERENCES...131

CHAPTER 11 HEALTHCARE CHATBOTS **134**

11.1 INTRODUCTION 134
11.2 CONCEPT OF CHATBOTS..134
11.3 APPLICATIONS IN HEALTHCARE 136
11.4 GLOBAL HEALTHCARE CHATBOTS 139
11.5 BENEFITS 140
11.6 CHALLENGES...140
11.7 CONCLUSION 141
REFERENCE 141

CHAPTER 12 HEALTHCARE ROBOTICS **143**

12.1 INTRODUCTION 143
12.2 WHAT IS A ROBOT?...144
12.3 APPLICATIONS..145
14.4 GLOBAL HEALTHCARE ROBOTICS 148
12.4 BENEFITS 150
14.5 CHALLENGES...150
12.6 CONCLUSION 151
REFERENCES..152

CHAPTER 13 HEALTHCARE DRONES **155**

13.1 INTRODUCTION 155
13.2 CONCEPT OF DRONES 156
13.3 APLICATIONS 157
13.4 GLOBAL HEALTHCARE DRONES..160
13.4 BENEFITS 162
13.5 CHALLENGES 163
13.6 CONCLUSION 164
REFERENCES..164

CHAPTER 14 AMBIENT INTELLIGENCE IN HEALTHCARE.................................**166**

14.1 INTRODUCTION 166
14.2 CONCEPT OF AMBIENT INTELLIGENCE...167
14.3 ENABLING TECHNOLOGIES..168
14.4 APPLICATIONS..169
14.5 GLOBAL AMBIENT INTELLIGENCE IN HEALTHCARE 171
14.6 BENEFITS 172
14.7 CHALLENGES...172

14.8 CONCLUSION...173

REFERENCES..174

CHAPTER 15 HEALTHCARE BLOCKCHAIN...**176**

15.1 INTRODUCTION...176

15.2 OVERVIEW OF BLOCKCHAIN...177

15.3 TYPES OF BLOCKCHAINS...179

15.4 APPLICATIONS..180

15.5 GLOBAL BLOCKCHAIN HEALTHCARE....................................182

15.6 BENEFITS...182

15.7 CHALLENGES..184

15.8 CONCLUSION..185

REFERENCES..185

CHAPTER 16 NANOMEDICINE..**188**

16.1 INTRODUCTION...188

16.2 OVERVIEW OF NANOMEDICINE...190

16.3 APPLICATIONS..190

16.4 NANOMEDICINE FOR GLOBAL HEALTHCARE......................193

16.5 BENEFITS...195

16.6 CHALLENGES...196

16.7 CONCLUSION..197

REFERENCES..198

CHAPTER 17 VIRTUAL AND AUGMENTED REALITY IN HEALTHCARE........**201**

17.1 INTRODUCTION...201

17.2 CONCEPT OF VIRTUAL REALITY...202

17.3 CONCEPT OF AUGMENTED REALITY......................................203

17.4 RELATIONSHIP BETWEEN VIRTUAL AND AUGMENTED REALITY...........205

17.5 APPLICATIONS OF VIRTUAL REALITY IN HEALTHCARE......206

17.6 APPLICATIONS OF AUGMENTED REALITY IN HEALTHCARE......208

17.7 GLOBAL AUGMENTED REALITY AND VIRTUAL REALITY........209

17.7 BENEFITS...209

17.8 CHALLENGES...210

17.9 CONCLUSION..211

REFERENCES..211

CHAPTER 18 HEALTHCARE BUSINESS INTELLIGENCE.......................**214**

18.1 INTRODUCTION 214
18.2 BUSINESS INTELLIGENCE CONCEPT 215
18.3 BUSINESS INTELLIGENCE IN HEALTHCARE....................216
18.4 APPLICATIONS..217
18.5 GLOBAL HEALTHCARE BUSINESS INTELLIGENCE 219
18.6 BENEFITS 220
18.7 CHALLENGES...221
18.7 CONCLUSION 222
REFERENCES..223

CHAPTER 19 HEALTHCARE 4.0...**225**

19.1 INTRODUCTION 225
19.2 FUNDAMENTALS OF INDUSTRY 4.0...................................226
19.3 CONCEPT OF HEALTHCARE 4.0 227
19.4 APPLICATIONS..228
1.5 GLOBAL HEALTHCARE 4.0..230
19.6 CHALLENGES..232
19.7 HEALTHCARE 5.0 232
19.8 CONCLUSION 233
REFERENCES..234

CHAPTER 20 3D PRINTING IN HEALTHCARE...........................**236**

20.1 INTRODUCTION 236
20.2 CONCEPT OF 3D PRINTING 236
20.3 APPLICATIONS..239
20.4 BENEFITS..242
20.5 CHALLENGES 243
20.6 GLOBAL 3D PRINTING 245
20.7 4D PRINTING 245
20.8 CONCLUSION 247
REFERENCES.. 248

CHAPTER 21 HEALTHCARE SOCIAL MEDIA.............................**250**

21.1 INTRODUCTION 250
21.2 SOCIAL MEDIA BASICS 251
21.3 POPULAR SOCIAL MEDIA..253
21.4 APPLICATIONS..254

21.5 BENEFITS 256

21.6 CHALLENGES...258

21.7 GLOBAL SOCIAL MEDIA IN HEALTHCARE 260

21.8 CONCLUSION 261

REFERENCES...261

CHAPTER 22 HEALTHCARE GAMIFICATION **264**

22.1 INTRODUCTION 264

22.2 CONCEPT OF GAMIFICATION 265

22.3 COMPONENTS OF GAMIFICATION 265

22.4 APPLICATIONS..267

22.5 BENEFITS..271

22.6 CHALLENGES 271

22.7 GLOBAL HEALTHCARE GAMIFICATION 273

22.8 CONCLUSION 275

REFERENCES...275

CHAPTER 23 FUTURE OF HEALTHCARE TECHNOLOGIES 278

23.1 INTRODUCTION 278

23.2 TRENDS IN HEALTHCARE TECHNOLOGIES............................279

23.3 FUTURE OF TECHNOLOGY IN HEALTHCARE..........................279

23.4 GLOBAL HEATHCARE TRENDS 283

23.5 FUTURE OF GLOBAL HEALTHCARE TECHNOLOGY 284

23.6 CHALLENGES 285

23.7 CONCLUSION... 288

REFERENCES... 288

INDEX **291**

ABOUT THE AUTHORS

A. **Matthew N. O. Sadiku** received his B. Sc. degree in 1978 from Ahmadu Bello University, Zaria, Nigeria and his M.Sc. and Ph.D. degrees from Tennessee Technological University, Cookeville, TN in 1982 and 1984 respectively. From 1984 to 1988, he was an assistant professor at Florida Atlantic University, Boca Raton, FL, where he did graduate work in computer science. From 1988 to 2000, he was at Temple University, Philadelphia, PA, where he became a full professor. From 2000 to 2002, he was with Lucent/Avaya, Holmdel, NJ as a system engineer and with Boeing Satellite Systems, Los Angeles, CA as a senior scientist. He is presently a professor emeritus of electrical and computer engineering at Prairie View A&M University, Prairie View, TX.

He is the author of over 990 professional papers and over 90 books including *Elements of Electromagnetics* (Oxford University Press, 7th ed., 2018), *Fundamentals of Electric Circuits* (McGraw-Hill, 7th ed., 2021, with C. Alexander), *Computational Electromagnetics with MATLAB* (CRC Press, 4th ed., 2019), *Principles of Modern Communication Systems* (Cambridge University Press, 2017, with S. O. Agbo), and *Emerging Internet-based Technologies* (CRC Press, 2019). In addition to the engineering books, he has written Christian books including *Secrets of Successful Marriages*, *How to Discover God's Will for Your Life*, and commentaries on all the books of the New Testament Bible. Some of his books have been translated into French, Korean, Chinese (and Chinese Long Form in Taiwan), Italian, Portuguese, and Spanish.

He was the recipient of the 2000 McGraw-Hill/Jacob Millman Award for outstanding contributions in the field of electrical engineering. He was also the recipient of Regents Professor award for 2012-2013 by the Texas A&M University System. He is a registered professional engineer and a fellow of the Institute of Electrical and Electronics Engineers (IEEE) "for contributions to computational electromagnetics and engineering education." He was the IEEE Region 2 Student Activities Committee Chairman. He was an associate editor for IEEE Transactions on Education. He is also a member of Association for Computing Machinery (ACM) and American Society of Engineering Education (ASEE). His current research interests are in the areas of computational electromagnetic, computer networks, and engineering education. His works can be found in his autobiography, *My Life and Work* (Trafford Publishing, 2017) or his website: www.matthew-sadiku.com. He currently resides in West Palm Beach, California. He can be reached via email at sadiku@ieee.org

B. **Rotimi A. K. Jaiyesimi,** a 1978 medical graduate of the University of Ibadan, Nigeria, is the Associate Medical Director for Patient Safety and Consultant Obstetrician and Gynaecologist at Mid and South Essex University Hospitals, England. He is a Fellow of the West African College of Surgeons and Fellow of Royal College of Obstetricians and Gynaecologists. He holds a master's degree in Business Administration from the Newcastle Business School and a master's degree in medical law from Northumbria University Law School, England. He is an International Health expert and medical expert witness. He has an interest in the use of technologies to improve patient care and experience. An innovator and a member of the Faculty of Clinical Informatics, he was the brain behind the development of a nouvelle real time electronic tool utilized for mortality review of in-hospital deaths, aiding learning from clinical decisions. This innovative tool won the HSJ National Award for the Value and Improvement in Patient Information Management. He is a Fellow of the Institute of Information Management (FIIM) and Senior Fellow of the Faculty of Medical Leadership and Management. He was a member of the College of Experts of the UK National Institute of Health Research Health Technology Assessments Trials Board. Though a full time clinician, he had an interest in academia and has published 60 scientific papers, chapters in books and presented at international scientific conferences. He was appointed visiting professor, Faculty of Health Sciences, University of Sunderland (2014-2017) and is currently visiting professor, Faculty of Law, University of Ibadan, Nigeria. A multi-award winner, he was the recipient of the Excellence Award, celebrating excellent contribution to the UK National Health Service at 70 years, Nigerian National Health Care Professionals (UK) and a Lifetime Achievement Award, University of Ibadan, Nigeria. His email address is jaiyesimi@obs-gyn.org.

C. Joyce B. Idehen graduated from Prairie View A&M University in 2014 with a Bachelor of Science in Nursing and worked as a Registered Nurse for 2.5 years in Houston, Texas. She is currently a 4th year medical student at American University of Antigua – College of Medicine. Her wish is to specialize in Family Medicine. Passionate about health equity, diversifying the face of medicine, preventative care, women's health, and mental health, she eventually intends to implement such things while advocating for her patients in private practice. Joyce is currently working on research projects on the relationship between the COVID-19 virus and psychiatry and the impact of systematic racism on black women with breast cancer.

D. Sarhan M. Musa is a professor in Electrical and Computer Engineering Department at Prairie View A&M University. He holds a Ph.D. in Electrical Engineering from the City University of New York. He is the founder and director of Prairie View Networking Academy (PVNA), Texas. He is LTD Sprint and Boeing Welliver Fellow. Professor Musa is internationally known through his research, scholarly work, and publications. He has given several invited talks at international conferences. He has received several prestigious national and university awards and research grants. He is a senior member of the IEEE. He has served as the member of technical program committee and steering committee for several major journals and conferences. Professor Musa has written more than a dozen books on various areas in Electrical and Computer Engineering. His current research interests include artificial intelligence, machine learning, data analytics, Internet of things, wireless network, data center protocols, energy and power system, and computational methods.

CHAPTER 1

INTRODUCTION

*"Modern technology has become a total phenomenon for civilization, the
defining force of a new social order in which efficiency is no longer an option
but a necessity imposed on all human activity."* – Jacques Ellul

1.1 INTRODUCTION

We live in the digital age where everything is touched and connected by technology. Our homes, our cars, and our jobs are all connected to technology. Technology is getting better, smaller, and faster. It is becoming more and more in demand in every sector of the economy, particularly in healthcare. Technology drives healthcare more than any other force. It has always been an integral part of healthcare delivery, enabling health care providers to use various tools to detect, diagnose, treat, and monitor patients. Typical examples of medical technologies include medications, medical devices, and biotechnology products. Technologies in the healthcare change at a fast pace from cutting edge to ubiquity [1].

The pace of change in healthcare technology is unprecedented, but human nature does not change at these technological timescales. There have been dramatic technological changes in healthcare. Any sufficiently advanced technology is indistinguishable from magic. Most of these new technologies are modern magic: new pharmaceuticals that change moods, infusion pumps, and robotic keyhole surgery [2].

Health technologies comprise of all the devices, medications, vaccines, processes, procedures, and systems designed to streamline healthcare operations, lower costs, and enhance quality of care. Technology is drastically changing and improving healthcare, from anesthetics and antibiotics to MRI scanners and radiotherapy. Although emerging healthcare technologies will not fix all healthcare problems, they can improve the practice, decision making, and management of healthcare. Some of these technologies will change the practice of healthcare and transform our whole approach to disease management. It is well known that hospitals adopt new technologies that enhance their service capabilities and enable them to attract and retain physicians who use the technologies [3].

This chapter provides introduction on emerging technologies in healthcare and also an introduction to the book. It begins by discussing the concept of emerging technology. Then it covers several emerging technologies in healthcare. It discusses some of the applications of the emerging technologies. It presents some of the benefits and challenges of the emerging technologies. The last section concludes with some comments.

1.2 CONCEPT OF EMERGING TECHNOLOGY

We live in the digital age where everything is touched and connected by technology. Our homes, our cars, and our jobs are all connected to technology. Technology is getting better, smaller, and faster. It is becoming more and more in demand in every sector of the economy, particularly in healthcare. The pace of change in healthcare technology is unprecedented, but human nature does not change at these technological timescales. The main stakeholders in healthcare include insurance companies, big pharma, doctors, managers, suppliers, builders, and the government. There have been dramatic technological changes in healthcare.

Emerging technology (ET) lacks a consensus on what classifies them as "emergent." It is a relative term because one may see a technology as emerging and others may not see it the same way. It is a term that is often used to describe a new technology. A technology is still emerging if it is not yet a "must-have" [4]. An emerging technology is the one that holds the promise of creating a new economic engine and is trans-industrial.

ET is used in different areas such as media, healthcare, business, science, or education. Emerging healthcare technologies cannot be fully exploited without a clinical team to shape the therapeutic response, where management within hospitals have been able to do over the years with their multidisciplinary clinical workforce. How hospitals and policymakers respond to these emerging technologies will help determine whether hospitals remain at the center of the US healthcare system. Some US hospitals have remarkably responded to these new technologies and adapted their services to incorporate them.

1.3 EMERGING HEALTHCARE TECHNOLOGIES

Emerging technologies in healthcare include information technology, nanotechnology/nanomedicine, biotechnology, cloud computing, cognitive computing, Internet of things, augmented/virtual reality, global positioning system (GPS), radio frequency identification (RFID), microwave, voice search, voice recognition, chatbots, social media, blockchain, 3D telepresence technology, 3D printing, wireless technology, mobile technology, 3D ultrasound, biometrics, genetics and genomics, electronic health records, magnetic resonance imaging (MRI), wearable computing devices, drones, robotics, and artificial intelligence. Of the several emerging technologies, the following examples stand out [5,6]:

- *Wireless Technology:* Wireless computing devices cover the healthcare landscape. They appear to be a natural emerging technology for healthcare professionals. This includes laptops, wireless phones, tablets/ipads, and personal digital assistants will find their way into the hands of the caregivers as well as the patients. Wireless-equipped healthcare systems can remotely and continuously monitor the patients' health condition at home. These systems can improve patients' life quality by decreasing the dependability on caregivers and reduce healthcare expenses. Advances in wireless technology and smart devices are creating a pervasive wireless environment that can address a wide range of health-related challenges and provide health monitoring without constraining the activities of the user. Wireless body area network (WBAN) is in the early stages of development, but it is promising for future healthcare applications.

It has the potential to revolutionize healthcare delivery in ambulances, emergency rooms, operation rooms, outpatient clinics, and home health [7].

- *Mobile Technology:* This technology would allow medical practice from anywhere, any time, and from any device. It is touching virtually every aspect of our lives. Mobile devices include tablets and smartphones. The use of mobile devices in the healthcare is recent and it is still in the infancy stage. It has the potential for managing chronic illnesses of the aging population [8]. The rise of the Internet age and the proliferation of smart devices have brought profound changes for the practice of medicine. Mobile health (or mHealth) refers to the practice of medicine via mobile devices such as mobile phones, tablet computers, personal digital assistants (PDAs), and wearable devices. It integrates mobile technology with the health delivery with the promise of promoting a better health and improving efficiency. Patients are beginning to use mobile technology to monitor and track their health.

- *Wearable Technology:* This technology allows wearing light weight sensors unobtrusively using regular clothes. Wearable devices can monitor individual's physiological functions 24 hours a day. 3-D printing technology is reaching the development of wearable devices. The major concern is that wearable devices pose issues with user privacy and security [9].

- *Microwave:* Microwave is an emerging technology that is used to treat biohazardous waste that comes from healthcare facilities. There are four major processes for the treatment of biohazardous components in healthcare waste: thermal (e.g. incineration, microwave), chemical, irradiative, and biological. Microwave technology has the potential to save energy costs in comparison to the more widely used technologies [10].

- *Artificial intelligence* (AI): This is a field of computer science that is concerned with designing systems to do things that would require intelligence of humans. Today, artificial intelligence is shorthand for any task a machine can perform just as well as, if not better than, humans. AI technologies are now increasingly being been adopted in many areas of the public sector such as education, social interventions, and healthcare. AI in healthcare refers to the application of AI technology in the diagnosis and treatment of patients. AI is being applied in healthcare to review mammograms, monitor early stage heart disease, and enable accurate decision-making among medical providers. Today, AI is already being used in medicine in several other areas such as decision support systems, laboratory information systems, robotic surgical systems, therapy, and reducing human error [11].

- *Robotics:* Robots have been playing an increasingly important role in our daily life. They are indispensable in many industries. Robotics deals with the design, construction, operation, and application of robots. Robots are becoming an integral part of the healthcare toolkit. Robots play an important role in healthcare as they can improve diagnosis, lower the number of medical errors, and improve the overall quality and effectiveness of healthcare delivery. They hold the promise of addressing major healthcare issues in surgery, diagnostics, prosthetics, physical and mental therapy, monitoring, and support. Robots have the potential to provide assistance to healthcare providers in daily caregiving tasks, such as transportation, telemedicine, and providing services that can create a new level of quality healthcare by providing experts to patient. A wide range of robots are developed to serve different purposes within the healthcare environment. This results in various kinds of healthcare robots such as surgical robots, logistics robots, disinfectant robots, cleaning robots, pill robots, laboratory robots, rehabilitation robots, nursing robots, telepresence robots, therapy robots, assistive robots, robotic prosthetic limbs, diagnostics robots, and many other types [12]. Robotics can perform the following tasks [13]:

- ➢ Help with surgeries, e.g. position a digital microscope or cut bone.
- ➢ Monitor patient vital signs and alert medical staff when there are issues.
- ➢ Disinfect patient rooms and operating environments.
- ➢ Deliver medical supplies, meals, and health records.
- ➢ Automatically enter information into an EHR.
- ➢ Scan health records to assist with the detection, diagnosis, and treatment of diseases.
- ➢ Locate a vessel and draw blood.
- ➢ Take samples and then transport, analyze, and store them.
- ➢ Prepare and dispense medications in labs.
- ➢ Do repetitive tasks like performing blood tests.
- ➢ Package medical devices to reduce risk of contamination.
- ➢ Help paraplegics move and administer physical therapy.
- ➢ Help with personal care and training.
- ➢ Converse and interact with people.

A typical robot for surgery is shown in Figure 1.1 [14].

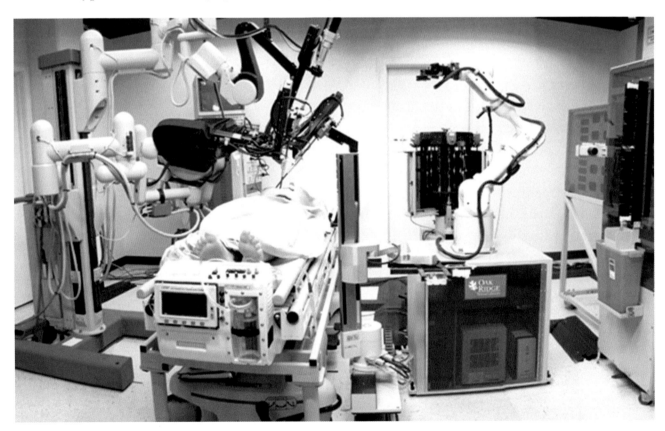

Figure 1.1 A robot for surgery [14].

- *3D Printing:* 3D printing, also known as additive manufacturing (AM) or rapid prototyping (RP), is the means of producing three dimensional solid objects from a digital model. It has been regarded as one of the pillars of the third industrial revolution. It was invented by Charles Hull in the early 1980s. Since then it has been used in manufacturing, automotive, electronics, aviation, aerospace, consumer products, education, entertainment, medicine, space missions, the military, chemical and jewelry industries. It is a technology perfectly tailored for the healthcare industry. It offers a range of precision healthcare solutions, including tissue and organ fabrication, creation of customized prosthetics, implants, and anatomical models, drug delivery, and testing, as well as in clinical practice. Benefits of 3DP in healthcare include the customization and personalization of medical products, drugs, and equipment; cost-effectiveness; increased productivity; the democratization of design and manufacturing; and enhanced collaboration. Hospitals could potentially create items on demand and this would significantly alter the healthcare supply chain [15]. Figure 1.2 illustrates 3D printed drug [16].

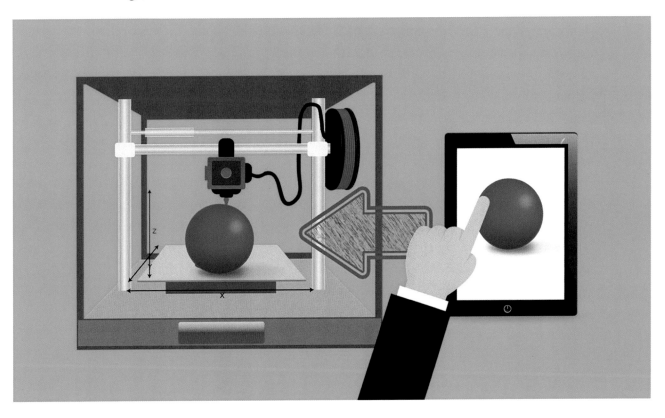

Figure 1.2 3D printed drug [16].

- *Augmented/Virtual Reality:* Virtual reality (VR) is a highly interactive, computer-based multimedia environment in which the user becomes the participant in a computer-generated world. For example, surgical residents can use virtual overlays of the circulatory system to help direct them during procedures. It can be used to train surgeons in a realistic and low-risk simulated environment. Billing agents can use "smart glasses" to see patient insurance and billing information when they are away from their computers. It can help reduce the amount of anxiety a patient is feeling before and after surgery, and offers therapeutic potential and rehabilitation for acute pain and anxiety disorders [17].

- *Nanomedicine*: Nanomedicine, a marriage of nanotechnology and medicine, is taking the place of nanotechnology in the fight against unmet diseases. Nanotechnology is the science of small things or the manipulation of matter on an atomic or molecular scale. Nanomedicine is essentially the medical application of nanotechnology to the diagnosis, management, and treatment of disease. It is regarded as one of the most promising technologies of the 21st century. It seeks to manufacture drugs and other products that are packaged into nanoscale systems for improved delivery. The most prominent area of nanomedical research and drug approvals is cancer treatment. The application of nanomedicine, particularly in cancer treatment, promises to have a profound impact on health care. Medications can be more efficiently delivered to the site of action using nanotechnology [18].

- *Cloud Computing:* This is an on-demand and self-service Internet infrastructure that offers large scalable computing and storage, data sharing, on-demand anytime and anywhere access to resources. The healthcare industry has been hesitant in embracing the cloud computing because of the concern of data privacy and integrity. Cloud computing is changing the way healthcare providers to deliver services to their patients. It may provide scalable and cost-effective healthcare services. Healthcare providers are increasingly facing keen competition and are compelled do more for less. They are rapidly turning to the cloud to address the business and patient needs. On the patient side, people are accustomed with managing their own healthcare needs. Application areas include emergency healthcare, home healthcare, assistive healthcare, telemedicine, storage, sharing and processing of large medical resources [19].

- *Internet of Things* (IoT): This allows all entities to be connected to each other through wired or wireless communication means. IoT has been gaining popularity rapidly since its inception into the IT world and is being used in healthcare, education, gaming, finance, transportation, and several more. The healthcare industry is among the fastest to adopt the Internet of things. Applications of IoT in healthcare are numerous, ranging from remote monitoring to smart sensors and medical device integration. The applications benefit patients, families, nurses, and physicians. IoT healthcare is applicable in many medical instruments such as ECG monitors, glucose level sensing, and oxygen concentration detection. It has been long predicted that IoT healthcare will revolutionize the healthcare sector in terms of social benefits, penetration, accessible care, and cost-efficiency [20]. A typical IoT-based healthcare system is shown in Figure 1.3 [9]. As an extension of IoT, the Internet of Medical Things (IoMT) is the technology that connects the medical devices to the healthcare IT systems. It is an infrastructure consisting of connected medical devices, sensors, software applications, and healthcare IT systems that focus on medical testing, monitoring, and diagnostics. IoMT devices often run autonomously since they are programmed to operate within a specific workflow and to send and receive data automatically. IoMT is transforming healthcare operations [21].

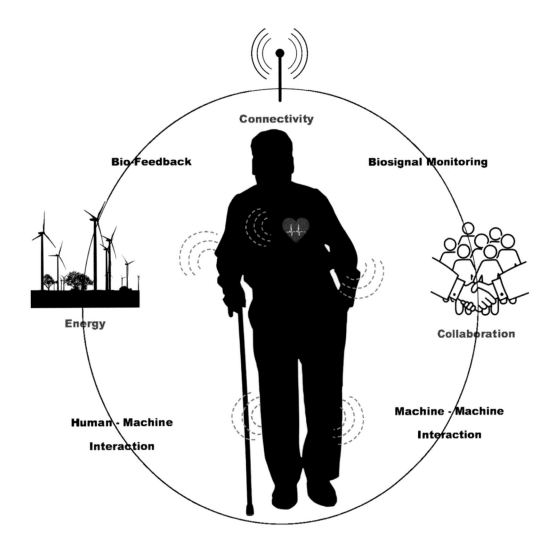

Figure 1.3 A typical IoT-based healthcare system [9].

- *Blockchain*: This technology consists of a shared or distributed database used to maintain a growing list of transactions called blocks. With blockchain (BC), transaction records are stored and distributed across all network participants rather than at a central location. Blockchain in healthcare will be in clinical trial records, regulatory compliance, and medical records. The technology can help medical practitioners make better and more accurate diagnoses and prescribe more effective treatments. The goal of BC is to give patients and their providers one-stop access to their entire medical history across all providers. Blockchain is able to securely, privately, and comprehensively track patient health records. It makes electronic medical records more efficient, disintermediated, and secure. It also makes health information exchanges (HIE) more secure, efficient, and interoperable [22].

- *Social media*: Advances in technology are impacting the future of healthcare, being more social than ever before. Social media refers to Internet-based and mobile-based tools that allow individuals to communicate with things. This is king in healthcare marketing. The Internet has empowered individuals to share health information and interact using social media. Social media are basically web-based tools used for computer-mediated communication. It is a powerful tool that healthcare professionals can use to communicate and interact with patients. It has become an undeniable force that healthcare industry must reckon with. Although social media is still evolving, it has made a profound impact on the healthcare industry [23].

These technologies are selected because they pose both the risk of disruption and reward of reducing costs. Some of them are illustrated in Figure 1.4 [24].

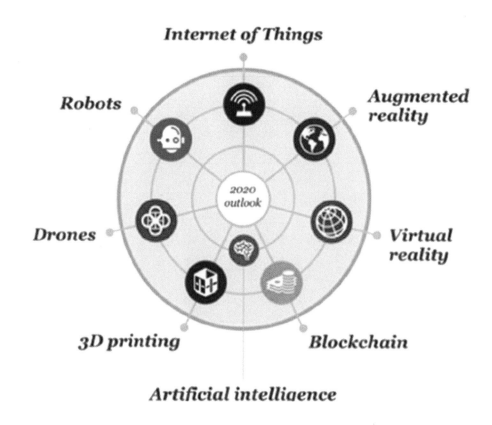

Figure 1.4 Some emerging healthcare technologies [24].

1.4 APPLICATIONS OF EMERGING HEALTHCARE TECHNOLOGIES

Emerging technologies are usually more accessible, less expensive, and easier to learn than their predecessors. The technologies can be used for prevention of diseases, diagnostics, effective healthcare delivery, rehabilitation, improving quality of life for patients, reducing morbidity and fatality rates, treating chronic deceases, and enhancing healthcare access [25]. Emerging technologies have been noted as potential mechanisms for reducing medication errors. An amalgamation of these technologies will be needed to have an end-to-end solution for emerging healthcare applications.

The emerging technologies presented above can be applied to every aspect of healthcare. Some popular areas include the following [26]:

- *Regenerative Medicine:* This basically involves culturing and grafting human tissues, both artificial and cultured. Remarkable advances have already been made in culturing and grafting human cells to repair burn damage. Regenerative medicine has the potential to heal or replace tissues and organs due to age, disease, damage, trauma, or congenital defects. This field tends to regenerate damaged tissues and organs in the body by stimulating previously irreparable organs to heal themselves [27].

• *Remote Patient Monitoring:* A rapidly emerging area of service in healthcare is in remote monitoring of patients with some degree of unstable clinical risk. It involves having small sensors placed on body of a patient to monitor various health parameters like blood pressure, heart beat, temperature, and prolonged electrocardiogram. The potential advantages of remote monitoring of implantable devices could include timely monitoring of clinical events and symptoms. The time spent by medical staff can be saved [28].

• *Personalized Healthcare*: Personalized healthcare is healthcare tailored to suit individual patients. It is one of the areas that benefit from IoT. Emerging technologies that provide personalized healthcare services to patients include [29]: (1) Pattern recognition methods for prediction and diagnosis of diseases, (2) Body sensor networks. (3) Algorithms for the analysis of patient-specific physiological signals, (4) Ontologies and context-based electronic health records (EHRs), (5) Modeling of physiological systems, (6) Monitoring and treatment support tools for chronic diseases, (7) Patient-specific multiscale modeling, (8) Integrated e-health solutions. Personalized healthcare offers numerous benefits to medical professionals and patients especially elderly people. It makes it possible for doctors and medical staff to monitor patients remotely and for patients to receive instant treatment [30]. They can obtain patient's body parameters remotely and at regular interval. The IoT devices gather information from patients and share the information with medical professionals. Also, 3D printed pharmaceuticals could accelerate mass customization of medicine and innovation.

• *Chronic Diseases:* A chronic disease is a persistent disease process that has a long-lasting effects on the human body. Common chronic diseases include hypertension, rheumatoid arthritis, diabetes mellitus, and Human Immunodeficiency Virus (HIV). The aging population is growing rapidly and emerging technologies can meet the healthcare needs of the elderly. The aging population has led to an increase prevalence of chronic diseases. Besides aging, other major causes of chronic diseases are unhealthy lifestyles which include poor food choices, tobacco use, lack of exercise, and mental stress. The escalated costs of treatment poses the need to focus on prevention and improved management of chronic diseases. Using emerging technologies to study chronic diseases is a new trend, because they allow for deeper analysis, more accurate predictions, and better performance than traditional tools [31].

• *Electronic Health Records* (EHR): The electronic health record (EHR) is a digital record of a patient's health history, and is most likely the simplest application of healthcare technology. EHR may be made up of records from many sources such as hospitals, providers, clinics, and public health agencies. Health records continue to evolve as a result of technology. Any changes in documentation of care have a significant impact on nursing practice. EHR is available 24/7 and has built-in safeguards to assure patient health information confidentiality and security [6]. Emerging technologies have been recommended as potential mechanisms for reducing medication errors.

• *Telemedicine:* Telemedicine literally means "healing at a distance." This is an important core technology for healthcare delivery. Telemedicine's major goal is to bring medical services to isolated, geographically dispersed, and physically confined persons unable to reach a physician within reasonable time or distance. This new modality of healthcare delivery is gradually finding its way into the mainstream medicine. Telemedicine uses existing (or enabling) technologies (PCs, virtual networks, etc.) to send electronic messages and deliver medical data from one place to another. Telemedicine applications span the areas of telecare, telecardiology, teleradiology, telepathology, teledermatology, teleophtlalmology, teleoncology, telepsychiatry or "teleeveryting" in general [32,33]. Wireless telemedicine (or "m-health") is an important and emerging area in telemedical and telecare systems. It uses current mobile communication systems to provide medical services with a high degree of mobility. The effective utilization of telemedicine and related technologies will be able to assist with, but is not limited to [34]:

> ➢ support more types of services
> ➢ bring services to more people in more regions
> ➢ make healthcare more affordable for the poor and the elderly
> ➢ optimize health for all ages
> ➢ on-scene treatment for medical professionals on the move
> ➢ provide preventive care in addition to emergency treatment
> ➢ remote rehabilitation monitoring
> ➢ chronic disease relief and care
> ➢ ascertain service reliability and eliminate human errors
> ➢ safeguard patients' information and medical history.

Other applications include surgery, cancer treatment, healthcare education, and wearable devices.

1.5 BENEFITS

Advancements in science and technology have brought healthcare services to virtually all corners of the world. Healthcare technologies can be used in a several beneficial ways. The benefits that emerging technologies have brought to healthcare include [35]:

- Reducing healthcare costs
- Providing greater patient care
- Avoiding preventable deaths
- Improving quality of life
- Improving public health
- Increasing average life expectancy
- Reducing healthcare waste
- Improving efficiency and quality of care
- Developing new drugs and treatments
- Changing the practice of nursing in the coming decade

A growing number of healthcare organizations are embracing new technologies to increase their efficiency and effectiveness. Adopting these technologies will help healthcare facilities provide higher quality patient care at a lower cost.

1.6 CHALLENGES

While these technologies offer countless benefits, there are some major concerns and drawbacks. It is well known that current healthcare systems are stuck with the equation [36]:

Current Organization + New Technology = Expensive Current Organization.

Other challenges include:
* Some patients may not be savvy with technology
* Implementing a new technology may be a prohibitive and uphill task
* When technology fails to work, it can be frustrating
* A single mistake in using technology can cause disastrous consequences
* New technology can be complex or expensive, causing a slow rate of adoption
* Security and privacy risks are of paramount importance
* Medical information is very sensitive; its misuse could have serious consequences
* Shrinking budgets inhibits innovations
* Expenditure generated by healthcare technology will increase but may be expensive to the patients
* Healthcare technology providers are mostly interested in their bottom line (what does this mean?)
* Wireless devices are difficult to adopt because products from different vendors do not always work well together
* Easy for unauthorized user to collect and analyze any personal or clinical data
* Strict adherence with the regulations of Health Insurance Portability and Accountability Act (HIPPA) due to increasing patient data breaches and identity theft

Much remains to be done before these technologies are incorporated into daily life of the elderly. In the future there will remain an enduring distinction between safety and security. The future trends should include tightening the culture of technology development. In spite of their advantages and disadvantages, emerging technologies really make our lives easier, especially in the healthcare sector.

1.7 CONCLUSION

There are a lot of issues within the field of healthcare: health equity and equality, expensive costs are rising and performance is declining. If we want healthcare to improve in the future, we must continuously plan for it.

Today, emerging technologies are booming. They are developed and implemented in healthcare organizations at a rapid rate. Future technological innovations (new drugs, new treatments, new devices, etc.) will keep transforming healthcare delivery. Since technology drives healthcare, the fundamental problems of wellbeing, health and happiness, will remain. We need to be aware of the drivers, align with them, and work with them to ensure the best outcomes for society as a whole.

The emerging healthcare technologies discussed in this chapter have several things in common: large, fixed-cost expenditures to acquire the technologies, and a need for highly trained clinical operators [24]. The technologies will have a great impact on delivering better and safer healthcare services. More information on emerging health technologies can be found in the books in [34,37-43].

REFERENCES

[1] H. Thimbleby, "Technology and the future of healthcare," *Journal of Public Health Research,* vol. 2, no. 3, December 2013.

[2] S. M. Davet et al., "A framework to manage the early value proposition of emerging healthcare technologies," *Irish Journal of Management,* vol. 31, no. 1, 2011, pp. 59-75.

[3] M. N. O. Sadiku, Y. P. Akhare, and S. M. Musa, "Emerging technologies in healthcare: A tutorial," *International Journal of Advances in Scientific Research and Engineering,* vol. 5, no. 7, July 2019, pp. 199-204.

[4] M. Halaweh, "Emerging technology: What is it?" *Journal of Technology Management & Innovation,* vol. 8, no. 3, 2013, pp. 108-115.

[5] "5 Technology trends impacting healthcare," March 2018, https://cbcommunity.comcast.com/browse-all/details/5-technology-trends-impacting-health-care

[6] C. Huston, "The impact of emerging technology on nursing care: Warp speed ahead" *The Online Journal of Issues in Nursing,* vol. 18, no. 2, May 2013.

[7] M. Patel and J. Wan, "Applications, challenges, and prospective in emerging body area networking technologies," *IEEE Wireless Communications,* February 2010, pp. 80-88.

[8] M. Bajwa, "Emerging 21st century medical technologies," *Pakistan Journal of Medical Sciences,* vol. 30, no. 3, May-June, 2014, pp. 649-655.

[9] C. F. Pasluosta et al., "An emerging era in the management of Parkinson's disease: Wearable technologies and the Internet of things" *IEEE Journal of Biomedical and Health Informatics,* vol. 19, no. 6, November 2015, pp. 1873-1881.

[10] K. Zimmermann, "Microwave as an emerging technology for the treatment of biohazardous waste: A mini-review," *Waste Management & Research,* vol. 35, no. 5, 2017, pp. 471 –479.

[11] M. N. O. Sadiku, T. J. Ashaolu, and S. M. Musa, "Artificial intelligence in medicine: A primer," *International Journal of Trend in Research and Development,* vol. 6, no. 1, Jan.-Feb. 2019, pp. 270-272.

[12] M. N. O. Sadiku, Y. Wang, S. Cui, and S.M. Musa, "Healthcare robotics: A primer," *International Journal of Advanced Research in Computer Science and Software Engineering,* vol. 8, no. 2, Feb. 2018, pp. 26-29.

[13] "10 Emerging trends in healthcare technology for 2020 and beyond," March 25th, 2020 https://www.syberscribe.com.au/blog/10-emerging-trends-healthcare-technology-2019-beyond/

[14] "Robots in medical applications," https://www.rsipvision.com/robots-in-medical-applications/

[15] M. N. O. Sadiku, J. Foreman, S. M. Musa, "3D Printing in healthcare," *International Journal of Scientific Engineering and Technology,* vol. 7, no. 7, July 2018, pp. 65-67.

[16] "New trending report on 3D printed drugs market with high CAGR in coming years by 2025 with focusing key players like - Aprecia, BV, LLC, 3D printer drug machine, FabRx," March 2020, https://www.openpr.com/news/1956271/new-trending-report-on-3d-printed-drugs-market-with-high-cagr

[17] M. O. Onyesolu and F. U. Eze, "Understanding virtual reality technology: Advances and applications," https://www.semanticscholar.org/paper/Understanding-Virtual-Reality-Technology%3A-Advances-Onyesolu-Eze/12c4294ce620ec062e8dad1acb738b7cc9d211ba

[18] M. N. O. Sadiku, T. J. Ashaolu, and S. M. Musa, "Nanomedicine: A primer," *International Journal of Trend in Research and Development,* vol. 6, no. 1, Jan.-Feb. 2019, pp. 267-269.

[19] M. N. O. Sadiku, S. R. Nelatury, and S.M. Musa, "Cloud computing in healthcare," *Journal of Scientific and Engineering Research*, vol. 5, no. 9, 2018, pp. 202-205.

[20] M. N. O. Sadiku, S. Alam, and S.M. Musa, "IoT for healthcare," *International Journal of Electronics and Communication Engineering*, vol. 5. no. 11, November 2018, pp. 5-7.

[21] M. N. O. Sadiku, S. M. Musa, and S. Binzaid, "Internet of things in medicine," *International Journal of Research in Engineering*, vol. 1, no.2, April 2019, pp. 15-17.

[22] M. N. O. Sadiku, K. G. Eze, and S.M. Musa, "Block chain technology in healthcare," *International Journal of Advances in Scientific Research and Engineering*, vol. 4, no. 5, 2018, pp. 154-159.

[23] M. N. O. Sadiku, N. K. Ampah, and S. M. Musa, "Social media in healthcare," *International Journal of Trend in Scientific Research and Development*, vol. 2, no. 5, June/July 2018, pp. 665-668.

[24] A. Datta,"Top eight disruptive technologies and how they are relevant to geospatial," 2018, https://www.geospatialworld.net/blogs/top-disruptive-technologies-relevant-geospatial/

[25] M. Ilyas, "Emerging technologies for healthcare," *Proceedings of International Symposium on High Capacity Optical Networks and Enabling Technologies*, 2008, pp. 15-18..

[26] J. Goldsmith, "Technology and the boundaries of the hospital: Three emerging technologies," *Health Affairs*, vol. 23, no. 6, November/December 2004, pp. 149-156.

[27] A. S. Maoa and D. J. Mooney, "Regenerative medicine: Current therapies and future directions," *PNAS*, vol. 112, no. 4, November 2015, pp. 14452–14459.

[28] D. Panescu, "Wireless communication systems for implantable medical devices," *IEEE Engineering in Medicine and Biology Magazine*, March/April 2008, pp. 96-101.

[29] M. Akay et al., "Emerging technologies for patient-specific healthcare," *IEEE Transactions On Information Technology In Biomedicine*, vol. 16, no. 2, March 2012, pp. 185-189.

[30] M. M Alam et al., "Survey on the roles of communication technologies in IoT-based personalized healthcare applications," *IEEE Access*, vol. 6, 2018, pp. 36611-36631.

[31] D. Gu et al, "Discovering and visualizing knowledge evolution of chronic disease research driven by emerging technologies," *IEEE Access*, vol.7, 2019.

[32] M. N. O. Sadiku, M. Tembely, and S.M. Musa, "Telemedicine:: A primer (Part 1)," *International Journal of Advanced Research in Computer Science and Software Engineering*, vol. 9, no. 6, June 2019, pp.43-46.

[33] M. N. O. Sadiku, M. Tembely, and S.M. Musa, "Telemedicine: Teleeverything phenomena (Part 2)," *International Journal of Advanced Research in Computer Science and Software Engineering*, vol. 9, no. 6, June 2019, pp.35-38.

[34] B. Fong, A.C.M. Fong, and C. K. Li, *Telemedicine Technologies Information Technologies in Medicine and Telehealth*. John Wiley & Sons, 2011.

[35] B. Banova, " The impact of technology in healthcare," June 2019, https://www.aimseducation.edu/blog/the-impact-of-technology-on-healthcare/

[36] R S. H. Istepanian and Jose C. Lacal, "Emerging mobile communication technologies for health: Some imperative notes on m-health," *Proceedings of the 25the Annual International Conference of the IEEE EMBS*, Cancun, Mexico, September 2003, pp. 1414-1416.

[37] S. Jones and F. M. Groom (eds.), *Information and communication Technologies in Healthcare.* Boca Raton, FL: CRC Press, 2012.

[38] J. M. Boyce, *Measuring Healthcare Worker Hand Hygiene Activity: Current Practices and Emerging Technologies.* Cambridge University Press, 2015.

[39] J. A. Jacko (ed.), *The Human-Computer Interaction Handbook: Fundamentals, Evolving Technologies, and Emerging Applications.* Boca Raton, FL: CRC Press, 3rd edition, 2012.

[40] S. M. Ricchins, *Emerging Technologies in Healthcare.* Boca Raton, FL: CRC Press, 2015.

[41] J. M. Winters et al. (eds.), *Emerging and Accessible Telecommunications, Information and Healthcare Technologies.* Resna Press, 2002.

[42] D. N. Le et al. (eds.), *Emerging Technologies for Health and Medicine: Virtual Reality, Augmented Reality, Artificial Intelligence, Internet of Things, Robotics, Industry 4.0.* Scrivener Publishing, 2018.

[43] W. M. Carroll (ed.), *Emerging Technologies for Nurses: Implications for Practice.* Productivity Press, 2015.

CHAPTER 2

WEARABLE HEALTHCARE TECHNOLOGIES

"It is not the strongest of the species that survives, nor the most intelligent, but the one most responsive to change." - Charles Darwin

2.1 INTRODUCTION

Digitalization is changing every area of human behavior. The digital healthcare revolution provides an opportunity to transform healthcare and empower patients to take charge of their own health. At the core of the rapid evolution is the wearable healthcare devices, which are designed to enhance the quality of human life.

Health is regarded as one of the global challenges for mankind. A modernized healthcare system should provide healthcare services to people at any time and from anywhere. The emergence of wearable devices has transformed the face of healthcare. The healthcare industry is employing wearable technologies in order to improve efficiency and quality. There is no denying that wearable devices or gadgets are gradually becoming more and more mainstream. The possibilities are endless for wearable technology in healthcare. Wearable devices may be the future of healthcare.

This chapter provides introduction on the applications of wearable technologies in healthcare. It begins by providing a general background on wearables. Then it discusses wearables in healthcare and their various applications. It presents the benefits and challenges of wearable devices in healthcare. The last section concludes with comments.

2.2 WEARABLES

A wearable device is any device that is worn comfortably on the body and enables user interaction. It is typically integrated into the clothing or attached to the body of a person to enhance human performance. It often includes smart devices that can be worn on the body or attached to clothes. Wearable devices have been around for centuries. The first one was introduced in the 1660s by the Qing Dynasty. Since then the popularity of wearables has shifted from royalty to the healthcare industry. Wearable computing is a natural evolution of the smartphone technology that has become so ubiquitous and indispensable in education, business, and medicine. We wear wrist watches to know the time. Perhaps the most crucial bit of wearable tech accessible today is Google Glass. There has been a proliferation of wearables from consumer gadgets to medical devices that are approved by the Food and Drug Administration (FDA).

Wearable devices or systems are usually lightweight, miniature electronic or digital devices that are worn by a user, including clothing, watches, glasses, shoes, and similar items. A wearable computer is computer-powered device that is never-sleeping ever-present network-connected electronic system that can be used at anytime and anywhere and does not in any way disturb the user's interaction with the real world. It should be worn, much as eyeglasses or clothing are worn, and interact with the user [1]. It includes all manner of technology that is on or in the body such as fitness trackers, smartwatches, smart clothing, smart rings, smart glasses, wearable mobile sensors, smart jewelry, and smart ECG (electrocardiogram) monitors. Typical wearable devices are shown in Figure 2.1 [2]. Wearables are always ready, unrestrictive, not monopolizing of user attention, observable and controllable by the user, attentive to the environment, useful as a communication tool, and personal devices [3]. Wearables are being used across healthcare, insurance, interactive systems, safety critical settings, wearable cameras, baby and pregnancy monitors, entertainment, fitness and sports, emergency responders, and military. Some of these applications are illustrated in Figure 2.2 [4]. Due to it wide range of applications, international corporations such Google, Apple, and Intel are investing heavily on wearable technology research and development [5]. As with any new technology, one must exercise caution when using a wearable device.

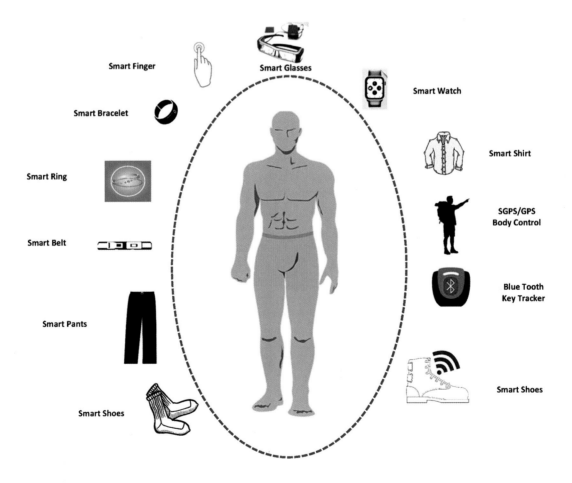

Figure 2.1 Different types of wearable devices on human body [2].

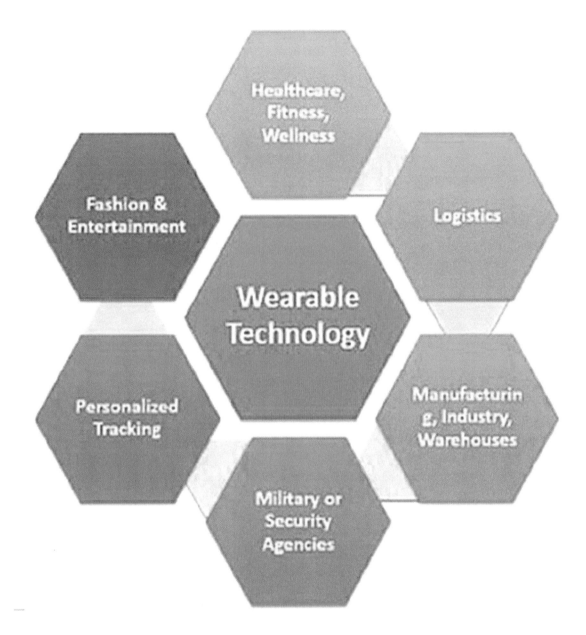

Figure 2.2 Different applications of wearable technology [4].

2.3 WEARABLES IN HEALTHCARE

Wearable technologies are apparatuses that can be worn in different parts of the body. They are often used in the healthcare industry, specifically in hospitals. With advances in technology, wearable techs are becoming smaller, smarter, more lightweight, mobile, invisible, and more convenient. Over the past decade, companies have created wearable devices for patients, nurses, and doctors. From patient homes to hospital beds, there is a multitude of uses for wearable devices [6]. Wearables can help individuals with a fitness regime. The doctors use them in diagnosing or treating patients. A doctor can wear Google Glass while performing surgery.

Wearable devices include wristbands, smartwatches, wearable mobile sensors, and other mobile hub medical devices that collect a large range of data. These devices can help patients and providers manage chronic conditions such as diabetes and heart conditions [7].

To be useful, wearable devices must collect data. Wearable devices interface with smartphones and personal computer software to collect a wide variety of data. Examples of data include location through GPS, quality of surrounding air, body temperature, heart rate, blood pressure, humidity, atmospheric pressure, etc. [8].

A wearable healthcare technology (WHT) essentially consists of two different components: wearable and body sensors. It incorporates sensors, memory, solar cells, and batteries. It stays in contact with the body for extended periods of time. Wearable technologies are characterized by body-worn devices, as smart clothing, e-textiles, and accessories. Sensors are an important part of wearable devices, and continue to become smaller and more sophisticated. Common sensors include pressure, temperature, position and humidity, GPS, and gyroscopes to detect movement. They can allow blood glucose level, blood pressure, heartbeat rate, and other biometric data to be constantly measured and sent to the healthcare providers [9].

Wearable devices can be classified into major three categories based on their application [10]: (1) Lifestyle and Healthcare, periodically monitoring, for sports and activity monitors; (2) E-textiles, also called as smart garments, smart clothing, smart textiles, or smart fabrics, that contain components like battery and computers; and (3) E-Patches, placed on to the skin to monitor specific dose of medication.

Examples of wearable healthcare devices include [11]:
- Ambulatory Pumps & Monitors
- Glucose Monitoring and Insulin Dispensing
- Sleep Tracking Wearables
- Pain Management Wearables
- Mobile EKG Heart Monitors
- Mobility Analysis Wearables
- Blood Pressure Monitors
- Smart Sensor Patches
- Smart Clothing
- Wearable Defibrillator
- Wristband Activity Trackers
- Vital Connect's Healthpatch MD

2.4 APPLICATIONS OF WEARIABLES IN HEALTHCARE

Wearable healthcare devices are increasing in popularity. Mobile healthcare apps and wearable technologies are numerous. Common applications of healthcare wearable technologies include the following [12]:
- *Remote Monitoring:* Monitoring systems enable continuous measurement of critical biomarkers for medical diagnostics and health monitoring. They monitor patients post-hospitalization, including wearable glucose monitors, ECG monitors, pulse oximeters, and blood pressure monitors. They play a crucial role in patient-centered preventive care. The most common wearables to monitor your health are Fitbit, Garmin, and Apple Watch. Using wearable devices can expand the range of communication between patient and physicians. These wearable devices for patients track daily steps, exercise levels, heart rate, and sleep schedules.

A typical monitoring system is shown in Figure 2.3 [13]. Monitoring systems can be used to monitor body temperature, bodily fluids, safety, health and wellness, cardiovascular signals or Parkinson's disease (PD) patients.

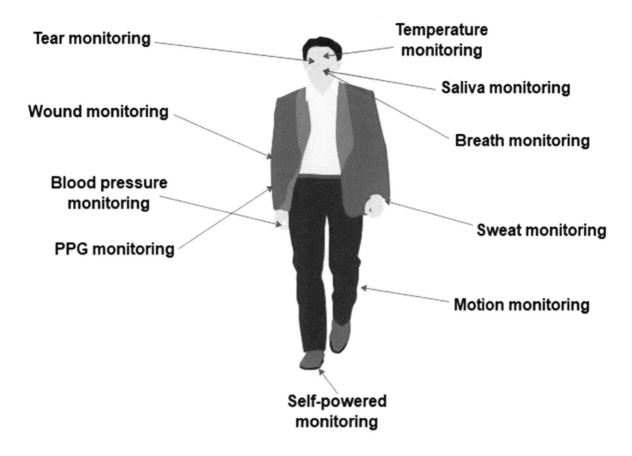

Figure 2.3 A typical monitoring system [13].

- *Diagnosis:* This describes the assessment of the patient's status that sends an alarm when vital parameters exceed a predefined threshold. Wearable devices can provide data that can help nurses diagnose problems quickly. Sleep apnea can be easily diagnosed, and sleep quality improved with a wearable measuring electrocardiogram (ECG).
- *Fitness:* Wearable fitness devices are a popular topic in health and wellness. They can be used to track physical activity, sleep, heart rate, and even provide on-screen workouts. Wearable fitness devices, such as the FitBit and Nike+, have appeared on the market. Incorporating wearable technology into a weight loss program would yield marked results [14]. Obese and overweight individuals who use trackers can experience noticeable improvements in their body mass index and significant reductions in feelings of anxiety, depression, anger, fatigue, and confusion.
- *Elderly Care:* The geriatric population has placed heavy demands on the current healthcare system. They have more medical issues such as vision or hearing loss, limited mobility, and other comorbidities. They need personal attention and assisted living. Wearable devices are among the tools that can aid the continuous monitoring of the elderly.

- *Cardiology:* The field of cardiology has been using wearable devices to monitor heart rate and rhythm, blood pressure. Several new wearable devices have been widely adopted by both physicians and patients.

- *Diabetics:* The wearable technology is potentially life-changing for many diabetics and provides new opportunities to help patients. The device would measure blood glucose levels and send the data wirelessly to a mobile device. Wearable devices help patients monitor their own health, thereby lowering the costs of managing chronic diseases.

- *Wireless Body Area Networks* (WBANs): These are a special purpose wireless sensor networks (WSNs) that can provide ubiquitous real-time monitoring of human physiology. A WBAN is a network formed by low-power devices that are located on, in or around the human body. In these networks, various sensors are attached on clothing, the body or even implanted under the skin. WBAN unobtrusively envelops the body to capture health data. It is primarily responsible for collecting the data either directly from the body through sensors. Figure 2.4 shows a typical WBAN [15].

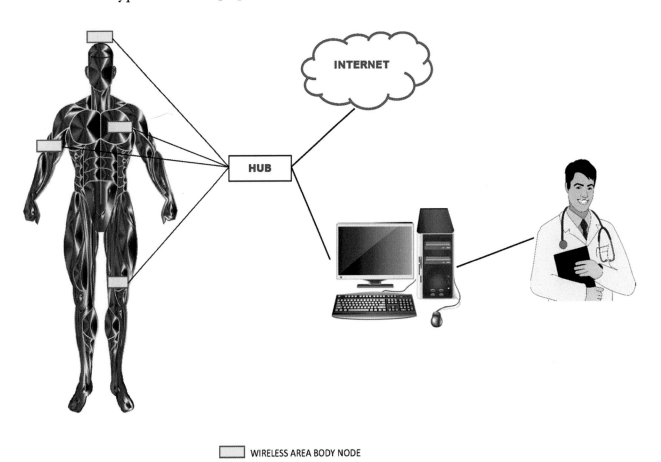

WIRELESS AREA BODY NODE

Figure 2.4 A typical WBAN [15].

- *Wearable Biosensor:* This is an important development in healthcare technology. It is a combination of wearable objects and biosensors, which can be worn on the body like bandages, rings, clothes, smart watches, tattoos, jewelry, etc. Biosensors enable real-time monitoring, prevention and personalized medicine for various chronic and acute diseases. It can allow blood glucose level, blood pressure, heart rate, and other biometric data to be constantly measured and sent to the healthcare providers.

- *Electronic Health Records:* In connected hospitals, every medical device is connected with the Electronic Health Records (EHR) for communicating accurate patient records and automatically sending data from devices to the EHR. With the advances in digital technology, healthcare is getting more access to patient information to understand patient medical conditions for better collaborative care. Modern health systems integrate EHR and medical devices, including wearable health and fitness tracking devices. They are increasingly interdependent on EHR capabilities, offerings, and innovations to better capture patient data [16].

Other areas of applications of WHT include infant safety and care, elderly care, epilepsy, chronic disease management, military support, law enforcement, sports medicine, and preventive medicine. Health systems and organizations that are interested in wearable healthcare technology includes NYU Langone Health, Penn Medicine, Duke Health, Novant Health, and Icahn School of Medicine at Mount Sinai.

2.5 BENEFITS

The benefits of using WHT are many: to reduce medical errors, reduce costs, increase patient engagement, improve efficiency and healthcare quality. Wearable healthcare technology that is integrated into the EHR produces massive data that may be useful for patients and providers. Wearables are used in the military for security purposes and they allow one to work from everywhere. Other benefits include [17,18]:

- *Hands-free experience or connectivity*– Wearables can receive incoming calls, while allowing the user to remain "hands-free." Wearables can alert you of messages, incoming calls, emails, etc. without having to constantly be checking your phone.
- *Convenience & portability* – Wearables allow instant access to medical information and resources. They are easy for the patient to use and offer real-time data for physicians to analyze.
- *Personalized information* – Several wearables provide the option of customization according to the user's personal health.
- *Improved clinical decision-making* –Physicians can use these tools for looking up multiple medical sources and gaining access to drug reference databases.
- *Greater accuracy* – Wearables allow convenient tracking of a user's health and exercise habits for improving their overall well-being.
- *Improved efficiency* – Wearables help physicians to be more efficient in their work tasks.
- *Improved productivity* – Health-related apps have also increased the productivity of pharmacists by allowing them to access drug information quickly.
- *Increase employee satisfaction:* Wearables generally make it easier for people to perform specific tasks and improve employee job satisfaction.
- *Sports Medicine:* Wearables can help athletes or coaches to effectively manage athletic training and matches

- *Self-care:* Patients are digitally savvy today. Wearable technology allows patients to play a more active role in maintaining their health and making informed decisions. It can facilitate self-care through monitoring and prevention. With wearable healthcare devices, there is possibility for a more proactive approach to healthcare.
- *Monitors Vulnerable Patients:* Wearable technology can be used to monitor from a distance vulnerable patients, who may be prone to medical issues. For example, many elderly patients now wear heart monitors and GPS location devices that alert caregivers when something goes wrong.
- *No FDA approval:* Wearable devices are different from regular medical devices and they do not need to go through the strict FDA approval process. Wearable device manufacturers are self-regulated with no oversight from the FDA [19].

2.6 CHALLENGES

There are challenges and risks in all aspects of WHT, which need to be addressed before wearables are fully adopted in healthcare. These include system interoperability, information overload, confidentiality, and patient privacy [17,20]:

- *Privacy/Security* – Patient confidentiality and data security are major concerns when using wearable devices. The rapid expansion use of wearables continues to pose the greatest challenge to the growth of wearable health technology. Electronic health records raise potential privacy issues since wearable devices may lead to possible unauthorized access to private patient information. The collection of personal data in large quantities raises privacy and security concerns for the user [21].
- *Safety* – Lithium batteries can be dangerous when not handled properly. They can explode and catch fire when damaged. Wearable devices using these batteries pose a potential safety risk.
- *Battery life* – Battery life is one of the most crucial challenges of wearables. Most wearable batteries last for one to two days and this insufficient amount of time makes them unreliable. Wireless charger solves this problem to some degree.
- *Data accuracy* – Most wearables need to be better developed for actual accuracy and flexibility.
- *Theft* – Wearables need to be developed further in order to limit their use and prevent theft. Misuse of personal health data by third parties could lead to identity theft. Technology is a tool which can be used wisely or foolishly.
- *App Integration* – One of the most important aspects of wearables is their ability to connect to other systems. But due to countless apps being developed, facilities are having a difficult time keeping up, let alone integrating new system within their current one.
- *Excessive information* - It is easy to go astray in the jungle of healthcare gadgets that promise you a healthier lifestyle. Finding the right kind of healthcare wearable can be a challenge.
- *Distraction:* Just like smart phones, wearable technology provides plenty of distractions.
- *Wearables are expensive:* Although wearables are a great investment for healthcare, the high price for both patients and healthcare industry is one drawback for the wearable trend. Most

consumers still find wearable tech to be expensive, estimating $300-400, depending on the application.

- *Lack of Regulations:* The lack of transparency among manufacturers of wearable devices and the lack of regulations on the manufacturing of these devices is harmful to the healthcare industry. Wearable device manufacturers are presently self-regulated and operate with no oversight from the FDA in the US or MHRA in the UK [21].

To protect the confidentiality and privacy, healthcare systems may require setting up another secure network for wearable devices. The quality and validity of wearable gadgets is a matter of concern. There is a risk that patients become permanently dependent on the wearables. Most current wearable devices are at their premature stages and are not yet FDA approved. Wearable technologies have been banned in some casinos, movie theatres, and restaurants for security reasons [22]. These issues must be addressed in order to have a wide-scale adoption of WHT.

2.7 CONCLUSION

Wearable healthcare technology (WHT) has emerged as a promising technology to improve the wellbeing of individuals. A recent study shows that a significant percentage of US adults were willing to wear technology that monitors their health. The wearable healthcare technology is a rapidly evolving field and its market is booming. New technology, such as WHT, succeeds best when it fits enhances human behavior.

This rise of digital healthcare demands for specialized skills and a different type of employees. Future healthcare professionals must understand the implementation of wearable technologies, which require design decision across multiple concerns [23]. Due to the rapidly moving field of wearables, they are gradually becoming more and more mainstream. Wearable technologies will continue to make waves in the healthcare industry. They support the implementation of telemedicine in the patient's natural environment. They may be regarded as the next generation of personal portable devices for telemedicine practice. They are here to stay. More information about wearable healthcare technologies can be found in the books in [24-26].

REFERENCES

[1] M. N. O. Sadiku, S. Alam, and S. M. Musa, "Wearable computing," *International Journal of Engineering Research*, vol. 6, no. 10, Oct. 2017, pp. 445-447.

[2] https://www.researchgate.net/figure/Different-types-of-wearable-technology_fig5_322261039

[3] M. Kaiiali, "Designing a VM-level vertical scalability service in current cloud platforms: a new hope for wearable computers," *Turkish Journal of Electrical Engineering & Computer Sciences*, vol. 25, 2017, pp. 2555 – 2566.

[4] Canopus Infosystems, "What are the latest trends in wearable technology?" https://yourstory.com/ mystory/3073273d91-what-are-the-latest-trends-in-wearable-technology-

[5] M. Salahuddin and L. Romeo,"Wearable technology: Are product developers meeting consumer's needs?" *International Journal of Fashion Design, Technology and Education*, vol. 13, no. 1,2020, pp. 58-67.

[6] J. Mesh, "How wearables are changing the healthcare industry," August 2018, https://www.healthcareitleaders.com/blog/how-wearables-are-changing-the-healthcare-industry/

[7] C. Dinh-Le et al., "Wearable health technology and electronic health record integration: Scoping review and future directions," *JMIR Mhealth and Uhealth*, vol. 7. no. 9, September 2019.

[8] L. Cilliers, "Wearable devices in healthcare: Privacy and information security issues," *Health Information Management Journal*, 2019, pp. 1-7.

[9] H. A. Ali, "Sensors and wearable technology in healthcare," October 2018, https://techengage.com/sensors-wearable-technology-healthcare/

[10] K. Vijayalakshmi, "A demand for wearable devices in health care," *International Journal of Engineering & Technology*, vol. 7, 2018, pp. 1-4.

[11] "Wearable medical devices," http://www.polyonedistribution.com/files/2018%20HC%20Wearable%20Device%20Application%20Bulletin.pdf

[12] A. K. Witte and R. Zarnekow, "Transforming personal healthcare through technology - A systematic literature review of wearable sensors for medical application," *Proceedings of the 52nd Hawaii International Conference on System Sciences*, 2019, pp. 3848-3857.

[13] Z. Lou et al., "Reviews of wearable healthcare systems: Materials, devices and system integration," *Materials Science and Engineering*, vol. 140, April 2020.

[14] K. Eaton, "The impact of wearable devices in the healthcare industry," December 2016, https://www.fbabenefits.com/impact-wearable-devices-healthcare-industry/

[15] "PhD in wireless body area networks," http://phdinfo.org/PhD_in_WirelessBodyAreaNetwork.html

[16] C. D. Le et al., Wearable health technology and electronic health record integration: Scoping review and future directions," *JMIR Mhealth Uhealth*, vol. 7, no. 9, September 2019.

[17] "Pros and cons of wearable technologies," December 2017, https://www.clodoc.com/blog/pros-and-cons-of-wearable-technologies/

[18] M. Wu and J. Luo, "Wearable technology applications in healthcare: A literature review," *Online Journal of Nursing Informatics*, vol. 23, no. 3, November 25, 2019.

[19] C. Erdmier, J. Hatcher, and M. Lee, "Wearable device implications in the healthcare industry," *Journal of Medical Engineering & Technology*, vol. 40, no. 4, 2016, pp. 141-148.

[20] L. Cilliers, "Wearable devices in healthcare: Privacy and information security issues," *Health Information Management Journal*, 2019.

[21] C. Erdmier, J. Hatcher, and M. Lee, "Wearable device implications in the healthcare industry," *Journal of Medical Engineering & Technology*, vol. 40, no. 4, 2016, pp. 141-148.

[22] Technavio, "Exploring five challenges in the wearable technology market," July 2014, https://blog.technavio.com/blog/exploring-five-challenges-in-the-wearable-technology-market

[23] J. Tanai, M. Forssi, and T. Hellsténi, "The use of wearables in healthcare – Challenges and opportunities," *Arcada Working Papers*, vol. 6, 2017.

[24] R. Tong (ed.), *Wearable Technology in Medicine and Health Care*. Academic Press, 2018.

[25] N. Dey et al. (eds.), *Wearable and Implantable Medical Devices: Applications and Challenges*. Academic Press, 2019.

[26] B. Furht and A. Agarwal, *Handbook of Medical and Healthcare Technologies*. Springer, 2013.

CHAPTER 3

TELEMEDICINE

"Time and health are two precious assets that we don't recognize and appreciate until they have been depleted." - Anonymous

3.1 INTRODUCTION

Applications of information and communications technologies (ICT) have become widespread due to the rapid development of microelectronics, computers, and Internet. One of the most important applications of ICT is its use to improve healthcare services and systems. Telemedicine (TM) is a technological response to bring health services to people wherever it is not possible or feasible to bring people to health services. It is simply "healing at a distance" using telecommunication system. It may be regarded as the virtual physician visit. TM will do for healthcare what the personal computer (PC) has done for the office.

The marriage between information technology and science-based medical knowledge has given birth to telemedicine (also known as telehealth or ehealth). Telemedicine (TM) is typically the transmission of medical images between healthcare centers for diagnosis across distance.

It is an opportunity to meet people where they are at and ensure that they are receiving the care they need. It has been used to overcome distance barriers and to save lives in critical care and emergency situations.

Telemedicine's primary goal is to bring medical services to isolated, geographically dispersed, and physically confined persons unable to reach a physician within reasonable time or distance. This new modality of healthcare delivery is gradually finding its way into the mainstream medicine. Telemedicine should now be regarded as an integrated component of the care continuum [1,2].

Telemedicine is closely related to telehealth; the two are often used interchangeably. Telehealth is an umbrella term that covers the technologies that provide support for long distance clinical healthcare. Telemedicine, on the other hand, refers to the remote delivery of clinical care through communication technologies. Telemedicine applications and services include email, video, wireless tools, smart phones, etc. Examples of telemedicine include group therapy, nursing interactions, education and training, televisits to community health workers, follow-up visits, management of chronic conditions, medication management, specialist consultation, and medical image transmission [3].

This chapter provides an introduction to telemedicine. It begins by discussing the concept of telemedicine and its different types. It describes various applications of telemedicine. It presents the benefits and challenges of telemedicine. The last section concludes with comments.

3.2 CONCEPT OF TELEMEDICINE

Telemedicine literally means "healing at a distance." The rise of the Internet age and the proliferation of smart devices have brought profound changes for the practice of telemedicine. Telemedicine is now regarded as the use of electronic information and communications technology (ICT) to provide medical services when distance separates the patient and healthcare provider. It allows healthcare professionals to evaluate, diagnose. and treat patients at a distance using telecommunications technology. It uses video cameras and monitors to connect the patient and the health care providers. A typical example of telemedicine is shown in Figure 3.1 [4].

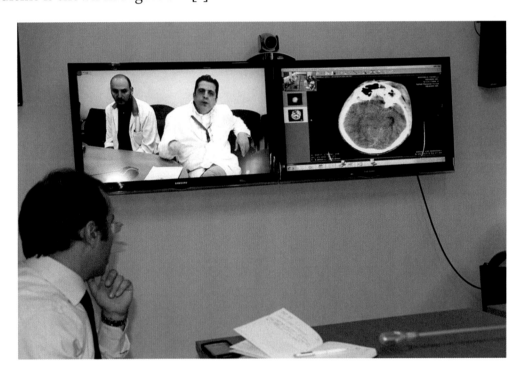

Figure 3.1 A typical example of telemedicine [4].

Modern telemedicine began in the early 1900s in the Netherlands with the transmission of heart rhythms over the telephone. Today, telemedicine is used in a variety of specialties including radiology, neurology, and pathology. It is rapidly expanding to serve millions of people and providing health services for individuals living in remote and rural areas. Telemedicine manifests itself in a number of ways, all of which are centered around data transfer and communications. It seeks to improve a patient's health by allowing real time interactive communication between the patient and the practitioner at the remote site. It does not represent a separate medical specialty; it is a tool that can be used by health practitioners to extend the traditional practice of medicine to a distant location.

Demand of affordable and quality health care is increasing daily. Telemedicine is the use of technologies to provide clinical services when patients are far away. Telemedicine is a win-win for healthcare providers seeking to improve patient access. It provides quality health care to the people at the cost that they can afford, as well as patients looking for more convenient ways to engage with care providers. Four main goals of telemedicine [5]:

(1) Its purpose is to provide clinical support.;

(2) It is intended to overcome geographical barriers, connecting users who are not in the same physical location;

(3) It involves the use of various types of ICT;

(4) Its goal is to improve health outcomes.

Telemedicine is a hybrid system, which involves the medical as well as ICT domain. It is a combination of expertise and technology to deliver medical services over distance. There are basically three conditions under which telemedicine should be considered [6]: (1) when there is no alternative (e.g. in emergencies in remote environments), and (2) when it is better than existing conventional services (e.g. teleradiology for rural hospitals) (3) when it is safer to meet online than in person for a non-emergent situation (ie, a patient who may be high risk of contracting coronavirus during the 2020 covid-19 pandemic)

Technological infrastructures are important for the implementation of telemedicine systems. The rise of the Internet age brought with it profound changes for the practice of telemedicine. The key enabling technologies for telemedicine include digital communications, videotelephony, and information technologies. Telemedicine has used various terrestrial and space-based (satellite) transmission media.

3.3 TYPES OF TELEMEDICINE

Telemedicine is an umbrella term that encompasses any medical activity involving distance between care provider and patient. According to the Center for Connected Health Policy (CCHP), there are four categories for telemedicine use today. In other words, the practice of telemedicine can be broken down into four types of solutions: store-and-forward, patient telemonitoring, real-time telemedicine, and mobile health [7].

- *Store-and-Forward Telemedicine:* This is also known as "asynchronous telemedicine." It is a method by which healthcare providers share patient medical data. It is asynchronous in the sense that the consulting specialist, patient, and primary doctor do not need to all be communicating simultaneously. Store-and-forward solutions enable healthcare providers to forward and share patient medical data with a provider at a different location. All sorts of medical data (e.g. lab results, medical images, bio-signals) can be transmitted across vast distances. Pathology, radiology, dermatology, and other medical fields rely on this form of telemedicine on a daily basis.

- *Remote Patient Telemonitoring:* Remote patient monitoring, or "telemonitoring" allows healthcare providers to monitor patients' health data from a far, usually while the patient is at home. It allows healthcare professionals to track a patient's vital signs and activities at a distance. It is effective for chronic conditions such as heart disease, diabetes, and asthma. It can also be used by elderly patients. It can also be used in the inpatient hospital setting for those patients who are at high risk for falls, but there might not be sufficient amount of staff to have a 1 to 1 sitter and can be monitored via technology from a central location in the hospital.

- *Real-time Telemedicine:* Real-time or live telemedicine refers to any two-way communications that let providers and patients communicate in real-time. This makes it easy to do a doctor-patient visit anytime, anywhere. Using the method, patients and providers use video conferencing software to hear and see each other. It is popular for primary care, urgent care, follow-up visits, and the management of medications, and chronic illness. This may involve the use of robots and other technologies to allow a medical practitioner to perform a procedure at a certain location.
- *Mobile health:* mHealth (or Mobile health) refers to the practice of medicine via mobile devices such as mobile phones, tablet computers, personal digital assistants (PDAs), and wearable devices. It integrates mobile technology with the health delivery with the promise of promoting a better health and improving efficiency. MHealth services propose healthcare delivery anytime and anywhere overcoming geographical barriers with low and affordable costs. Challenges such as privacy concerns have limited the impact of mHealth, but it has enormous potential to reshape healthcare delivery in the future [8]. Patients are beginning to use mobile technology to monitor and track their health.

One can choose from these four types of telemedicine.

3.4 APPLICATIONS OF TELEMEDICINE

Telemedicine, as practiced today, is a major new development in medicine. It allows healthcare practitioners to diagnose, treat, and monitor patients at a distance using telecommunications technology. It is a process, not a technology. It is not a new branch of medicine; it is integrated in many different medical fields. Practitioners from a various medical specialties have claimed success in their telemedicine pursuits. Telemedicine is a "teleeverything" (or tele-X) phenomenon as evident in various applications and services which include telehealth, telecare, telenursing, telepharmacy, telesurgery, teleradiology, telepsychiatry, teledermatology, teleconsultations, telenephrology, teleobstetrics, teleoncology, teledentistry, teleaudiology, telerehabilitation, teleophthalmology, teletrauma, teleneuropsychology, telecardiology, and telepediatrics, Figure 3.2 summarizes a number of services that telemedicine supports. The frequency of application of telemedicine to the various specialties is given as follows [9]:

- Radiology - 37%
- Emergency Medicine - 22%
- Pathology - 11%
- Cardiology - 9%
- Internal Medicine - 7%
- Dermatology 4%

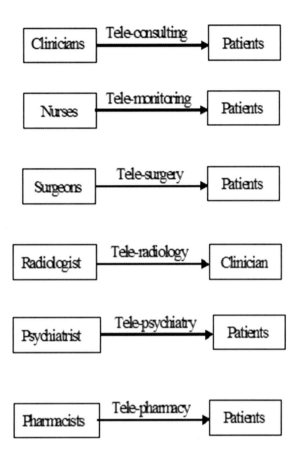

Figure 3.2 Some services that telemedicine support [9].

Some of the most popular teleeverything solutions are presented as follows [10-14].

- *Telehealth*: This is the use of information and telecommunication technology (ICT) to provide patients with healthcare at a distance. It is an opportunity to meet people where they are at, be it home, office, school, in an inpatient and outpatient setting, as well as scheduled and on-demand appointments. Telehealth programs can address the needs of patients in a way that traditional care delivery cannot. They provide opportunities to make healthcare more efficient, better coordinated, and closer to home.

- *Telecare:* Telecare allows home nursing services (especially for the elderly) to be delivered more cheaply. Home nursing visits by video are substantially cheaper than sending a nurse in person. Telecare may be used to provide support to healthcare providers of older adults, thereby increase the quality of patient care.

- *Teleconsultation*: This is basically the provision of knowledge or experience of an expert across distance. Telemedicine technology enables virtual consultations between healthcare professionals and patients. It makes real-time medical consultation via two-way videoconferencing. It may also involve diagnosis at distance of a patient by a physician at distance (e. g. telecardiology). Provider-to-provider consultation may take place within the same healthcare system. It is estimated that the number of telemedicine consultations will reach 160 million cases by 2020.

- *Telemonitoring:* Remote patient monitoring (RPM) has become a popular form of telemedicine. Patient monitoring is the collection of personal medical data from a connected patient in one location that is transferred electronically to a caregiver at a different location for monitoring purposes. This involves the supervision of a patient and his data at distance, who may or may not be in the hospital and/or clinic (e. g. diabetes patients, veterans, patients with heart insufficiencies). For example, patients with irregular heart rhythms would be continuously connected to an electrocardiography (ECG), and be monitored elsewhere in the hospital by other personals.

- *Teleradiology:* This is the practice of radiology from a distance. It is the ability to send radiographic images (X-Rays, CT, etc.) from one location to another. Digital imaging modalities include computer tomography (CT), magnetic resonance imaging (MRI), single-photon emission computer tomography (SPECT), and positron emission tomography (PET). Teleradiology may require three essential components: an image sending station, a transmission network, and a receiving-image review station. Today the Internet enables the use of new technologies for teleradiology. Teleradiology solutions offer providers at one location to send a patient's x-rays and records securely to a qualified radiologist at another location. Teleradiology is the transfer of radiological images. X-Rays, MRIs, and CTs, which may be used for consultation, diagnosis or interpretation. They can be transferred through satellite connections, local area networks, or even telephone lines. Teleradiology is the most popular use for telemedicine.

- *Telepsychiatry:* This allows qualified psychiatrists to provide treatment to patients remotely. It basically uses videoconferencing for patients residing in underserved areas to access psychiatric services. It is undertaken in real time (synchronous) or asynchronously. Telepsychiatry can connect patients and mental health professionals, allowing effective diagnosis, treatment, consultation, and transfer of medical data. It is incredibly popular, in part because of the nation-wide shortage of available psychiatrists. It offers wide range of services to the patients and medical practitioner such as consultation between the psychiatrists, therapists, educational clinical programs, diagnosis and assessment, medication management, and routine follow-up [15].

- *Teledermatology:* This allows the practice of dermatology over a distance using communication networks. In clinical teledermatology, dermatologists evaluate video or still images of skin disorders along with patient information. Teledermatology solutions are usually store-and-forward technologies that allow a general healthcare provider to send a patient photo of a rash, a mole, or another skin anomaly, for remote diagnosis. They have been found to improve efficiency. Applications comprise health care management such as diagnoses, consultation, and treatment as well as (continuing medical) education. The dermatologists Perednia and Brown were the first to coin the term "teledermatology" in 1995. Mobile teledermatology refers to the use of mobile telemedicine in dermatology [16].

- *Telerehabilitation:* This is the delivery of rehabilitation services over communications networks such as the Internet for rehabilitation patients. This allows medical professionals to deliver rehab services (such as physical therapy) remotely. Telerehabilitation also allows experts in rehabilitation to engage in a clinical consultation at a distance. Telerehabilitation practice embraces other areas such as neuropsychology, speech-language pathology, audiology, occupational therapy, and physical therapy. For example, a physician might use telerehabilitation as therapeutic interventions for persons with disabilities. The use of telerehabilitation has grown over the years.

- *Telepharmacy:* This refers to the provision of pharmacy services to the patients with the use of communication technology when direct contact with a pharmacist is not possible. Telepharmacy services include drug therapy monitoring, prior authorization, and refill authorization. Telepharmacy services can be delivered at retail pharmacy sites, through hospitals, nursing homes, or other medical care facilities. Remote dispensing of medications by automated packaging and labeling systems is a typical example of telepharmacy.

- *Telepathology:* This is the practice of pathology at a distance, using telecommunications technology to transfer pathology data between distant locations. A pathologist, Ronald S. Weinstein, coined the term "telepathology" in 1986, when he published the first scientific paper on robotic telepathology. Two essential techniques currently used in telepathology are static imaging and dynamic imaging. In static telepathology, one or more microscope images are captured and transmitted to a pathologist for interpretation. In dynamic telepathology, the pathologist receives real-time pictures from the remote microscope. Telepathology has been successfully used for many applications including tissue diagnoses, education, and research.

- *Telesurgery:* This is also known as remote surgery, where the physical distance between the surgeon and the patient is immaterial. This is the ability for a doctor to perform surgery on a patient at a distant location. In telesurgery, a surgeon carries out an operation at a distance from the patient. Telesurgery combines elements of robotics and communication technology. The US military have been using telesurgery, mainly for improving surgery on the battlefield. A major limitation is the speed, latency, and reliability of the communication system between the surgeon and the patient. Figure 3.3 shows an example of telesurgery [17].

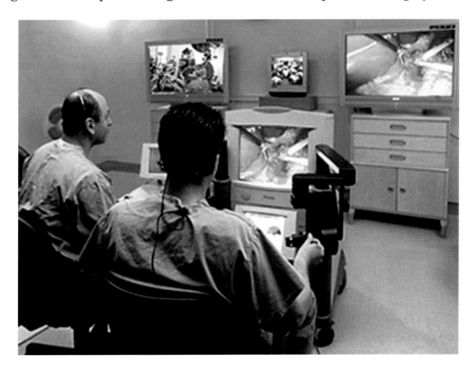

Figure 3.3 An example of telesurgery [17].

- *Teleophthalmology:* This is a branch of telemedicine that delivers eye care through medical equipment and telecommunications technology. Teleophthalmology solutions allow ophthalmologists to examine patients' eyes from a distance. It also allows disease screening, diagnosis, and monitoring. The importance of visual information in ophthalmology makes it obvious that telemedicine will offer benefits in terms of ophthalmological consultations. Teleophthalmology can be practiced, for example, between primary healthcare practitioners and specialists. A typical example is an ophthalmologist diagnosing and treating an eye infection [18].

- *Telenursing:* This refers to the use of information technology in order to provide nursing services when a large physical distance exists between patient and nurse. As a field it is part of telehealth, and has many points of contacts with other medical applications, such as teleconsultation, telemonitoring, etc. Telenursing may help solve increasing shortages of nurses; to reduce distances and save travel time, and to keep patients out of hospital.

- *Teletrauma care:* This helps improve the effectiveness of the delivery of care in a trauma environment. Using telemedicine, trauma specialists can interact with personnel to determine the severity of injuries just as a trauma specialist located physically with the patient. The trauma practitioners can watch a live video stream from the patient's bedside. For example, trauma surgeons can observe and consult on cases from a remote location using video conferencing.

- *Telepediatrics:* This is a technological tool that is improving the health of children around the world. It enables pediatricians to use telemedicine for a broad range of applications such as teleeducation, teleconsultation, telepractice, and teleresearch. Using this technology overcomes the barriers of time and distance, allowing specialists to bring their skills to the bedside of the child in need [19].

- *Teleneuropsychology:* This is another form of telemedicine. It is the use of telemedicine technology for the remote administration of neuropsychological tests, which are used to evaluate the cognitive status of individuals.

- *Telenephrology:* This is nephrology practiced at a distance. Telenephrology solutions are most commonly used interprofessionally, when a family physician needs to consult a nephrologist about a patient with kidney disease.

- *Teleobstetrics:* This allows obstetricians to provide prenatal care from afar. A typical example may involve recording a baby's heart at one location and forwarding it to an obstetrician for diagnosis at another facility.

- *Teledentistry:* This is the use of ICT for dental care, consultation, and education. It can be used to assist general dentists and improve services to underserved populations. It can also be used to help children with dental screenings, treatment, and referral.

- *Teleaudiology:* This is the application of telemedicine to provide audiological services and practice. Teleaudiology program can be combined with an existing hearing care practice.

- *Teleoncology:* This provides more accessible and convenient care to patients with cancer. Teleoncology can enhance both access to and the quality of clinical cancer care. Implementation of teleoncology should be based on the needs of local communities and introduced to potential stakeholders.

- *Telementoring:* This involves the use of video and telecommunication technologies to offer individual guidance. For example, a physician may telementor a local healthcare provider who is new in the field.

- *Telecardiology:* This involves real-time transmission of an ECG from a patient to a cardiologist. Telecardiology has the potential to change the way cardiac care is being delivered in the primary care setting. Telemedicine benefits in almost all areas in the continuum of cardiovascular disease. For example, the monitoring center can dispatch a mobile intensive care unit if necessary.
- *Tele-education*: This involves education and training of patients and/or professionals at distance. Online information sources are currently available over the Internet. When the information is oriented towards medicine or healthcare it fits into our definition of tele-medicine. Telemedicine can also facilitate medical education by allowing workers to observe experts in their fields and share best practices easily. For example, some trauma centers are delivering trauma lectures to hospitals and healthcare providers worldwide

These services are helpful in improving accessibility of healthcare to all patients, particularly those living in rural areas with limited local health professionals.

Besides teleeverything, other applications of telemedicine include [20]:

- *Remote Clinics*: Governments have taken the lead in setting up telemedicine clinics around the world. This is a new way of providing specialty medical services to people living in remote, usually rural communities. Video clinics have also been reported to be well received by the patients.
- *Stroke Telemedicine*: Telemedicine service for stroke is an effort to lower cost and improve quality of care. It facilitates care of patients with acute stroke by specialists at stroke centers.
- *Space Shuttle*: During Space Shuttle missions, telemedicine is used daily to ensure the sound health of the crew. Right from the beginning of its operation, NASA has incorporated telemedicine into routine space operations. NASA has undertaken a telemedicine technology development program to develop the necessary systems, protocols, and training to deal with the in-flight problems [21].
- *Online Booking:* Outpatient clinic appointment bookings can improve patient experience. The booking can be done using emails or texting. Appointment confirmation is sent now by text messages rather than the traditional letter.
- *Home-monitoring:* Care services at the home of the patient (e. g. for elderly patients, diabetics). Home-monitoring may confer improvement in cost-effectiveness and quality of care.
- *Developing Countries:* Telemedicine allows a rapid deployment of healthcare in developing nations. Instead of building and staffing large number of facilities, telemedicine allows clinics to consult at anywhere in the world.

Other clinical applications of telemedicine include teleburn services, intensive care unit, emergencies, abortion, obesity, otolaryngology, cardiovascular disease, disaster medicine, and tele-epidemiology. The nonclinical applications of telemedicine include continuing medical education, online healthcare information resources, coordinating research at multiple sites, and video conferencing for administrative meetings. Telemedicine makes it easier for providers to follow-up with patients. Telemedicine can help patients adhere to their medication regiments.

3.5 BENEFITS

Telemedicine is a new fascinating development that enhances the level of medical services. It holds the promise of significant changes within the healthcare industry since it offers an opportunity to attract and retain consumers. It can transform the future of medicine in both rural and urban settings. Appropriate deployment of telemedicine technologies can increase efficiency of care delivery, reduce expenses of caring for patients, and keep patients out of the hospital. It can provide access to scarce specialist care and improve the quality of care in rural areas. Telemedicine should support and enhance traditional face-to-face medicine. A strong doctor-patient relationship is the foundation for high-quality patient care and reducing health care costs.

With the related fields of mobile health and health IT, telemedicine is changing faster than ever before. It is rapidly expanding to serve millions of consumers. The following benefits for both patients and healthcare providers have greatly contributed to the rapid spread of telemedicine [21].

- *Convenience*: Telemedicine service is a convenient, accessible, affordable alternative to traditional in-office care. Telemedicine is increasingly becoming a tool for convenient medical care. It reduces the cost and inconvenience of traveling for patients.
- *Cost Saving*: It may save money for both patients and physicians. With a full suite telemedicine software, physicians may not need to spend as much time in their clinic.
- *Affordability*: The patients need no transportation time or costs. Thus, telemedicine is regarded as a cost-effective alternative to the more traditional face-to-face way of providing medical care.
- *Accessibility:* It has the ability to provide healthcare to a patient, regardless of the patient or provider's location. It is easier for patients to access care when they need it, where they are at, whether that's at home, office, school, etc. in a way that traditional care delivery settings cannot.
- *Improves Care Quality:* The quality of healthcare has risen whenever telemedicine is deployed. Telemedicine can provide access to scarce specialist care (shortage of health professionals) and improve the quality of care in rural areas.
- *Shortage of Clinicians*: Telemedicine systems are regarded as a necessary measure to alleviate the shortfall in skilled medical specialists in developing countries [22].
- *Rural Health:* For people living in the rural/remote areas and underserved communities in developing countries, access to healthcare services is limited. Telemedicine can be of a great help in the remote areas. It connects patient and specialized doctors remotely. It can facilitate the delivery of healthcare services to rural areas. For rural and underserved areas in particular, telemedicine can reduce transportation problem [23].
- *Cross-border Telemedicine:* Telemedicine eliminates geographic barriers and traditional barriers and matches supply with demand in real time. It allows the transmission of health information across the borders of nation states. International telemedicine is attracting the attention of private firms and hospitals operating in South America, Africa, Asia, and the Arab world [24].

3.6 CHALLENGES

In spite of these benefits, telemedicine is yet to become the go-to place for healthcare. Critics of telemedicine argue that it overpromotes the role of nonphysician health care providers, decreases the value of credentials, changes the patient-physician relationship, redistributes income among specialists and generalists, and will increase the surplus of physicians and specialists [25]. Challenges related to telemedicine may range from technical limiting barriers to ethical and patient confidentiality concerns.

- *Technical Training and Equipment:* Like most technology solutions, telemedicine requires some training and equipment purchases. Some critics of telemedicine argue that online interactions are impersonal. Many physicians and patients alike still like a "personal touch."

- *License Restriction:* Healthcare providers currently obtain their medical licenses to practice in a specific state. A specialist based in Texas is not legally allowed to treat a patient in Florida. This creates a problem for telemedicine.

- *Limited reimbursement:* Its widespread use has been limited by low reimbursement rates and interstate licensing issues. State legislation determines the restrictions and reimbursement rates for telemedicine services. Telemedicine reimbursement is a major challenge.

- *Malpractice:* There is risk of data breach with any Internet-based service. Can a bad audio connection still make a doctor liable?

- *Inpatient management:* It is difficult to take full responsibility for hospital type care from a distance. Many practitioners are not willing to provide care or consultation without face-to-face contact and a physical examination that can only be done in person.

- *Cultural barriers:* A major challenge is a complex of human and cultural barriers. This may occur from the lack of desire, or unwillingness, of some physicians to adapt clinical paradigms for telemedicine applications.

- *Legal considerations:* These are a major obstacle to telemedicine uptake. These include an absence of an international legal framework to allow health professionals to deliver services in different states or countries.

- *Expensive Technology:* It requires a lot of time and financial investment to implement a telemedicine unit. Telemedicine is expensive in the beginning. It is an endeavor that requires up-to-date equipment, trained staff, and familiarization to telemedicine laws. It is difficult for the developing countries to allocate huge budget for the investment in telemedicine. There is lack of convincing scientific evidence of the clinical and cost effectiveness of many telemedicine applications.

- *Complexity:* It is regarded as a technology that is hard to use. Since medicine and technology have become sophisticated over the years, telemedicine has become complex. Needless to say, telemedicine requires patients to be familiar with the Internet. There is also the problem of incompatibility of telemedicine systems.

- *Privacy and Confidentiality:* In all nations, issues related to confidentiality, dignity, security, and privacy are of ethical concern. Although security, privacy, and confidentiality issues also exist in traditional healthcare, the electronic recording, storage, and retrieval of patient sensitive data in a telemedicine system increase opportunities for infringing on patients' rights. Financial cost also poses a barrier to the adoption of telemedicine in developing countries.

- *No standardization:* There is no standardization in the practice of telemedicine, which poses accreditation problem. There is lack of definite regulatory policy and guidelines in the practice of telemedicine across the world.

3.7 CONCLUSION

Telemedicine is the use of information and telecommunication technology (ICT) to provide patients with clinical services at a distance. Telemedicine is not a single technology. Instead, it is an integration of many communications and information technologies with medical field. Telemedicine is a tool for comprehensive care. There are great opportunities for telemedicine to improve diagnostics, therapeutics, and education in healthcare. Although telemedicine is still medicine at a distance, the technology and range of applications have changed it considerably. It is a fertile field that has dramatically altered the face of healthcare in a relatively short amount of time. It is revolutionizing traditional healthcare. If properly designed, implemented, marketed, and used appropriately, telemedicine can enhance the quality of life, independence, and quality of care of many persons with disabilities. More is still expected, especially when it comes to providing telemedical service for developing countries.

In spite of so much development and progress in the field of telemedicine, it has yet to become integral part of healthcare system due to cost associated and lack of technical expertise required. As technology continues to improve and decrease in cost, telemedicine will improve. Telemedicine will continue to benefit the healthcare system in developing nations in terms of preventive care and disease treatment. As a technology that is transforming the entire healthcare infrastructure, telemedicine is here to stay.

In the United States, the American Telemedicine Association (http://www.americantelemed.org/) and the Center of Telehealth are the most respectable places to go for information about telemedicine. More information about telemedicine can be found in the books in [10, 26-36] and the following journals devoted to it:

- *Journal of Telemedicine and Telecare*
- *International Journal of Telemedicine and Applications*
- *Telemedicine Journal*
- *Telemedicine Journal and e-Health*
- *Telemedicine Today*

REFERENCES

[1] M. N. O. Sadiku, M. Tembely, and S.M. Musa, "Telemedicine: A primer (Part 1)," *International Journal of Advanced Research in Computer Science and Software Engineering,* vol. 9, no. 6, June 2019, pp.43-46.

[2]. M. N. O. Sadiku, M. Tembely, and S.M. Musa, "Telemedicine: Teleeverything phenomena (Part 2)," *International Journal of Advanced Research in Computer Science and Software Engineering,* vol. 9, no. 6, June 2019, pp.35-38.

[3] H. A. Aziz And H. Abochar, "Telemedicine," *Clinical Laboratory Science,* vol. 28, no. 4, October 2015, pp. 256-258.

[4] J. Trader, "Why telemedicine needs secure patient identification," November 2015, https://www.rightpatient.com/blog/why-telemedicine-needs-secure-patient-identification/

[5] WHO, "Telemedicine: opportunities and developments in Member States," 2009.

[6] J. Craig and V. Petterson, "Introduction to the practice of telemedicine,"*Journal of Telemedicine and Telecare,* January, 2005.

[7] "Types of telemedicine," https://chironhealth.com/definitive-guide-to-telemedicine/about-telemedicine/types-of-telemedicine/

[8] M. N. O. Sadiku, A. E. Shadare, and S.M. Musa, "Mobile health," *International Journal of Engineering Research,* vol. 6, no. 11, Oct. 2017, pp. 450-452.

[9] L. J. Moore, "An investigation into the impact of telemedicine on the veterinary practitioner," *Doctoral Dissertation,* Auburn University, 2001.

[10] A. C. M. Fong, B. Fong, and C. K. Li, *Telemedicine Technologies: Information Technologies in Medicine and Telehealth.* John Wiley & Sons, 2011.

[11] "Examples of telemedicine," https://www.dgtelemed.de/de/telemedizin/anwendungsbeispiele.php

[12] "The ultimate telemedicine guide | What is telemedicine?" May 2018, https://evisit.com/resources/what-is-telemedicine/

[13] "Telemedicine," *Wikipedia,* the free encyclopedia https://en.wikipedia.org/wiki/Telemedicine

[14] R. Wootton, "Telemedicine: The current state of the art," *Minimally Invasive Therapy & Allied Technologies,* vol. 6, no. 5-6, 1997, pp. 393-403.

[15] S. Norman, "The use of telemedicine in psychiatry," *Journal of Psychiatric and Mental Health Nursing,* vol 13, 2006, pp. 771–777.

[16] E. M.T. Wurm et al., "Telemedicine and teledermatology: Past, present and future," *Journal der Deutschen Dermatologischen Gesellschaft,* vol. 6, no. 2, Feb. 2008, pp.106-112.

[17] F. G. La Rosa, "Telehealth and telemedicine: A new paradigm in global health," November 2016, http://www.ucdenver.edu/academics/colleges/PublicHealth/research/centers/globalhealth/events/Documents/GHLS%20Fall%202016/F-La_Rosa-Telehealth-Telemedicine-11-23-2016.pdf

[18] H. Lamminen et al., "Telemedicine in ophthalmology," *Acta Ophthalmologica Scandinavica,* vol. 81, 2003, pp. 105–109.

[19] B. L. Burke and R. W. Hall, "Telemedicine: Pediatric applications," *Pediatrics,* vol. 136, no. 1, July 2015.

[20] "Examples of telemedicine," https://www.dgtelemed.de/de/telemedizin/anwendungsbeispiele.php

[21] S. C. Simmons, "Telemedicine: A technology with space flight and terrestrial health care applications," *SAE Transactions,* vol. 104, 1995, pp. 915-920.

[22] K. I. Adenuga, N. A. Iahad, and S. Miskon, "Towards reinforcing telemedicine adoption amongst clinicians in Nigeria," *International Journal of Medical Informatics,* vol. 104, 2017, pp. 84-96.

[23] A. C. Smith et al., "Telemedicine and rural health care applications," *Journal of Postgraduate Medicine,* vol. 51, no. 4, October-December, 2005, pp.:286-293.

[24] L. Jarudi, "Doctors without borders: The advent of telemedicine and society," *Harvard International Review,* vol. 22, no. 1, 2000, pp. 36-39.

[25] H. K. Li, "Telemedicine and ophthalmology," *Survey of Ophthalmology,* vol. 44, no. 1, July–August 1999, pp. 61-72.

[26] A. C. Norris, *Essentials of Telemedicine and Telecare.* John Wiley and Sons, 2002.

[27] A. Kamenca, *Telemedicine: A Practical Guide for Professionals.* MindView Press, 2017.

[28] S. B. Bhattacharyya, *A DIY Guide to Telemedicine for Clinicians.* Springer, 2017.

[29] G. W. Shannon and R. Bashshur, *History of Telemedicine: Evolution, Context, and Transformation.* Mary Ann Liebert, 2009.

[30] A. W. Darkins and M.A. Cary, *Telemedicinae and Telehealth: Principles, Policies, Performance and Pitfalls.* London, UK: Springer, 2000.

[31] R. Wootton, J. Craig, and V. Patterson (eds), *Introduction to Telemedicine.* Boca Raton, FL: CRC Press; 2nd edition, 2017.

[32] S. Gogia (ed.), *Fundamentals of Telemedicine and Telehealth.* Academic Press, 2019.

[33] M. M. Maheu P. Whitten, and A. Allen, *E-Health, Telehealth, and Telemedicine: A Guide to Startup and Success.* San Francisco, CA: Jossey-Bass, 2001.

[34] Information Resources Management Association, *E-Health and Telemedicine: Concepts, Methodologies, Tools, and Applications.* IGI Global, 2015.

[35] M. J. Field (ed.), *Telemedicine: A Guide to Assessing Telecommunications for Health Care.* National Academies Press, 1996.

[36] The Coding Institute, *Telemedicine and Telehealth Handbook for Medical Practices 2019.* The Coding Institute, 2019.

CHAPTER 4

ELECTRONIC AND MOBILE HEALTH

"One kind word can warm three winter months." - Japanese Proverb

4.1 INTRODUCTION

Electronic health (ehealth) and mobile health (mhealth) are emerging concepts in healthcare. They both explore telemedicine. Next to using emails, search engines, and social media, looking for health information is the most important activity among Internet users. As more and more people use Internet-based and mobile health resources and as the Internet becomes a major channel for socialization and source of health information, ehealth and mhealth become important. The Internet continues to be in invaluable resource in providing information that is of use to health professionals. This includes information about diagnoses, medications and their side-effects, treatment options. The Internet facilitates access to health information [1].

The advent of mobile technology is transforming the way healthcare is delivered and managed. Mobile phones came on the market in the 1980s and only a few other technologies have had a comparable popular success. Advanced mobile phone technologies are enabling mobile healthcare delivery. These technologies, along with mobile Internet, offering anywhere and anytime connectivity, play a key role on modern healthcare solutions. Doctors, nurses, and other health professionals use mobile devices to access patient information, databases, and resources.

Mobile health is the creative use of emerging mobile devices to deliver and improve healthcare practices. It includes the use of cell phones, tablets, and integrated monitoring devices to support healthcare. It integrates mobile technology with the health delivery with the premise of promoting a better health and improving efficiency. Mobile health has become an increasingly important issue in a number of disciplines such as health communication, public health, and health promotion [2].

Mobile technologies can facilitate access to healthcare professionals and provide instant access to multiple wireless networks. They can increase the speed of decision making, especially for emergency situations. The rapid and wide-scale introduction of mobile technologies in healthcare is resulting in an emerging area of mobile health [3].

This paper provides a brief introduction to electronic health and mobile health. It begins by discusses the two concepts of ehealth and mhealth. It covers some applications of ehealth and mhealth.

It addresses the challenges faced by the adoption of ehealth and mhealth technologies. The last section concludes with comments.

4.2 CONCEPT OF ELECTRONIC HEALTH

Electronic health (ehealth) is a new concept which refers to the use of information and communication technology (ICT) to enable health care. It is the delivery of health information and services over the Internet and related technologies. E-health literacy is the ability to seek and gather health information from digital sources and apply the information to solve health problems. Individuals with high ehealth literacy frequently search the Internet for health information. They are savvy shoppers in the health marketplace and are effective managers of their own care. Government agencies such as the National Institutes of Health and Centers for Disease Control continually put health information online so that people can benefit and learn from it. The Internet has the potential for improving ehealth literacy. Ehealth is closely related to health informatics. It can also include health applications and links on mobile phones, referred to as mHealth.

Ehealth is an interdisciplinary field involving information technology, bioengineering, medical treatment, and healthcare. Technologies for ehealth include health monitoring, ubiquitous solutions for healthcare, games for health, real-time access of medical records and services, medical assisted systems for elderly people, and medical data over wireless body sensor networks. Ehealth cannot be separated from electronic health records (EHRs), which is the core part of an ehealth system. EHealth in general, and telemedicine in particular, is an important tool for extending healthcare services to remote regions of emerging and developing countries [4].

4.3 CONCEPT OF MOBILE HEALTH

Mobile health (or mHealth) refers to the practice of medicine via mobile devices such as mobile phones, tablet computers, personal digital assistants (PDAs), and wearable devices. It has emerged as a subdiscipline of electronic health (or eHealth). While eHealth can be regarded as technology that supports the delivery of healthcare and provides healthcare services online, mHealth essentially provides access to healthcare [5]. Several factors contribute to this trend, especially the continuous adoption of mobile devices and the need of providing care and support for an aging society. A typical m-Health services architecture is shown in Figure 4.1 [6]. Mhealth architecture includes many settings, devices, and operational features—all of these facilitate access, timeliness, and integration, as shown in Figure 4.2 [7].

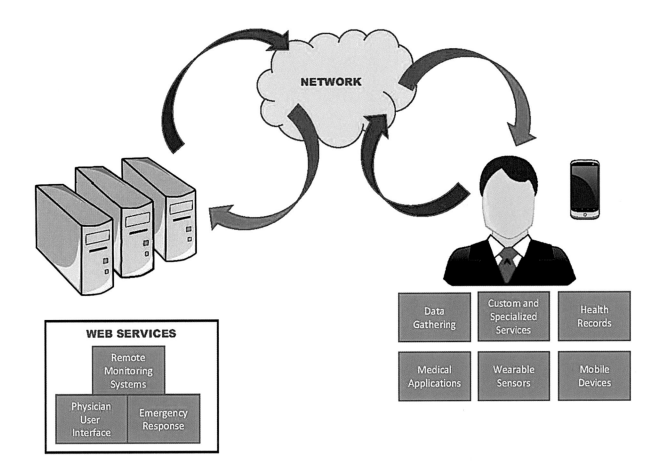

Figure 4.1 A typical mHealth architecture [6].

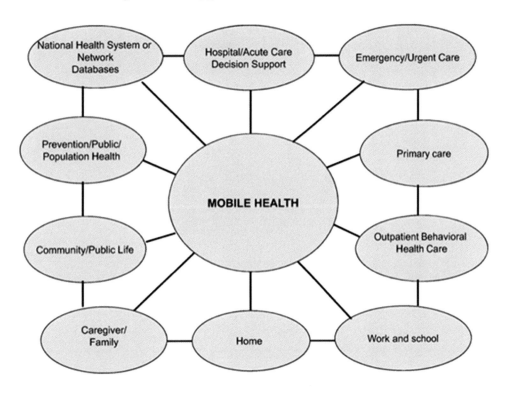

Figure 4.2 How mobile health, smartphone, and apps integrate information in the digital age [7].

Worldwide, mobile technologies have demonstrated the power of communication as an agent for social change. As advances in capabilities of mobile devices are made, significant benefits can be achieved in the delivery of health care services. Integrating use of GIS and GPS with mobile technologies adds a useful geographical mapping component.

Mhealth technologies include mobile/smartphone applications, wearable devices, handheld devices, health text messaging, remote monitoring, and portable sensor devices. There is an increase rise in the usage of mobile health sensors in wearable devices and smartphones. Mhealth can be implemented as automated or human-assisted. Mhealth technologies, when linked to cloud computing, provide several advantages. Mhealth applications often take advantage of a smartphone's features such as touch screens, cameras, gyroscopes, lights, sounds, and wireless connectivity, as well as software that processes interactive questionnaires, algorithms, formulae, calculators, and clinical decision support tools. Smartphones are replacing stethoscopes and pagers as the most ubiquitous physician accessory [8]. Figure 4.3 shows a mobile health unit [9].

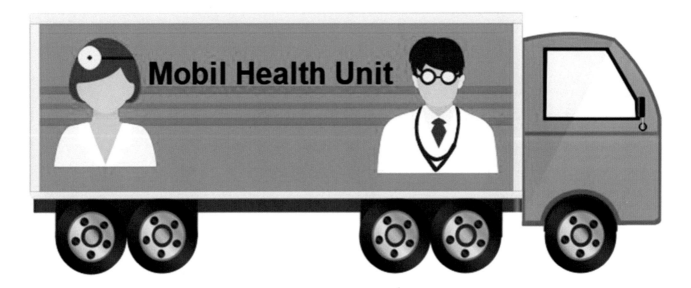

Figure 4.3 Mobile health unit [9].

Such a mobile health unit typically provides primary care from a specialty equipped medical vehicle with full clinic services and electronic medical records on board.

Important characteristics of mHealth include [10]:

- *Accessibility:* Mobile technology overcomes time-related, geographic, and location-specific constraints.
- *Inclusivity:* The high penetration of mobile apps and the free availability of many health apps increase the uses of mHealth.
- *Patients' Autonomy:* This is one of the most important defining characteristics of mHealth. mHealth technologies empower patients to monitor their health conditions on a continuous base.
- *Increasing Accuracy of Diagnostics and Treatment:* Chronic disease patients often need continuous supervision and personalized support which is difficult through traditional methods. Continuous

patient monitoring also enhances the knowledge and abilities of healthcare providers to identify the problems and provide better solutions to the needs of their patients.

- *Improvement in Service Quality:* mHealth can be used to manage human resources effectively in healthcare organizations in a number of ways such as continuous training and education of the workforce, work-planning, scheduling, supervising, and improving health workers' adherence to treatment guidelines

- *Testability:* With mobile technology, the concept of test marketing can be transmitted to the healthcare context. Test marketing enables researchers to test a new product in a typical target population.

4.4 APPLICATIONS

Ehealth systems are typically sustained on EHR-system, which is essentially a repository of information regarding the health records of patients. At present, the most commercialized ehealth technologies include a fetal heart rate monitoring, portable hemoglobin meter, medical data communication system, mobile technology to connect patients to remote doctors, and treatment response software application [6]. Some of these are ehealth commercial telemedical systems. For an example, data has shown that ehealth technology can strongly impact asthma self-management in children and adolescents and their families, which can improve patient compliance[11]. E-mental health has been gaining attention in a wide variety of disciplines such as psychology, clinical social work, family and marriage therapy, and mental health counseling. Ehealth and mhealth technologies have found many applications such as monitoring vital physiological parameters. Some applications target patient, while others target healthcare professionals.

Many innovative mHealth applications exist. Applications can deal with disease prevention and wellness, monitoring and remote care, smoking cessation, weight loss, diet and physical activity, medication adherence, chronic disease management, mobile decision making, and emergency interventions. In 2011, the World Health Organization (WHO) identified several emerging health technologies that present the potential for being solutions for unmet medical needs. Google Android and Apple iOS dominate the OS market.

The market of mhealth technology is directed toward patients, clinicians, and healthcare practitionerls. Mhealth applications have an impact on all healthcare services such as hospitals, urgent care centers, and outpatient clinics. Common applications of mhealth include the following:

- *Disease management*: Mhealth is particularly beneficial for chronic disease patients who require long-term and regular services. There are presently more than 165,000 mHealth applications (apps) publicly available in major app stores. The top 2 categories are wellness management and disease management apps, whereas other categories include self-diagnosis, disease management, well management, mental heatlh, medication reminder, patient education, and electronic patient portal. These apps can provide free or low-cost, around-the-clock access to high-quality, evidence-based health information [12].

- *Teleconsultation:* Mhealth has promoted the development of teleconsultation, which is basically cross-regional medical consultation by means of computer and communication technology between medical institutions. This application may change the disease intervention to prevention, keeping healthy people away from disease [13].

- *Mammography Screening:* Mhealth is increasingly utilized to assist in providing mammography screening. Providing these services can be effective in increasing access and decreasing barriers to screening hard-to-reach populations [14].
- *Diabetes Monitoring:* Mobile diabetes monitoring could be an effective tool to functionally address the clinical needs of rural communities and healthcare centers. This may involve insulin and medication recording, data export and communication, diet recording, and weight managements. Even physicians prefer that their patients be able to monitor their health at home, particularly their weight and blood sugar levels [15].

Other applications of mhealth technology includes obesity, smoking cessation, elderly care, cardiopulmonary disease, and educational applications. The rapid growth of mHealth applications has forced many healthcare organizations to treat employees as shared owners of end user technologies such as smartphones, iPads, and tablets. Many mHealth apps promote themselves through advertising on social media channels, thereby increasing their use.

4.5 BENEFITS

Ehealth connects medical informatics, public health, and business through associated technologies, such as the Internet. It provides health information to medically undeserved populations. It is committed to enhancing the quality and efficiency of healthcare services both locally and globally while reducing the escalating cost. Effective ehealth initiatives can benefit both patients (through better education, information and self-management) and healthcare systems (through resource sparing, data-analysis and computer-aided decision making) [16].

Mhealth aims to deliver healthcare anytime and anywhere, overcoming geographical and organizational barriers with reasonable and affordable costs. Both technologies were useful for adherence, diagnosis, disease control mechanisms, information provision, and decision-making [17].

Healthcare systems are increasingly using mHealth to provide better services with less financial and human resources. This technology represents an advantage especially for reaching patients who otherwise would have no access to healthcare. Its benefits include 24/7 availability, equity, immediate support treatment, continuous health monitoring, anonymity, networking, patient's knowledge/ education, and low cost [18]. Mhealth technologies enable social networking to promote healthy behaviors and awareness among patients. Today, social networks are playing an important role on the people's daily life.

4.6 CHALLENGES

Despite the benefits and widespread use of ehealth and mhealth technologies, healthcare leaders need to resolve a number of unique challenges for ehealth and mHealth to significantly contribute to healthcare service delivery.

Rapid advances in ehealth present both opportunities and challenges. A range of barriers prevent people from fully benefiting from the spectrum e-health provisions. Unequal access to the Internet continues to be responsible for the digital divide [19]. Although inequality of Internet access has declined in developed nations, access is still prohibitively expensive for the elderly and people in low income. As the web evolves, an increasing amount of information is available on the Internet, which causes information overload. As the number of websites continues to grow, their poor organization may make obtaining relevant information difficult. Many websites provide information that is inaccurate, questionable or hard to understand. Health consumers may have difficulties in identifying quality, trustworthy, credible, useful health information online. Most people still prefer receiving health information through face-to-face physician-patient interaction. The issues of privacy and security remain an ongoing major concern, especially in areas involving sensitive behavior or treatment (alcohol, drug use, mental or sexual health) and possibly illegal behavior. Privacy, confidentiality, and security are considered as essential freedom of an individual [20].

The success and widespread adoption of mHealth depend on meeting some challenges. These challenges include protecting the privacy of patient information shared on mobile devices, concerns about the unregulated status of mHealth, and legal issues especially in developing countries that lack privacy and data protection laws. Concerns about safety revolve around privacy risks. Mobile devices such as smartphones, tablets, and wearable devices that contain healthcare information are targets for thieves.

To address the privacy and security concerns, we now have the Health Insurance Portability and Accountability Act (HIPAA), the Health Information Technology for Economic and Clinical Health (HITECH), and other federal and state laws. In the US, mHealth devices come under the regulatory authority of the Food and Drug Administration (FDA). Healthcare providers that transmit patient information electronically must comply with the rules [21].

Mobile devices have limited computation, storage, and battery powers. It is not economical and feasible for a hospital to equip thousands of healthcare staff with mobile devices. Lack of operating system (OS) neutrality is another challenge in the development and adoption of mhealth applications. There are multiple operating systems for mobile phones such as iOs, Microsoft Windows, Palm OS, Blackberry, Linux, and the Android.

Different mhealth initiatives in different countries do not adopt globally due to lack of accepted standards or interoperable infrastructures, making future integrations difficult if not impossible. The mHealth intervention app market has long been isolated, unregulated, and patient-driven. There is little information on which of mHealth apps are effective, or how well they compare with face-to-face treatments.

The mHealth transformation has been disruptive in the developing countries, where the growth of mHealth has been rather slow. In those nations, healthcare systems are facing major challenges in providing affordable and better quality of care due to the increase in chronic and communicable diseases. There remains hurdles like low literacy, poor infrastructure, shortage of doctors and other skilled healthcare professionals, lack of continuous power supply, and cultural issues hindering the large-scale adoption of mHealth [22].

Other challenges include administrative, architectural, implementation, and balancing the productivity, cost benefits, or scientific value of new information technologies with the security risks [23]. Despite these challenges, mhealth has the potential of improving health outcomes, and it should be given priority by governments and non-governmental organizations (NGOs).

4.7 CONCLUSION

Ehealth refers to health services delivered through ICT, while mhealth refers to the use of mobile and wireless communication technologies to provide healthcare delivery and support wellness. The demand for self-monitoring health devices is skyrocketing primarily due to wireless and mobile health technologies.

Mhealth is an innovative means of providing healthcare services and is a promising frontier that can be used to solve health inequality and health coverage. Mhealth services propose healthcare delivery anytime and anywhere overcoming geographical barriers with low and affordable costs. Challenges such as privacy concerns have limited the impact of mhealth, but it has enormous potential to reshape healthcare delivery in the future. Mhealth continues to climb in popularity and it definitely represents the future trend of health care due to its great potential in improving health care efficiency and accessibility [24]. More information about ehealth and mhealth can be found in the books in [25-28] and the following related journals:

- *mHealth*
- *Journal omHealth*
- *Journal of Healthcare Communications*
- *Journal of Mobile Technology in Medicine*
- *JMIR (Journal of Medical Internet Research) mHealth and uHealth*
- *Telemedicine and e-Health*
- *Medical Technologies Journal*
- *Technology and Health Care*

REFERENCES

[1] M. N. O. Sadiku, M. Tembely, S.M. Musa, and O. D. Momoh, "eHealth literacy," *International Journal of Advanced Research in Computer Science and Software Engineering*, vol. 7, no. 6, June 2017, pp. 68-69.

[2] M. N. O. Sadiku, A. E. Shadare, and S.M. Musa, "Mobile health," *International Journal of Engineering Research*, vol. 6, no. 11, Oct. 2017, pp. 450-452.

[3] U. Varshney, "A model for improving quality of decisions in mobile health," *Decision Support Systems*, vol. 62, 2014, pp. 66–77.

[4] "eHealth," *Wikipedia*, the free encyclopedia, https://en.wikipedia.org/wiki/EHealth

[5] "mHealth," *Wikipedia*, the free encyclopedia https://en.wikipedia.org/wiki/MHealth

[6] B. M. C. Silva et al., "Mobile-health: A review of current state in 2015," *Journal of Biomedical Informatics*, vol. 56, 2015, pp. 265–272.

[7] D. M. Hilty et al., "A telehealth framework for mobile health, smartphones, and apps: competencies, training, and faculty development," *Journal of Technology in Behavioral Science*, vol. 4, April 2019, pp. 106–123.

[8] N. Cortez, "The mobile health revolution?" https://lawreview.law.ucdavis.edu/issues/47/4/Articles/47-4_Cortez.pdf

[9] "Mobile health unit," https://www.bayclinic.org/locations/administrative-office-2

[10] C. Sahin," Rules of engagement in mobile health: What does mobile health bring to research and theory?" *Contemporary Nurse,* vol. 54, no. 4-5, 2018, pp. 374-387.

[11] A. Licari, "What is the impact of innovative electronic health interventions in improving treatment adherence in asthma? The pediatric perspective," *The Journal of Allergy and Clinical Immunology: In Practice*, vol. 7, no. 8,November–December, 2019, pp. 2574-2579.

[12] C. K. Kao and D. M. Liebovitz, "Consumer mobile health apps: Current state, barriers, and future directions," *Physical Medicine and Rehabilitation* (PM R), vol. 9, 2017, pp. S106-S115.

[13] H. Li et al., "Mobile health in China: Current status and future development," *Asian Journal of Psychiatry*, vol. 10, 2014, pp. 101–104,

[14] S. E. Brooks et al., "Mobile mammography in underserved populations: Analysis of outcomes of 3,923 women," *Journal of Community Health,* vol. 38, 2013, pp. 900–906.

[15] S. Okazaki et al., " Physicians' motivations to use mobile health monitoring: A cross-country comparison," *Behaviour & Information Technology*, vol. 36, no. 1, 2017, pp. 21-32.

[16] M. R. Cowie, "Electronic and mobile health in chronic heart failure," *European Journal of Arrhythmia & Electrophysiology*, vol, 4, no. 2, 2018, pp. 45–45.

[17] B. Bervell and H. Al-Samarraie, "A comparative review of mobile health and electronic health utilization in sub-Saharan African countries," *Social Science & Medicine*, vol. 232, July 2019.

[18] M. Olff, "Mobile mental health: A challenging research agenda," *European Journal of Psychotraumatology*, vol. 6, no. 1, 2015, pp. 1-8.

[19] A. Chesser et al., "Navigating the digital divide: A systematic review of eHealth literacy in underserved populations in the United States," *Informatics for Health and Social Care*, vol. 41, no. 1, 2016, pp. 1-19.

[20] N. Werts and L. Hutton-Rogers, "Barriers to achieving e-health literacy," *American Journal of Health Sciences*, vol. 4, no. 3, 2013, pp. 115-120.

[21] B. Liss, "HIPAA and mobile health: Where's the app for that?" *The Computer & Internet Lawyer*, vol. 34, no. 9, September 2017, pp. 9-12.

[22] S. Latif *et al.*, "Mobile health in the developing world: Review of literature and lessons from a case study," *IEEE Access*, vol. 5, 2017, pp. 11540-11556.

[23] M. J. Harvey and M. G. Harvey, "Privacy and security issues for mobile health platforms," *Journal of the Association for Information Science and Technology*, vol. 65, no. 7, 2014, pp. 1305–1318.

[24] R. Miao et al., "Factors that influence users' adoption intention of mobile health: A structural equation modeling approach," *International Journal of Production Research*, vol. 55, no. 19, 2017, pp. 5801-5815.

[25] H. Marston, S. Freeman, and C. Musselwhite (eds.), *Mobile e-Health.* Springer, 2017.

[26] R. S. H. Istepanian, S. Laxminarayan, and C. S. Pattichis (eds.), *M-Health: Emerging Mobile Health Systems.* Springer, 2005.

[27] E. Sezgin et al. (eds.), *Current and Emerging mHealth Technologies: Adoption, Implementation, and Use.* Springer, 2018.

[28] S. Adibi, *Moble Health: A Technology Road Map.* Springer, 2015.

CHAPTER 5

INTERNET OF THINGS IN HEALTHCARE

"The Internet of Things is not a concept; it is a network, the true technology-enabled Network of all networks." — Edewede Oriwoh

5.1 INTRODUCTION

Healthcare is an essential part of the modern life. As they say, "Health is wealth." Healthcare is an essential service sector which has ubiquitous demand worldwide. It meets the basic need of every individual in the modern society. The healthcare system consists of patients, medical institutions, and healthcare resources to deliver healthcare services to meet human health needs. Unfortunately, the system is overwhelmed with problems such as expensive services, overworked doctors and nurses, illegitimate patient diagnoses, the growing rate of the aging population, increasing global demand for medical services, rise in the number of chronic diseases, and living environments with poor health [1]. Some of these problems are illustrated in Figure 5.1. In addition, present approaches used for monitoring a patient in hospitals are time consuming. The Internet of things (IoT) (also known as Future Internet) can resolve these issues quite well.

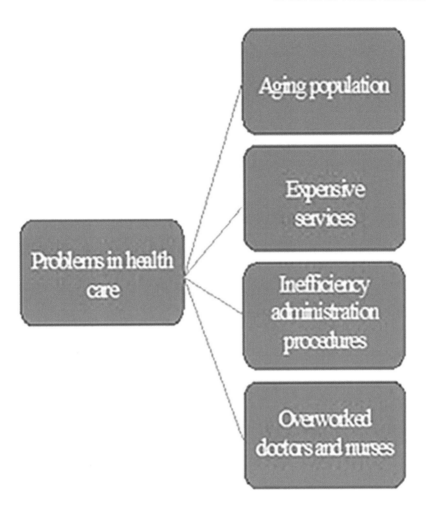

Figure 5.1 Some problems in healthcare [2].

Internet of things (IoT) is the global interconnection of several heterogeneous devices. The Internet has evolved to be an ever more pervasive and critical infrastructure connecting society and enabling global commerce. It allows people and "things" to connect anytime, anywhere using a variety of wired or wireless communication networks. It has become an integral part of modern society. It will have its presence in all sectors of human lives including healthcare. The market for the IoT in healthcare is growing steadily. IoT healthcare helps in effectively managing health and thus improving the quality of life. The central concept of the Internet of Things is to connect anything, anytime, and anywhere through Internet. The emergence of Internet of things has attracted the attention of governments, research scholars, and business community all over the world [2].

This chapter provides a brief introduction into IoT healthcare or the use of IoT in the healthcare domain. It begins by presenting an overview on IoT. It explains why healthcare needs IoT. It discusses Internet of medical things. It covers various applications of IoT in healthcare. It addresses some benefits and challenges of IoT in healthcare. The chapter concludes with some comments.

5.2 OVERVIEW ON INTERNET OF THINGS

The term "Internet of things" was introduced by Kevin Ashton from the United Kingdom in 1999. Internet of things (IoT) is a network of connecting devices embedded with sensors. It is a collection of identifiable things with the ability to communicate over wired or wireless networks. The devices or things can be connected to the Internet through three main technology components: physical devices and sensors (connected things), connection and infrastructure, and analytics and applications.

The IoT is a worldwide network that connects devices to the Internet and to each other using wireless technology. IoT is expanding rapidly and it has been estimated that 50 billion devices will be connected to the Internet by 2020. These include smart phones, tablets, desktop computers, autonomous vehicles, refrigerators, toasters, thermostats, cameras, pet monitors, alarm systems, home appliances, insulin pumps, industrial machines, intelligent wheelchairs, wireless sensors, mobile robots, etc.

There are four main technologies that enable IoT [3]:

1. Radio-frequency identification (RFID) and near-field communication.
2. Optical tags and quick response codes: this is used for low cost tagging.
3. Bluetooth low energy (BLE).
4. Wireless sensor network: they are usually connected as wireless sensor networks to monitor physical properties in specific environments.

Other related technologies are cloud computing, machine learning, and big data.

The Internet of things (IoT) technology enables people and objects to interact with each other. It is employed in many areas such as smart transportation, smart cities, smart energy, emergency services, healthcare, data security, industrial control, logistics, retails, government, traffic congestion, manufacturing, industry, security, agriculture, environment, and waste management. Figure 5.2 shows the Internet of things and its application areas [4].

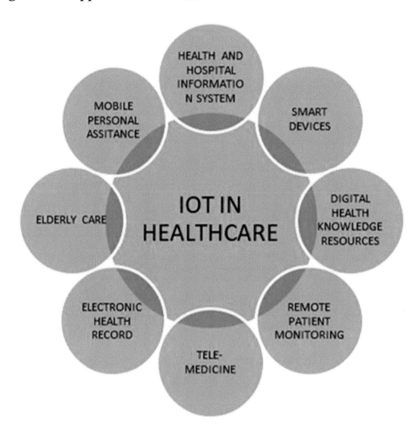

Figure 5.2 Applications of IoT in healthcare [4].

IoT supports many input-output devices such as camera, microphone, keyboard, speaker, displays, microcontrollers, and transceivers. It is the most promising trend in the healthcare industry. This rapidly proliferating collection of Internet-connected devices, including wearables, implants, skin sensors, smart scales, smart bandages, and home monitoring tools has the potential to connect patients and their providers in a unique way. Today, smartphone acts as the main driver of IoT. The smartphone is provided with healthcare applications.

The narrowband version of IoT is known as narrowband IoT (NBIoT). This is an attractive technology for many sectors including healthcare because it has been standardized [5]. The main feature of NBIoT is that it can be easily deployed within the current cellular infrastructure with a software upgrade.

5.3 WHY HEALTHCARE NEEDS IOT

In healthcare system, the motivation of using modern technologies such as IoT is to offer promising solutions for efficiently delivering all kinds of medical healthcare services to patients at affordable cost. IoT could be a game changer for the healthcare services [6]. It makes it now possible to process data and remotely monitor a patient in real time. IoT has been identified as a technological solution to some medical challenges. Through the IoT, anything in the healthcare system can be identified and monitored anytime anywhere. A typical IoT healthcare system is shown in Figure 5.3 [7]. Such system is also known as health-IoT or H-IoT.

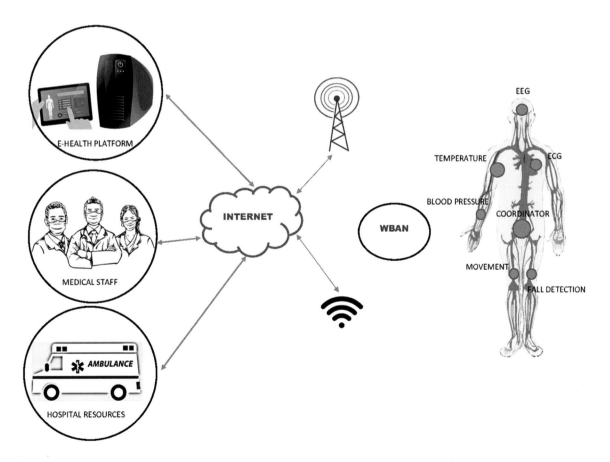

Figure 5.3 A typical IoT healthcare system [7].

IoT is important in healthcare because of the following services it provides.

- *Connectivity:* The major aim of IoT is to connect smart objects/things/devices to the Internet in a transparent way. IoT connects the entities of the real world with the virtual world, thus enabling anytime, any place connectivity for anything. It enables all medical devices to be connected to each other by some communication means. Once connected to the Internet, ordinary medical devices can collect invaluable data, give extra insight into signs, symptoms and trends, and enable remote care. Also, connected medical devices can exchange information or data.

- *Smart Devices:* IoT helps people and communities by making their systems smarter and their lives easier, more secure, and safer. IoT transforms ordinary products such as cars, buildings, and machines into smart, connected objects that can communicate with people and each other. These applications have given birth to smart everything, smart cars, smart homes, smart cities, smart parking, smart health, smart medicine, smart hospital, smart diapers, smart environment, smart transportation, smart lighting, smart grid, and smart energy. IoT also makes hospital networks smarter by monitoring critical infrastructure.

- *Effective Care:* The healthcare industry happens to be one of the fastest industry to adopt IoT. This is due to the fact that integrating IoT technologies into medical devices substantially improves the quality and effectiveness of service. The IoT can support treatments of illness to preventive care and wellbeing solutions. It enables practices in the area of healthcare for children, elderly, chronic care, real time monitoring of patients, operation theaters, and medicine dispenser. The application of IoT in healthcare can provide immediate treatment to the patient as well as monitor and keep track of health record for healthy people. IoT has enabled healthcare system to provide better healthcare services to people at any time and from anywhere in friendly manner.

- *Remote Patient Monitoring:* Before the advent of Internet of things, patients could only interact with doctors through visits. IoT-enables medical devices for remote monitoring., empowering physicians to deliver high quality care as well as increasing patient engagement and satisfaction. Monitoring in real time can significantly cut down unnecessary visits to doctors. Monitoring the health parameters (such as blood pressure, heart rate, temperature, etc.) of a patient remotely is achieved by IoT healthcare.

- *Tracking:* IoT devices tagged with sensors can be used to track real time location of medical equipment like wheelchairs, defibrillators, nebulizers, oxygen pumps, and other monitoring equipment. Deployment of medical staff at different locations can also be tracked.

- *Drug Management* : Drug management is always a challenge. It is one of the major expenses in the healthcare industry. With IoT along with smart devices, it becomes easier to manage. The usage of smart RFID tags in drug distribution and monitoring properly by smart devices provides a reasonable solution. This results in providing quality medications to patients.

These services enhance the quality and efficiency of care treatments which benefit patients, doctors, nurses, and hospitals in a great way. Besides the services above, IoT in healthcare also helps in [8]:

- Reducing emergency room wait time
- Keeping patients safe and healthy
- Ensuring availability of critical hardware

- Saving doctor's time and work
- Enabling nurses, doctors, and other team members to connect and communicate in real time.
- Receiving critical information at the point of care without unnecessary alerts

The healthcare sector has adopted various IoT solutions by creating the Internet of medical things (IoMT), be discussed next.

5.4 INTERNET OF MEDICAL THINGS

The Internet of things in healthcare is variably referred to as IoT-MD, IoMT, Medical IoT, mIoT, and IoHT. Internet of medical things (IoMT), a healthcare application of the IoT technology, has emerged as a combination of advanced medical sensing system, computer communication technologies. The sensing systems include RFID, GPS, and wireless sensor networks. IoMT enables machine-to-machine interaction and real time intervention solutions which are helping the healthcare industry increase its delivery, affordability, reliability, and productivity [9]. When connected to the Internet, ordinary medical devices become smart and can collect more data, give insight into trends, enable remote care, and give patients more control. For example, IoT devices can be used for reminding patients about appointments, when to take medications, changes in blood pressure, calories burnt, and much more [10]. An illustration of IoMT is shown in Figure 5.4 [11].

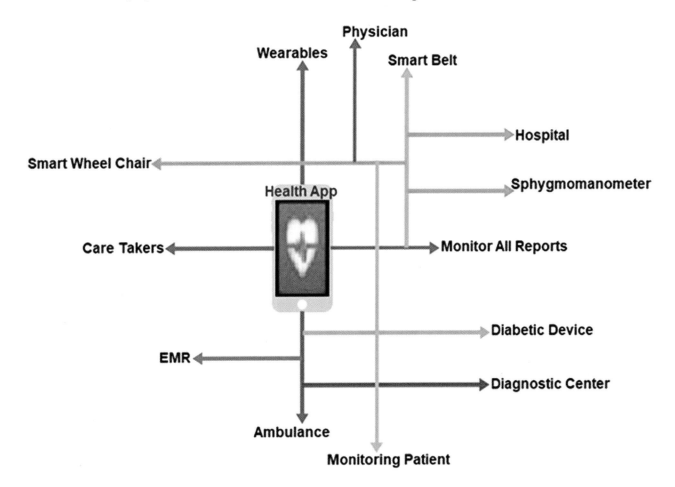

Figure 5.4 The Internet of medical things [11].

IoMT devices can sense real-time data for patient monitoring. Such devices are used to monitor parameters such as blood pressure, random blood sugar levels, and weight. IoMT will promote personalized care and high standard of living. Technologies used in IoMT can be divided into the three technical classes: local patient systems and controls; device connectivity and data management; and analytics solutions [12]. IoMT technology includes remote patient monitoring and medical system management. Smartphones are increasingly used as integral parts of IoMT. Various medical Internet of things platforms have been built for patient information management, telemedicine monitoring, and mobile medical [13].

IoMT is the technology that embeds wireless sensors in medical equipment, combines with the Internet and integrates with hospitals and patients. It is transforming healthcare industry by increasing efficiency, lowering costs, and improving patient quality of care and safety. The doctors can break the limit of the geographical scope and provide medical education for medical personnel in remote areas.

Medical devices present unique IoT challenges. These include the broad range of medical technologies, the diversity of network protocols, critical security and vulnerability, regulatory compliance imperatives resulting from the handling of patient data and stakeholders with varied interests. Security is crucial in healthcare applications, especially in the case of patient privacy. Wearable sensors, for example, are prone to expose patient information and patient privacy

5.5 APPLICATIONS OF IoT IN HEALTHCARE

Besides Internet of medical things, applications of IoT in healthcare are numerous, ranging from remote monitoring to smart sensors and medical device integration. The applications benefit patients, families, nurses, and physicians. IoT healthcare is applicable in many medical instruments such as ECG monitors, glucose level sensing, and oxygen concentration detection. These various applications provide solutions for the patient and health care professionals. Ten common applications are discussed here [14-16]:

1. Digital Hospital: Internet of things has broad application prospects in the field of medical information management. Currently, the demand for medical information management in hospitals is in form of identification, sample recognition, and medical record identification. Healthcare in hospitals is one way the medical is segment involved in IoT. With IoMT, hospital medical work is becoming increasingly intelligent, meticulous, and efficient.

2. Cancer Treatment: Smart technology helps simplify care for both cancer patients and their oncologists. By using smart monitoring system, patients were able to effectively communicate with their oncologists the adverse effects of chemotherapy and be quickly treated for them. [11]

3. Glucose Monitoring: Diabetes has been a fertile ground for developing smart devices. Such devices can help diabetics to continuously monitor their blood glucose levels for several days. Another smart device for diabetes patients is the smart insulin pen, which can automatically record the time, amount, and type of insulin needed to correct a patients blood sugar level [14].

4. Drug Anti-Counterfeiting: The amount of counterfeit medicines in the world has increased greatly and a lot of people die each year as a result of wrong medication. The label attached to a product will have a unique identity that is very difficult to forge and will serve as an effective counter-measure against medical fraud [17].

5. *Elderly Independent Living*: RFID sensor systems are being developed to support older people so that they can safely stay independent. This application is important in view of an aging population. IoT applications can provide support for the elderly by detecting the activities of daily living using wearable devices.

6. *Remote Monitoring:* Many patients continuously wear medical sensor-based devices to monitor their health statistics. Fitness, health electronics, and even smart watches have roles to play in monitoring, providing feedback, and in some cases a link to medical professionals. Remote monitoring translates into a greater number of patients worldwide having access to adequate healthcare. Continuous patient monitoring provides the real-time tracking, collects patient data, and wirelessly transmits for ongoing display. This increases operational efficiency. A typical real time remote monitoring system is shown in Figure 5.5 [18].

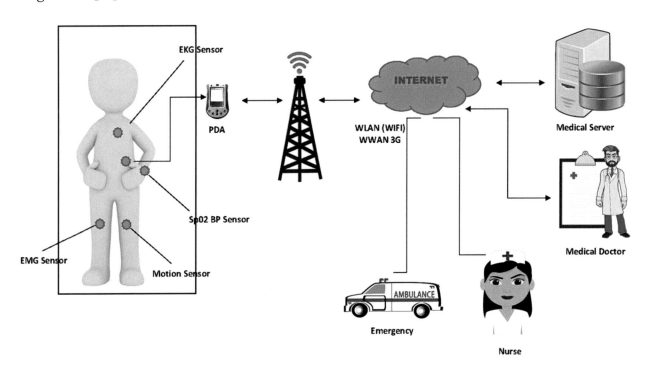

Figure 5.5 A typical real time remote monitoring system [18].

7. *Wearables Devices*: Innovative devices, such as wearable devices, implantable chips, and embedded systems in biomedical devices have been developed to continuously track continuous data on patient activity. Smart wearable devices allow the transfer of patient personal information between different devices. They support fitness, health education, symptom tracking, and disease management. They can be used to store health records especially for patients with diabetes, cancer, coronary heart disease, stroke, seizure disorders, and Alzheimer's disease [19].

8. *Body Sensor Network* (BSN): This technology is another IoT development in healthcare system, where a patient can be monitored using a collection of tiny-powered and lightweight wireless sensor nodes. It is essentially a collection of intelligent, miniaturized wireless sensor nodes used in monitoring the human body functions and surrounding environment. It opens the possibility for monitoring systems to operate wirelessly using low-cost wearable sensors [20,21].

9. *Smart Healthcare:* IoT is an enabling tool for the development of smart devices such as smart CGMs (Continuous Glucose Monitors), smart insulin pens, Smart Fridge for vaccines, smart watches for depression. More will be said about this in the next chapter.

10. *Robotic Surgery:* The combination of IoT and robot is giving new solutions in the healthcare industry. Doctors are using IoT enabled robotic devices to perform surgery. This enables doctors to perform the operation with more precision. The little robotic device can perform operations inside the body of the patient. Robots can also assist the nurse in the hospital, which is an extraordinary advancement of IoT and healthcare sector. Having robot in each patient's room can make the treatment more effective.

Other applications include people with disabilities, hearables, tracking and monitoring of objects and persons, identification and authentication, transport and data collection, smart contact lenses, clinical care, and continuous cardiac monitoring.

5.6 BENEFITS

Internet of things is a way of connecting devices to the Internet and to each other using wireless networks. It is injected into everything in healthcare, from X-ray machines to patient monitors. It creates new jobs and employment opportunities and bridges traditional engineering, computer sciences, and health care. It is transforming healthcare industry by increasing efficiency, lowering costs, and improving patient quality of care and safety. It ensures the personalization of healthcare services by providing digital identity for every patient. The doctors can break the limit of the geographical scope and provide medical education for medical personnel in remote areas. Figure 5.6 shows the most popular benefits of IoT in healthcare [22]. Besides these, other benefits include [23]:

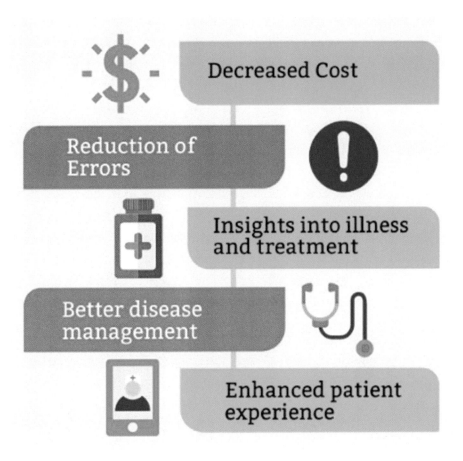

Figure 5.6 The most popular benefits of IoT in healthcare [22].

- *Quality:* Integrating IoT features into healthcare devices greatly improves the quality and effectiveness of service. It enables a radical improvement of health care and quality of life. IoT healthcare principles are already being applied to improve access to care, increase the quality of care, reduce the cost of care, reduce medical errors, to improve patient safety, and to optimize the healthcare processes.
- *Connectivity and Affordability:* Connectivity lies at the heart of Internet of things. It is the primary purpose of using IoT technology in healthcare, i.e. connect doctors with patients through smart devices, without restrictions. The IoT links the medical devices with the virtual worlds, thereby enabling anytime, anyplace connectivity for anything and not only for anyone. IoT opens doors of opportunity for greater connectivity in healthcare. It enables interoperability, machine-to-machine communication, information exchange, and data movement that makes healthcare service delivery effective. It allows nurses, doctors, and other medical practitioners to connect and communicate instantly and receive information proactively in real time inside and outside the hospital. IoT healthcare should provide better healthcare services to people at any time, from anywhere in friendly manner. The IoT promises to make healthcare cheaper and better.
- *Monitoring:* Applications deliver care to people in remote locations and real-time monitoring systems that provide a stream of accurate data for better care decision making [24]. IoT enables real-time monitoring of connected smart medical devices. Real-time monitoring can save

lives in event of a medical emergency like heart failure, diabetes, asthma attacks, etc. The IoT connected devices can collect health data (such as blood pressure, oxygen and blood sugar levels, weight, and ECGs) and use smartphone to transfer the data to a doctor who may be several kilometers away. This makes healthcare service effective. The healthcare remote monitoring systems have contributed to the improvement of the elderly people's quality of life [25].

- *Tracking:* An healthcare facility needs to be able track all the devices and applications on the network continuously. IoT is used in tracking patients, staff, and inventory. It is difficult to maintain maximum security without the ability to track assets (patients, medical staff, and hardware) throughout the hospital. The tracking may also include pharmaceutical inventory, helping elderly patients stay safe in their homes, and reminding patients when take their medications. IoT and real-time location systems facilitate asset tracking. This is an inexpensive, effective method of monitoring and tracking day-to-day activities in a hospital setting. The ability to enable location tracking of assets using sensor-based technology has created a service which is known as location-as-a-service.

5.7 CHALLENGES

Medical devices present some unique IoT challenges. These include the broad range of medical technologies, the diversity of network protocols, critical security and vulnerability considerations, regulatory compliance imperatives resulting from the handling of patient data, and stakeholders with varied interests. There is also an ambiguity about data ownership and a lack of EHR integration. This allows attackers/hackers to wreak havoc on the network. It is the responsibility of IT staff to bring more awareness to the health professionals about the challenges in supporting IoT devices. Besides these, other challenges include [8, 26-29]:

- *Data Security:* Security is one of the forefront challenges because any platform connected to IoT poses the risk of being insecure and open to hackers. Many businesses are wary of the security and privacy issues associated with IoT. IoT service providers need to be sure that their data is going to be safe. Increase in connected devices leads to an increase in endpoint vulnerability. Many IoT platforms consider security a core element and work to ensure that any potential leaks are stopped before hackers find them. Government, police, and IoT device manufacturers should find effective IoT security solutions. Security should be built in as the foundation of IoT systems, with rigorous validity checks, authentication, and data verification. Device manufacturers should build security into software applications and network connection that links the devices. Data security can be addressed by using a comprehensive governance mode, which provides secure access to sensitive data. Combining public and private infrastructure also can help protect data in transit. Companies have started to look at protecting their IoT ecosystem as well as their customers. When choosing security cameras, you should select the brand that has confidential encryption, such as SSL encryption.

- *Privacy:* A significant challenge that IoT poses is of data security and privacy. The data that is being shared across the IoT devices are sensitive. Wearable sensors, for example, are prone to expose patient information and patient privacy. Medical security and privacy issues directly influence patient life and the healthcare system all over the world. Privacy issues may include misuse of medical information, leakage of prescriptions, and eavesdropping on medical data. An enemy may obtain your health status while you are busy exercising in a fitness center since medical sensors may be placed on your body [30]. Many countries prohibit privacy violations.

- *Interoperability and Standards:* IoT consists of heterogeneous networks which connect all kinds of devices. Interoperability is the key to open markets to competitive solutions to IoT. The first requirement of Internet connectivity is that connected devices should be able to "talk the same language" of protocols. This makes interoperability the most basic core value. Recently, there has been a significant proliferation of Internet-capable devices and it is unlikely these devices are created by the same manufacturer. Implementing IoT often involves procuring devices that do not have IoT label. The complexity of procuring these devices and the lack of the IoT standard can make it difficult for stakeholders. Some IoT standards are still in development. The IEEE published its draft P2413 standard for IoT architecture, creating a universal language for IoT. Since IoT devices are usually purpose-built, universal security standards are difficult to develop. The use of open and widely available standards for IoT devices and services will provide greater user benefits.

- *Technology Infrastructure:* Infrastructure is critical for emerging IoT applications such as smart buildings, smart homes, smart cities, smart grid, intelligent transportation systems, and ubiquitous healthcare, to name a few. Most businesses lack the infrastructure and network components that huge volumes of IoT data require. For a new technology, there is no need to overinvest in infrastructure all at once. You can gradually get more sophisticated with your IoT solutions. The massiveness of connected devices to the Internet will pressure the adoption of IPv6, which is a technology considered most suitable for IoT.

- *Workforce:* It is challenging to change the mentality of the current workforce. It can be difficult to convince those in the upper levels about the opportunities of IoT projects. Sometimes, there is not enough technical skill to gain valuable insights from the huge amount of data collected from IoT. Healthcare industry should hire experts with the relevant IoT training.

- *Data Overload*: The medical IoT generate massive data which can be utilized to gain insights and make smart decisions. The big data accumulated by IoT devices is a challenge for the IoT data processing. Handling the data is becoming very difficult for doctors and this consequently affects the quality of their decision-making.

- *High Investment Cost:* The high initial costs in IoT investments can intimidate companies. But IoT costs are rapidly declining. IoT projects implementations with reasonable costs are recommended. Breakthroughs in the cost of sensors and processing power are enabling ubiquitous connections right now. The sensing devices such as RFID tags, sensors, actuator, etc. can be designed to minimize cost.

- *Energy*: IoT consists of various low-power embedded devices. IoT devices are resource-constrained. These devices are not full fledged resource-equipped, which inspired the concept of resource-constrained wireless sensor networks (WSNs). IoT uses low-power lossy networks, which complicates security issues by adding an additional constrain, energy. Since an energy source needs to supply each sensor in IoT, a tremendous amount of energy would be needed to run thousands of these sensors. This is a serious challenge that IoT has to handle. There are many ways to provide power such as main power supply, battery, solar system, etc. Smart devices may need to use smart battery.

These are some major challenges that influence the decision-making process of potential customers for a successful IoT implementation. Other challenges include cost, data integrity, data protection, laws and policies, insurance coverage, power consumption of devices, limited battery, global misinformation systems, global cooperation, intelligent data analytics, big data problems, and quality of service issues [31,32]. These challenges are being addressed by a vast range of organizations and government agencies around the world. In spite of the challenges, the adoption of IoT continues to expand.

5.8 CONCLUSION

The Internet of things (IoT) integrates physical objects, software, and hardware to interact with each other. The era of the Internet of things has already started and it will drastically transform our way of life. The central concept of the Internet of things is to connect anyone, anything, anytime, anyplace, any service, and any network. The Internet of things (IoT) is increasingly being recognized by different industries. Healthcare is one of the major sectors where IoT can have the most relevant economic and social impact. The impact of IoT in healthcare has been significant since it has opened up a world of possibilities in healthcare. From adherence to diagnosis, the applications are manifold. Due to these applications, the healthcare industry is changing at fast pace and is adopting the IoT rapidly. It has been long predicted that IoT healthcare will revolutionize the healthcare sector in terms of social benefits, penetration, accessible care, and cost-efficiency. The IoT revolution is redesigning modern healthcare with extended benefits.

However, the rapid growth of IoT has presented some significant challenges. IoT's development has been restricted by the challenges. Security happens to be the most prominent challenge for physicians interested in IoT applications in medicine. More information about IoT healthcare can be found in the books in [33-41]. and other books available on Amazon.

REFERENCE

[1] M. S. H. Talpur, The appliance pervasive of Internet of things in healthcare systems," *International Journal of Computer Science Issues,* vol. 10, no 1, January 2013, pp. 419-424.

[2] J. Illegems, "The Internet of things in health care," *Master's Thesis,* Universiteit Gent, 2017.

[3] M.N.O. Sadiku, S.M. Musa, and S. R. Nelatury, "Internet of things: An introduction," *International Journal of Engineering Research and Advanced Technology*, vol. 2, no.3, March 2016, pp. 39-43.

[4] A. Kakkar and Shaurya, "An IoT equipped hospital model: A new approach for e-governance healthcare framework," *International Journal of Medical Research & Health Sciences*, vol. 8, no. 3, 2019, pp. 36-42.

[5] S. Anand and S. K. Routray, "Issues and challenges in healthcare narrowband IoT," *International Conference on Inventive Communication and Computational Technologies,* 2017, pp. 486-489.

[6] A. S. Yeole and D. R. Kalbande, "Use of Internet of things (IoT) in healthcare: A survey," *Proceedings of the ACM Symposium on Women in Research*, March 2016.

[7] C. E. A. Zaouiat and A. Latif, " Internet of things and machine learning convergence: The e-healthcare revolution," *Proceedings of the 2nd International Conference on Computing and Wireless Communication Systems*, Larache, Morocco, November 2017.

[8] "Internet of things in healthcare: Applications, benefits, and challenges," https://www.peerbits. com/blog/internet-of-things-healthcare-applications-benefits-and-challenges.html

[9] M. N. O. Sadiku, S. M. Musa, and S. Binzaid, "Internet of things in medicine," *International Journal of Research in Engineering*, vol. 1, no.2, April 2019, pp. 15-17.

[10] G. J. Joyia et al., " Internet of medical things (IOMT): Applications, benefits and future challenges in healthcare domain," *Journal of Communications*, vol. 12, no. 4, April 2017, pp. 240-247.

[11] N. Dilawar et al., "Blockchain: Securing internet of medical things (IoMT)," *International Journal of Advanced Computer Science and Applications*, vol. 10, no. 1, 2019, pp. 82-89.

[12] "10 examples of the Internet of things in healthcare," February 2019 https://econsultancy.com/internet-of-things-healthcare/

[13] C. Yaoa et al., "A deep learning model for predicting chemical composition of gallstones with big data in medical Internet of things," *Future Generation Computer Systems*, vol. 94, 2019, pp. 140-147.

[14] "10 examples of the Internet of things in healthcare," February 2019 https://econsultancy.com/internet-of-things-healthcare/

[15] M. Hasan, "IoT in healthcare: 20 examples that'll make you feel better," https://www.ubuntupit.com/iot-in-healthcare-20-examples-thatll-make-you-feel-better/

[16] M. N. O. Sadiku, S. Alam, and S.M. Musa, "IoT for healthcare," *International Journal of Electronics and Communication Engineering*, vol. 5. no. 11, November 2018, pp. 5-7.

[17] L. Zhang, "Applications of the Internet of things in the medical industry (Part 1): Digital hospitals," https://dzone.com/articles/applications-of-the-internet-of-things-in-the-medi-1

[18] M. M. Dhanvijaya and S. C. Patil, "Internet of things: A survey of enabling technologies in healthcare and its applications," *Computer Networks*, vol. 153, April 2019, pp. 113-131.

[19] D. Bandyopadhyay and J. Sen, "Internet of things: Applications and challenges in technology and standardization," *Wireless Personal Communications*, vol. 58, no. 1, May 2011, pp. 49–69.

[20] T. Wu et al., "An autonomous wireless body area network implementation towards IoT connected healthcare applications," *IEEE Access*, vol. 5, 2017, pp. 11413-11422.

[21] P. Gope and T. Hwan, "BSN-care: A secure IoT-based modern healthcare system using body sensor network," *IEEE Sensors Journal*, vol. 16, no. 5, March 2016, pp. 1368-1376.

[22] "5 benefits of the convergence of IoT and healthcare," https://mailmystatements. com/2018/10/25/5-benefits-of-the-convergence-of-iot-and-healthcare/

[23] A. Rghioui and A. Oumnad, "Challenges and opportunities of Internet of things in healthcare," *International Journal of Electrical and Computer Engineering*, vol. 8, no. 5, October 2018, pp. 2753~2761.

[24] D. Niewolny, "How the Internet of things is revolutionizing healthcare," https://www.nxp.com/files-static/corporate/doc/white_paper/IOTREVHEALCARWP.pdf

[25] S. F. Khan, "Health care monitoring system in Internet of things (IoT) by using RFID," *Proceedings of the 6th International Conference on Industrial Technology and Management*, 2017., pp. 198-204.

[26] M. N. O. Sadiku, S. Binzaid, and S. M. Musa, "Internet of things: Challenges and solutions," *World Journal of Engineering Research and Technology*, vol. 3, no. 3, 2019, pp. 70-77.

[27] C. Maple, "Security and privacy in the Internet of things," *Journal of Cyber Policy*, vol. 2, no. 2, 2017, pp. 155-184.

[28] N. Dyness, "Six IoT implementation challenges and solutions," *Control Engineering*, October 2018, p. 21.

[29] L. Sears, "5 IoT challenges and solutions," August 2017 https://www.govloop.com/5-iot-challenges-solutions/

[30] P. Kumar and H. J. Lee, "Security issues in healthcare applications using wireless medical sensor networks: A survey," *Sensors*, vol. 12, 2012, pp. 55-91.

[31] R. Ajayi, "Adoption of Internet of things into healthcare enterprise systems: A phenomenological study," *Doctoral Dissertation*, Colorado Technical University, September, 2017.

[32] P. J. Ryan and R. B. Watson, "Research challenges for the Internet of things: What role can or play?" *Systems*, vol. 5, no. 1, 2017.

[33] C. Bhatt, N. Dey, and A. S. Ashour (eds.), *Internet of Things and Big Data Technologies for Next Generation Healthcare*. Springer, 2017.

[34] US Government, *A Study of the Internet of Things (IOT) and Radio Frequency Identification (RFID) Technology: Big Data in Navy Medicine – Healthcare Industry Transformation to Manage Costs and Increase Efficiency*, December 2017.

[35] A. P. B. Purushothaman, *IoT Technical Challenges and Solutions*. Boston, MA: Artech House, 2017.

[36] S. C. Mukhopadhyay (ed.), *Internet of Things: Challenges and Opportunities*. Springer, 2014.

[37] Q. F. Hasan, A. R. Khan, and S. A. Madani (eds.), *Internet of Things: Challenges, Advances, and Applications*. Boca Raton, FL: Taylor & Francis, CRC Press, 2018.

[38] M. S. Maximiano and C. I. Reis (eds.), *Internet of Things and Advanced Application in Healthcare*. Medical Information Science Reference, 2017.

[39] P. B. Pankajavalli and G. S. Karthick (eds.), *Incorporating the Internet of Things in Healthcare Applications and Wearable Devices (Advances in Medical Technologies and Clinical Practice* (AMTCP)). IGI Global, 2019.

[40] P. Raj et al. (eds.), *Internet of Things Use Cases for the Healthcare Industry*. Springer; 2020.

[41] C. Bhatt, N. Dey, and A. S. Ashour, *Internet of Things and Big Data Technologies for Next Generation Healthcare*. Springer 2017.

CHAPTER 6

SMART HEALTHCARE

"You treat a disease, you win, you lose. You treat a person, I guarantee you, you'll win, no matter what the outcome." - Patch Adams

6.1 INTRODUCTION

Healthcare is an indispensable part of life. It plays a major role in the growth and well being of any nation. The healthcare system is important because of its focus on human care. Its main purpose is to improve certain qualities such as availability, privacy, reliability, safety, and security. The healthcare industry sector can be divided into four segments [1]: (1) Health care services and facilities; (2) Medical devices, equipment, and hospital supplies manufacturers; (3) Medical insurance, medical services and managed care; (4) Pharmaceuticals.

Today, healthcare industry is experiencing several challenges including rapid increase in population, ageing population, rising burden of noncommunicable chronic diseases (such as diabetes and obesity), care costs skyrocketing, and the global shortage of medical personnel. Healthcare is under tremendous pressure to deliver superior health outcomes, comply with regulations, achieve customer satisfaction, reduce cost of care, ensure patient safety, and handle financial constraints and budget reductions. Also, people have become more interested in disease prevention and health promotion, rather than disease treatment. As a result, healthcare system is being transformed from traditional reactive and hospital-centered to preventive and personalized, from disease-focused to well being-centered. Thus, the healthcare industry is heading towards a more preventative, predictive, participatory, and personalized care. Figure 6.1 compares traditional healthcare with smart healthcare [2].

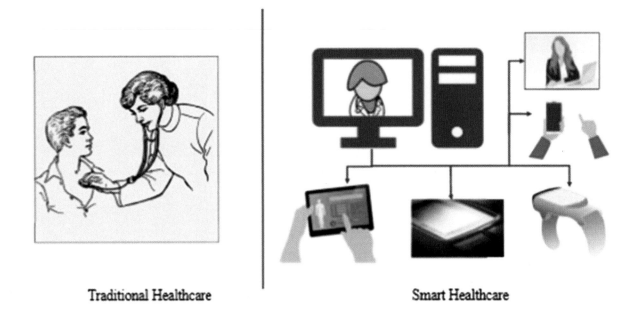

Traditional Healthcare   Smart Healthcare

Figure 6.1 Comparing traditional healthcare with smart healthcare [3].

The current technological advancements are leading to the emergence of a smart and realistic solution known as "smart healthcare" (SH). Smart healthcare should be regarded as a vital component of the smart city concept. It is one of the core infrastructure elements in building smart cities. The integration of smart healthcare and smart city involves the merging of information and technology with the aim of enhancing healthy living to all masses and improving medical services around the world. The Internet of things technology is rapidly being incorporated into homes and giving rise to the smart home, and into healthcare giving rise to smart healthcare [2]:

- IoT + Architecture = Smart Home
- IoT + Healthcare = Smart Healthcare Devices

This chapter provides an introduction on smart healthcare. It begins with discussing the concept of smart healthcare and the key enabling technologies. It highlights the seven major features of smart healthcare. It covers some applications and services of smart healthcare. It presents smart hospital and smart medication. It covers the benefits and challenges of smart healthcare. The last section concludes with comments.

6.2 CONCEPT OF SMART HEALTHCARE

The concept of "smart healthcare" originated from the related concept of "smart planet" proposed by IBM in 2009. Smart Planet is an intelligent infrastructure that uses sensors to perceive information, transmits information through the Internet of things (IoT), and processes the information using supercomputers [3]. Smart healthcare is one of ten priority areas in the development of smart city. Other components include smart government, smart education, smart transportation, smart grid/ smart energy, smart surveillance, smart environment, smart society, smart reporting, smart payment, and smart commerce [4]. The integration of healthcare and smart cities has led to the utilization of smart healthcare technology into medical practices around the world.

Smart healthcare involves using smart technologies for health purposes. It is using smart technologies for better diagnosis of the disease, improved treatment of the patients, and enhanced quality of lives. It uses a new generation of information technologies, such as the Internet of things (IoT), mobile and wireless networks, big data, cloud computing, blockchain, robotics, and artificial intelligence, to transform the traditional medical system into an intelligent healthcare system, which is more efficient, more convenient, and more personalized [5]. It provides healthcare services through smart gadgets (such as smartphones, smartwatch, wireless smart glucometer, wireless blood pressure monitor) and networks such as Wi-Fi, Zig-Bee, Bluetooth, 5G, body area network, and wireless local area network. Figure 6.2 shows the classification of the smart healthcare market, based on the services, medical devices, technologies used, applications, and end users [6].

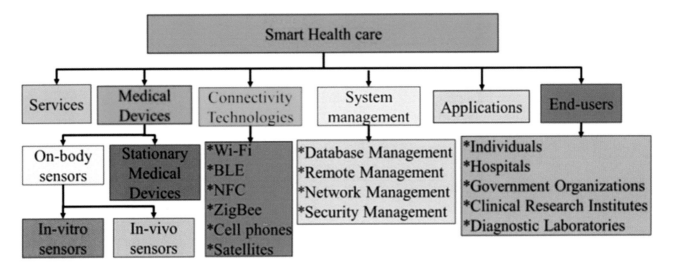

Figure 6.2 Classification of the smart healthcare market [6].

Smart healthcare enables a doctor to monitor a patient's vitals from the office while the patient remains in home care. Smart healthcare is a huge market opportunity because it improves lots of lives with the smart health solutions. Stakeholders around the globe are seeking innovative, cost-effective ways to deliver patient-centered, technology-enabled smart healthcare, both inside and outside hospital walls. SH empowers patients to self-manage some emergency situation [7]. Interactions between parties are efficient and patient centered.

Smart healthcare is an interdisciplinary field that includes sensing, networking, computing, radio frequency identification (RFID), wireless sensor network (WSN), and artificial intelligence. Internet of things (IoT) plays significant role in wide range of healthcare applications and serves as a catalyst for the healthcare. It is an enabler to achieve improved care for patients and providers. Smart healthcare technologies (mobile and electronic) include sensors, medicine dispensation, smart drugs, smart pills, smart surgeries, wearables, and early registration devices [8]. These technologies provide the opportunity to build novel and fascinating smart, connected healthcare systems. Smart healthcare combines smart technologies within the home, hospital, patient, and information exchange. A typical smart healthcare system is shown in Figure 6.3 [9].

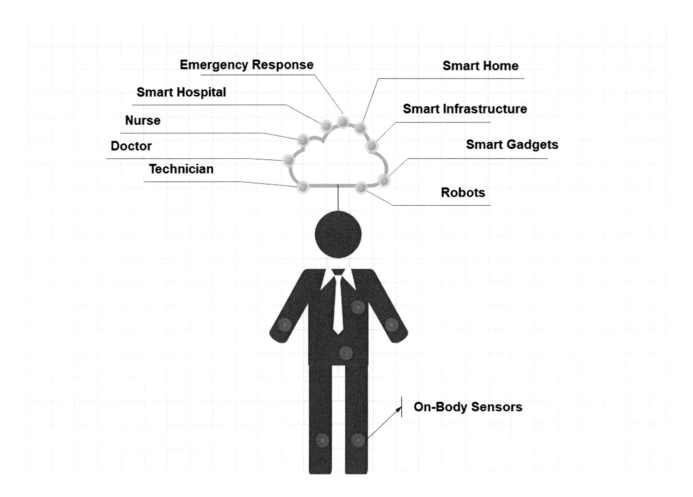

Figure 6.3 A typical smart healthcare system [9].

6.3 ENABLING TECHNOLOGIES

There are different ways technologies are changing smart healthcare. Top healthcare technologies such as IoT, cloud computing, big data, machine learning, and advanced analytics have turned the traditional healthcare into smart healthcare. These are major technological innovations which have added the element of "smartness" in the healthcare industry [10].

- *Wireless technologies:* These are the backbone of the smart healthcare systems. Different wireless technologies such as Wi-Fi, Bluetooth, radio frequency identification (RFID), wireless sensor network (WSN), wearable medical devices, smart mobile technologies, etc. play a vital role in exchanging the information among different physical elements RFID implant allows for user identification, movement detection, and automation, and enables the smart environment to react to the presence of the user. Wearable sensor nodes are those that measure vitals and other important signs, including pulse, respiratory rate, and body temperature, as these are the essential signs for determination of critical health. Mobile technologies will play a crucial role as they have become the patient's constant companion. Wearable sensors are capable of sensing even very small changes in vital signs, which a human cannot easily observe. The familiar technologies such as the smart phone and smart watch will be developed further to include reliable health technology sensors and abilities. These new technologies will allow remote monitoring of patients, health data collection, medication compliance, and access to medical records [11].

- *IoT in Healthcare*: IoT helps extend the benefits of Internet such as remote access, data sharing, and connectivity to various other application domains such as healthcare, transportation, parking activities, agriculture, and surveillance. IoT in healthcare technologies is also popularly known as Internet of Medical Things (IoMT). The Internet of things (IoT) allow all entities to be connected to each other through wired or wireless communication means. The healthcare industry is among the fastest to adopt the Internet of things. The primary goal of IoT in healthcare is to connect doctors with patients through a smart device. Healthcare providers are expecting the IoT to revolutionize the process of gathering healthcare data and care delivery [12]. Communications related to Internet of things for healthcare can be classified into two major categories: short-range communications and long-range communications. ECG data are gathered using a wearable monitoring node and are transmitted directly to the IoT cloud using Wi-Fi. IoMT is particularly a boon for a burdened healthcare system. IoMT devices help the elderly to keep a close track of their medications and vitals like heart rate, glucose levels, and sleep patterns. Designing a wearable sensor for continuously monitoring blood pressure remains a challenge in healthcare IoT [13].

- *Big Data in Healthcare:* The healthcare industry is responsible for generating an unprecedented amount of data on daily basis. This big data is partly related to patient healthcare and well-being. It is created by mass adoption of the Internet and digitization of healthcare information, including health records such as demographic data, historical data, illness related information, test results, imaging data, costs, discharge summaries, pharmacies, insurance companies, medical imaging, genomics, social media, smart phones, wearables, sensors, and other IoT devices. Big data is commonly characterized by the so-called 5 V's - volume, velocity, variety, veracity, and value. It has been noticed that the governments across the globe are working towards building an effective healthcare infrastructure, with big data being the very foundation. More will be discussed on big data in the next chapter.

- *Cloud computing in Healthcare:* Cloud computing is a new means of providing computing resources and services. It offers large scalable computing and storage, data sharing, on-demand anytime and anywhere access to resources. It encourages cost savings, scalability, and system flexibility. Application areas include emergency healthcare, home healthcare, assistive healthcare, telemedicine, storage, sharing and processing of large medical resources. There are three primary services that can be provided by cloud technologies in healthcare environments: Software as a Service (SaaS), Platform as a Service (PaaS), and Infrastructure as a Service (IaaS). Cloud computing can support healthcare organizations to share information such as EHR, prescriptions, insurance information, and test results. The cloud makes it easier to archive and use patient records and medical images. The cloud also makes it easier to collaborate and offer care as a team. The demand for cloud computing healthcare solutions has grown exponentially.

- *Machine Learning in Healthcare*: Machine learning (ML) is the discipline that gives computers the ability to learn without being explicitly programmed. In medicine, the bottom line is to use machine learning to augment patient care, save more lives, improve more care, while saving money at the same time. ML can automate the manual processes carried out by practitioners, which are usually time-consuming and subjective. Machine learning performs diagnostics or treatment plans would be extremely valuable in a healthcare scenarios. Thus, using ML can save time for practitioners and provide unbiased, repeatable results [14]. The application of machine learning in the healthcare systems has opened up new avenues in the smart healthcare market. Personalized care has been the hallmark of smart healthcare solutions, which can be easily gained through machine learning.

- *Nanomedicine:* This is a unique branch of medicine that involves the development and application of materials and technologies with nanometer length scales. It is an interdisciplinary discipline that combines nanoscience, nanoengineering, nanotechnology, nanoelectronics, and life sciences. The interest in nanomedicine spans a wide area in medicine such as drug delivery, vaccine development, antibacterial, diagnosis and imaging tools, wearable devices, implants, and high-throughput screening platforms. The most prominent areas of nanomedical research and drug approvals are cancer treatments, imaging contrast agents, and drug delivery. Nanodevices can repair DNA or replace the defective part of DNA. Nanomedicine will lead to many more exciting medical breakthroughs [15].

6.4 FEATURES OF SMART HEALTHCARE

Smart healthcare uses a new generation of information technologies to radically transform the traditional healthcare system, making it more efficient, more convenient, and more personalized. The important features of smart healthcare are depicted in Figure 6.4 and can be broadly summarized as 7Ps [16]:

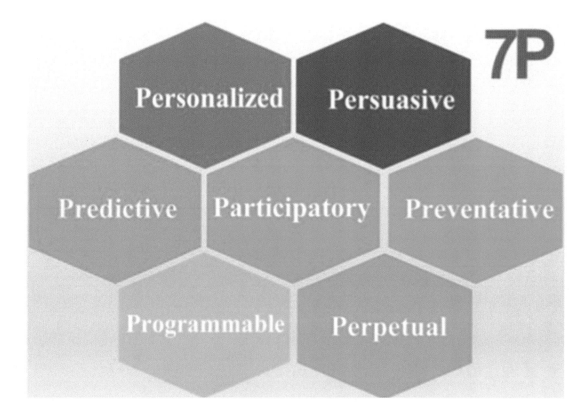

Figure 6.4 7Ps features of smart healthcare [16].

1. *Personalized:* The smart healthcare provides a unique and suitable treatment plan for each patient.

2. *Persuasive:* The smart healthcare system can change the behavior of the user for improving his/her healthcare management.

3. *Predictive:* Smart healthcare enables a kind of predictive maintenance for humans.

4. *Participatory:* The smart healthcare represents a new participatory care paradigm.

5. *Preventative:* The smart healthcare provides solutions to help people stay away from diseases rather than treatment (i.e., reminders of upcoming vaccinations)

6. *Perpetual:* The perpetual awareness system in smart healthcare is characterized by continuous monitoring.

7. *Programmable:* The smart healthcare systems should allow users to set programs when dealing with some sophisticated medical cases.

6.5 APPLICATIONS AND SERVICES

Healthcare is undergoing a transformation from traditional hospital focused approach to a distributed patient-centric approach. With the increasing demand for automated, remote, and real-time healthcare services in smart cities, smart healthcare monitoring is necessary to provide complete care to residents. Smart healthcare applications and services require collection and analysis of raw sensory data. Typical applications of smart healthcare technologies include the following:

- *Smart Home Healthcare:* This centers on providing care in the home for outpatients, the elderly, and those with disabilities. It allows patients to communicate their current health status to healthcare provider from home. It has the potential for managing chronic illnesses of the aging population. The technology is designed to assist the homes' residents accomplishing their daily-living activities. An elderly person should be monitored constantly if he/she has health-related issues. Smart homes can be cost-effective and allow greater independence and quality of life while reducing the chance of social-isolation. Robotics is an area that has merits in the field of home assistance. A robot at home is a robot which takes care of patients at home. The home of tomorrow will be substantially different and smart [17].

- *Patient Monitoring:* Smart healthcare monitoring is necessary to provide improved and complete care to residents. This allows the doctor to monitor patients' conditions for providing treatment even from remote locations. (This may be done using cognitive computing.) Wireless body area networks (WBANs) are the basic components of community healthcare monitoring. They entail having small sensors placed on body of a patient to monitor various health parameters like blood pressure, heart beat, temperature, and prolonged electrocardiogram (this sentence has been repeated at least 5-6x times by nowc) [18].

- *Pathology Detection:* A smart healthcare framework uses IoT sensors attached to a patient to acquire data, such as electrocardiogram (ECG), EEG, and body temperature, and determines the patient's state. An EEG-based pathology detection method uses scalp EEG recorded through EEG sensors. The EEG signal is transmitted to the deep learning system, which performs pathology detection. Healthcare specialists can study the result generated and monitor the patients [19].

- *Smart Hospitals:* Becoming a smart hospital involves embracing IoT technology throughout the entire facility. Smart hospitals rely on information and communication technology-based environments and increase efficiency and patient satisfaction. Due to cost pressure, hospitals are facing challenges like less financial resources. As a result, reduction of labor cost becomes the critical criterion for the implementation of smart items infrastructure in a stationary setting [20]. The main goal of smart hospitals is to deliver patient care by making the most of advanced ICT. More will be discussed on smart hospitals in the next section.

- *Virtual clinics:* These are online clinics that provide 24-hour online access for patients. Smart mobile devices now have an application called "Virtual Clinic" that allows doctors in the healthcare network to answer questions to patients in real time. This type of healthcare delivery is relatively new and can improve the experience of care for patients [21].

- *Pharmaceutical Industry*: Smart healthcare is employed in the pharmaceutical industry for drug production, inventory management, and other processes. Clinical trials of drugs may involve combining the use of the IoT, big data, and artificial intelligence.

- *Wearable Technologies:* These are becoming popular as patients use them to track their physical activities, heart rate, and sleep patterns daily. Wearable technology in healthcare is a clothing or accessory with advanced electronic devices that patients can wear. This includes fabrics, eyewear, smart watches, jewelry, smartphone apps, smart health watches, smart bandages, smart clothing, wearable monitors, and other monitoring sensors that can be worn on the body. Wearable technologies help fight health conditions that are difficult to manage. Smart watches help patients be in-charge of their health all the time. They also monitor people's sleep patterns and detect when they stop breathing. The wearable medical devices continuously generate big data.

6.6 SMART HOSPITALS

Since the advent of smart healthcare, various systems have been developed. Hospitals are traditionally the center of healthcare delivery systems with multiple facilities such as ICU, primary care providers, clinics, pharmacies, rehabilitation centers. Hospitals are mainly responsible for major surgeries, intensive critical care, the management of severe trauma, and treatment for other acute, severe, complicated conditions. Other services are delivered at clinics, at gyms, and even in patients' homes [22]. Rapidly evolving technologies, along with demographic and economic changes, are expected to affect hospitals worldwide. Integrating digital technologies into traditional hospital services will create a healthcare system without walls and a digital hospital of the future.

The concept of smart hospital (or intelligent hospital) is quickly becoming a reality because it can reduce healthcare costs, reduce risks, and increase patient satisfaction. The smart hospital is essentially a healing environment where the increasing digitization of the building means that the technology is working seamlessly to deliver benefits to the people connected to it. It is often patient-centered and offer a better patient experience. It embeds new technologies into its design and operations to improve the customer experience. Smart hospital rooms with smart beds are designed with a hospital's specific patient population mind. The rooms allow patients to view patient vitals. Figure 6.5 shows a room in a smart hospital [23].

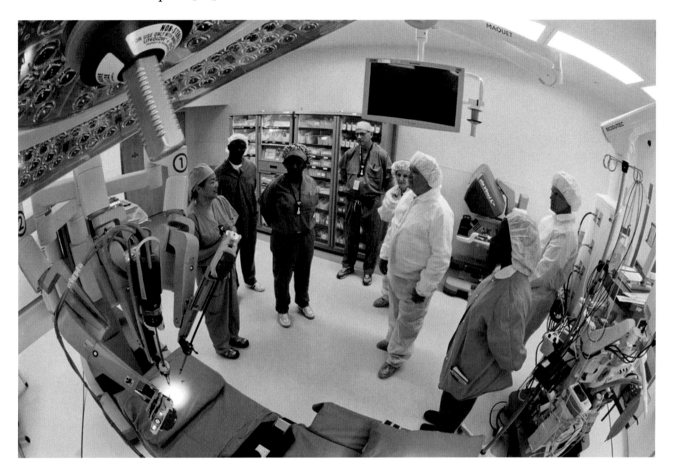

Figure 6.5 A room in a smart hospital [23].

Some objectives of a smart hospital are shown in Figure 6.6 [24]. Integration and automation are the future directions of smart hospitals. Smart hospital software development implies the use of smart technology systems, smart mobility systems, and smart systems for patients, staff, and equipment to provide functionality to devices such as smartphones, tablets, and medical devices. Commonly used smart technologies in smart hospital software include Wi-Fi, RFID, sensors, mobile apps, and wearables [25].

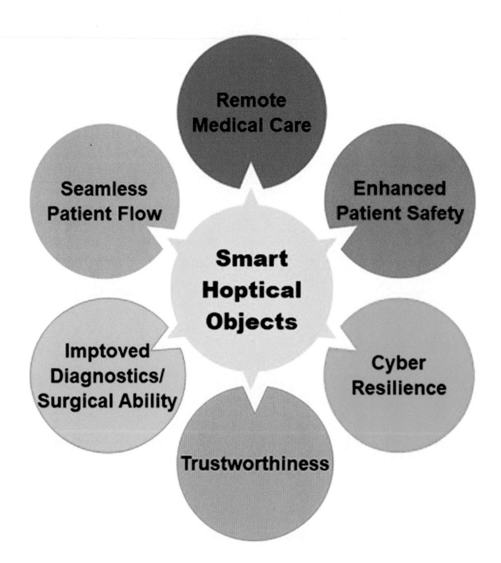

Figure 6.6 Some objectives of a smart hospital [24].

These technologies have been instrumental in changing the patient experience for the better inside and outside of the hospital. For example, while patients are taking the rehabilitation treatment in the hospital, they are monitored by the devices so that the real-time information can be obtained and checked by doctors.

Becoming a smart hospital requires the participation of all staff, including physicians, nurses, and management. It is important that the hospital staff continually improve patient outcomes by learning the innovative technologies smart hospitals require and be trained adequately to utilize it. Common benefits of smart hospital technology include: (1) all devices are integrated and interconnected, (2) streamline the work process, (3) store all patient records digitally in the cloud, (4) enhance administration, deliver superior patient care, and improve profitability. Smart healthcare systems no longer restrict their data collection to sources within the four walls of the hospital. Smart hospitals will have a major impact on global healthcare systems.

6.8 SMART MEDICATION

Medicines are the common solution for preventing and curing diseases. The majority of our efforts are focused on treating rather than preventing disease (but you said earlier how things are moving towards prevention rather than treatment, both cannot be true). Emerging technologies are making great strides in healthcare and medicine worldwide. Medicine is undergoing a sector-wide transformation due to the advances in computing and networking technologies. This is affecting medical research and practice. It is changing from reactive and hospital-centered to preventive and personalized, from disease-focused to wellbeing-centered. This is fundamentally changing medicine and making it to becoming smarter.

Rapid advances in medical and pharmaceutical technologies have led to more drugs that can cure previously incurable diseases and help people live longer with chronic diseases (i.e., HIV). However, medication error has been identified as one of the areas that pose the greatest risk of harm to a patient. Medication errors can occur throughout the medication use process of ordering, dispensing, and administration [26]. As the elderly (defined here as individuals 65 years or older) suffer from chronic disease, it is important to take medicine at the prescribed time. But often times, an elderly patient with cognitive decline (eg, dementia) may forget to take their medications on time or they may also forget that they have already taken it previously that day (doubling the dose) [27].

Medication nonadherence is a serious issue and major challenge in healthcare with severe consequences in terms of cost and quality of care. Medication adherence (MA) is taking medications as prescribed by healthcare providers. It is compliance with medication regiment. It is the key to achieving optimal medical treatment. It reduces the risk for complications from their illness and death and keeps healthcare costs under control. Adherence varies with patients. Unintentional non-adherence occurs when a patient simply forgets to take their medication. Intentional non-adherence happens when a patient makes a conscious decision not to take his medication. The geriatric population, those who are socioeconomic disadvantaged, those with disabilities should be assisted with MA so that they can function at their optimal health [28].

Various devices have been developed in both industry and academia on different platforms to improve medication adherence. These include smartphone apps, smart medication boxes, smart pills, wearable sensors, and implantable devices [29]. Smartphone apps for improving MA are already in the market for iPhone and Android devices. Smart medication boxes have programmable alarm to remind the patient to take medication at appropriate times. A typical medication system can dispense medication as specified by the caregiver. It can remotely monitor and regulate patients' medication adherence, and enable communication with healthcare professionals [30]. Smart medication system improves medication adherence for single and multiple medications even for patients with mild cognitive deficiency. A typical medication system is shown in Figure 6.7 [31]. The system is designed to be portable, generate personalized reminder to patients, monitor patient's medication adherence, and communicate with healthcare professionals if necessary.

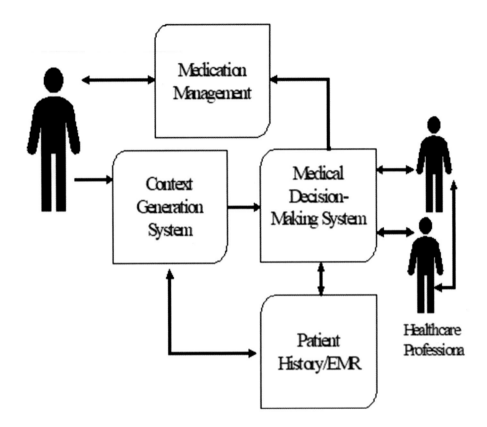

Figure 6.7 – A typical smart medication system [31].

6.9 BENEFITS

Smart healthcare technology has many obvious advantages in system integration, information sharing, and intelligent processing. Other benefits include the following [32].

1. *New Opportunities:* Smart healthcare can provide new opportunities and advantages. With the Internet of things, mutual sharing of information becomes easy and convenient. Smart healthcare systems can help improve security, simplify maintenance, make effective use of staff, and improve the user experience.

2. *Values:* Smart healthcare can add value for the patients, healthcare personnel, healthcare industry, and society in relation to early detection and intervention, and personalized treatment.

3.*Reduced Costs:* Smart healthcare systems analyze patient data to both enhance the quality of patient care and reduce the cost of care. They bring down the cost by cutting down unnecessary visits and utilizing better quality resources.

4. *Better Experience:* With Internet-enabled smart devices, smart healthcare has become reality in which patients receive medical treatment from anywhere across the globe. Smart healthcare can relieve personnel pressure, achieve unified management of information, and improve the patient's medical experience. It can decrease wait times at the emergency room. Being connected to the healthcare system through the Internet of things, both patients and physicians get more engaged in their treatment.

With Internet-enabled smart devices, smart healthcare has become reality in which patients receive medical treatment from anywhere across the globe.

5. Remote Monitoring: This is also known as telemedicine or telehealth. Using smart devices and connected medical devices enables healthcare providers to monitor patients in real time. It spares the patients the inconvenience of traveling to and from the doctor's office. Real-time monitoring can save lives in event of a medical emergency like heart attack, asthmatic attack, etc

6. Record Management: Before, the healthcare providers had access to only limited data of the patients and the healthcare practitioners may not have known how medications they prescribed affected their patients as quickly. Mobile devices have helped the healthcare industry go forward by leaps and bounds. Today, there are mobile devices and smart wearable devices that allow the people to check their vitals on a regular basis.

7. Improvement in Physician's Efficiency: The smart healthcare system improves the performance of healthcare practitioners. Since doctors are the backbone of a healthcare system, it is important to provide them with a smart and advanced system to improve their efficiency. Smart devices record the patients' data and make it readily available to doctors and improve their efficiency.

6.10 CHALLENGES

There remain definite technological and societal challenges to be addressed before smart healthcare technologies are widely adopted. The challenges include the following [33].

1. Security and Privacy: Security is one of the forefront challenges because any platform connected to IoT poses the risk of being insecure and open to hackers. Sharing patients' sensitive information over the Internet leads to serious security and privacy concerns. Security is a challenging requirement during data collection from patients. The blockchain is a potential technology that can be used to reinforce the security practice in the healthcare. It may eliminate the risks of user experience when they store their health information on their smartphone [34]. Confidentiality is an important security requirement in smart healthcare. The smart healthcare system is vulnerable to cyber-attack [35]. Government, police, and IoT device manufacturers should find effective IoT security solutions

2. Workforce: It is challenging to change the mentality of the current workforce. It can be difficult to convince those in the upper levels about the opportunities of technologies. A major challenge is practitioners' hesitation and unwillingness to use these new technologies in medical practice. Many of the health practitioners especially in developing economies may not have has much knowledge or experience of technology. Some have been flustered by the constant changing technologies. Today's shortages of nursing providers will become more acute as the population continues to grow and age.

3. Lack of Information Sharing. Hospitals are often reluctant to share information. This leads to lack of medical cooperation between hospitals. Privacy must be protected from misuse and violation so that patients and medical institutions will agree to release and share the data.

4. *Lack of Standards:* Standardization is a key issue limiting progress in smart healthcare. Medical institutions lack uniform standards across different regions and organizations. It's difficult to standardize delivery processes given the non-standardized nature of patients with different needs, preferences, personal characteristics, conditions, and medications. Companies are often encouraged to use global open standards,

5. *Integration of Technologies:* Integration of new technologies into existing healthcare systems can be challenging. There needs to be the infrastructure and competencies needed to incorporate smart health technologies in daily operations.

6. *Affordability:* Healthcare cost is increasing and becoming unaffordable, especially in the developed countries. IoT infrastructures are costly and not easy to acquire. The maintenance of smart healthcare system is also costly.

7.*Human Errors:* These often occur during the operation of devices or execution of processes. They may be due to insufficient training. Physician/patient errors are a major threat in the context of a smart hospital where there is heavy reliance on ICT assets.

The solutions to these challenges depend on technological progress and the joint efforts of patients, doctors, health institutions, and technology companies.

6.11 CONCLUSION

The rapidly advancing information technologies and emerging IoT technology have led to the development of smart healthcare systems. The integration of healthcare and smart cities has led to the utilization of information and communication technologies (ICT) into medical practices around the world. The integration has improved the quality of the residents in the smart cities [36]. Smart healthcare uses a new generation of information technologies, such as the Internet of things (IoT), big data, cloud computing, AI, blockchain, and 3D printing, to transform the traditional medical system, thereby making healthcare more efficient, more convenient, and more personalized [37]. The prospects for smart healthcare are vast. It can facilitate better health self-management for individual patient.

The smart healthcare systems are constantly developing and providing better healthcare services in smart communities. It is not an exaggeration to say that smart healthcare systems have become one of the most sought-after technological innovations by healthcare organizations. Smart health technologies will be commonplace in the near future. They are still in their infancy stage and their prevalence is still limited. The demand for smart healthcare engineers is anticipated to grow. There is a need to continuously adapt engineering curricula and foster future generations of smart healthcare engineers [38]. Currently, most medical schools do not incorporate AI technology into the curriculum.

The future of smart healthcare looks smart. More information about smart healthcare can be found in the books in [40-46] and the following related journals:
- *Global Health Journal*
- *Electronic Journal of Health Informatics*

- *International Journal of Medical Research & Health Sciences*
- *Technology and Health Care*

REFERENCES

[1] M. Bause et al., "Design for Health 4.0: Exploration of a new area," *Proceedings of the International Conference On Engineering Design*, Delft, The Netherlands, August 2019, pp. 887-896.

[2] D. Choi, H. Choi, and D. Shon, "Future changes to smart home based on AAL healthcare service," *Journal of Asian Architecture and Building Engineering,* vol. 18, no. 3, 2019, pp. 190-199

[3] P. Sundaravadivel, "Application-specific things architectures for IoT-based smart healthcare solutions," *Doctoral Dissertation,* University of North Texas, May 2018.

[4] Indrawati, R. Febriliantina, and H. Amani, "Identifying smart healthcare indicators for measuring smart city: An Indonesian perspective," *Proceedings of the 2017 International Conference on Telecommunications and Communication Engineering*, Osaka, Japan, October 2017, pp. 86-91.

[5] S. Tian et al., "Smart healthcare: making medical care more intelligent," *Global Health Journal*, vol. 3, no. 3, September 2019, pp. 62-65.

[6] P. Sundaravadivel et al., "Everything you wanted to know about smart healthcare," *IEEE Consumer Electronics Magazine,* vol. 7, no. 1, January 2018, pp. 18-28.

[7] K. Aziz." Smart real-time healthcare monitoring and tracking system using GSM/GPS Technologies," *Proceedings of the 3rd MEC International Conference on Big Data and Smart City*, 2016.

[8] "Smart health technology," https://path2025.dk/smart-health-technology/

[9] S. P. Mohanty, U. Choppali, and E. Kougianos, "Everything you wanted to know about smart cities: The Internet of things is the backbone," *IEEE Consumer Electronics Magazine*, vol. 5, no. 3, July 2016, pp. 60-70.

[10] P. Sundaravadivel et al., "Everything you wanted to know about smart healthcare," *IEEE Consumer Electronics Magazine,* vol. 7, no. 1, January 2018, pp. 18-26.

[11] M. N. O. Sadiku, A. A. Omotoso, and S. M. Musa, "Smart healthcare: A primer," *International Journal of Trend in Scientific Research and Development,* vol. 3, no. 4, May-June 2019, pp. 1356-1359.

[12] S. Anand and S. K. Routray, "Issues and challenges in healthcare narrowband IoT," *International Conference on Inventive Communication and Computational Technologies*, 2017, pp. 486-489.

[13] M. N. O. Sadiku, S. Alam, and S.M. Musa, "IoT for healthcare," *International Journal of Electronics and Communication Engineering*, vol. 5. no. 11, November 2018, pp. 5-7.

[14] M. N. O. Sadiku, S. M. Musa, and A. Omotoso, "Machine learning in medicine: A primer," *International Journal of Trend in Scientific Research and Development*, vol. 3, no. 2, Jan.-Feb. 2019, pp. 98-100.

[15] M. N. O. Sadiku, T. J. Ashaolu, and S. M. Musa, "Nanomedicine: A primer," *International Journal of Trend in Research and Development*, vol. 6, no. 1, Jan.-Feb. 2019, pp. 267-269.

[16] H. Zhu et al., "Smart healthcare in the era of Internet-of-things," *IEEE Consumer Electronics Magazine,* September/October 2019, pp. 26-30.

[17] J. Bennett, O. Rokas, and L. Chen, "Healthcare in the smart home: A study of past, present and future," *Sustainability,* vol. 9, 2017.

[18] M. S. Hossain, G.Muhammad, and A. Alamri, "Smart healthcare monitoring: A voice pathology detection paradigm for smart cities," *Multimedia Systems*, July 2017, pp. 1-11.

[19] S. U. Amin et al.; "Cognitive smart healthcare for pathology detection and monitoring," *IEEE Access*, vol. 7, 2019, pp. 10745- 10753.

[20] V. Stantchev et al., "Smart items, fog and cloud computing as enablers of servitization in healthcare," *Sensors & Transducers*, vol. 185, no. 2, February 2015, pp. 121-126.

[21] M. Bajwa, "Emerging 21st century medical technologies," *Pakistan Journal of Medical Sciences*, vol. 30, no. 3, 2014, pp. 649-655.

[22] B. Chen et al., "Finding the future of care provision: The role of smart hospitals," May 2019, https://www.mckinsey.com/industries/healthcare-systems-and-services/our-insights/finding-the-future-of-care-provision-the-role-of-smart-hospitals

[23] "Smart Hospitals Market Research Report 2020-2026 General Vision, Intel Corporation, IBM Corporation, Microsoft Corporation," February 18, 2020 https://galusaustralis.com/2020/02/466329/smart-hospitals-market-research-report-2020-2026-general-vision-intel-corporation-ibm-corporation-microsoft-corporation/

[24] ENISA, "Smart hospitals security and resilience for smart health service and infrastructures," November 2016, https://www.researchgate.net/publication/310844589_Smart_Hospitals_Security_and_Resilience_for_Smart_Health_Service_and_Infrastructures_NOVEMBER_2016_Smart_Hospitals_About_ENISA/link/583a114608ae3d91723f65a0/download

[25] "What is a smart hospital and how to build your own solution?" https://archer-soft.com/blog/what-smart-hospital-and-how-build-your-own-solution

[26] P. H. Tsai et al., "Smart medication dispenser: Design, architecture and implementation," *IEEE Systems Journal*, vol. 5, no. 1, March 2011, pp. 99-110.

[27] M. Lim et al., "A smart medication prompting system and context reasoning in home environments," *Proceedings of the Fourth International Conference on Networked Computing and Advanced Information Management*, 2008, pp. 115-118.

[28] M. N. O. Sadiku, A. E. Shadare, and S.M. Musa, "Smart medication," *International Journal of Trends in Research and Development*, vol. 5, no. 1, Jan.-Feb. 2018, pp. 246-247.

[29] G. Gimpel, U. Varshney, and P. Ahluwalia, "Emerging for medication adherence," *IT Pro*, May/June 2016, pp. 30-36.

[30] U. Varshney, "A smart approach to medication management," *Computer*, January 2013, pp. 71-76.

[31] U. Varshney, "Smart medication management system and multiple interventions for medication adherence," *Decision Support Systems*, vol. 55, 2013, pp. 538-551.

[32] J. Wilson, "Benefits of smart healthcare that we need to know," May, 2018, https://sybridmd.com/blogs/sybrid-news/benefits-of-smart-healthcare-that-we-need-to-know/

[33] M. N. O. Sadiku, S. Binzaid, and S. M. Musa, "Internet of things: Challenges and Solutions," *World Journal of Engineering Research and Technology*, vol. 3, no. 3, 2019, pp. 70-77.

[35] J. Qiu et al., "Towards secure and smart healthcare in smart cities using blockchain," *IEEE International Smart Cities Conference*, September. 2016.

[36] R. Chaudhary et al., "LSCSH: Lattice-based secure cryptosystem for smart healthcare in smart cities environment," *IEEE Communications Magazine*, April 2018, pp. 24-32.

[37] J. Qui et al., "Towards secure and smart healthcare in smart cities using blockchain," https://www.researchgate.net/publication/327142128_Towards_Secure_and_Smart_Healthcare_in_Smart_Cities_Using_Blockchain

[38] S. Tian et al., "Smart healthcare: Making medical care more intelligent *Global Health Journal,* vol. 3, no.3, September 2019, pp. 62-65.

[39] B. Rodić-Trmčić et al., "Designing a course for smart healthcare engineering education," *Computer Applications in Engineering Education*, vol.26, no. 3, May 2018, pp.484–499.

[40] S. U. Khan, A. Y. Zomaya, and A. Abbas (eds.), *Handbook of Large-Scale Distributed Computing in Smart Healthcare.* Springer, 2017.

[41] C. Röcker and M. Ziefle, *Smart Healthcare Applications and Services; Developments and Practices.* IGI Global, 2011.

[42] A. Sinha and M. Rathi, *Smart Healthcare Systems.* Chapman and Hall/CRC, 2019.

[43] L. V. Langenhove, *Smart Textiles for Medicine and Healthcare: Materials, Systems and Applications.* Boca Raton, FL: CRC Press, 2007.

[44] W. Zhao. X. Luo, T. Qiu (eds.), *Recent Developments in Smart Healthcare.* Mdpi AG, 2018.

[45] B. Shen (ed.), *Translational Informatics in Smart Healthcare.* Springer, 2017.

[46] P. Pronovost and E. Vohr, *Safe Patients, Smart Hospitals: How One Doctor's Checklist Can Help Us Change Health Care from the Inside Out (Pronovost, Safe Patients, Smart Hospitals).* Plume, 2010.

CHAPTER 7

HEALTHCARE BIG DATA

"Only a life lived in the service to others is worth living." – Albert Einstein

7.1 INTRODUCTION

Health plays a crucial role in people's lives. The healthcare industry comprises of in-patient services (i.e., hospitals), out-patient services (i.e., clinics, surgical centers),pharmaceutical companies, insurance, nursing homes, telemedicine, charity organizations, and medical equipment. The global healthcare industry is striving to lower the costs while improving the quality of care provided. With the ever-increasing cost for healthcare services and ever-increasing health insurance premiums, the healthcare industry is in need of proactive healthcare management and wellness. As the industry moves from a volume-based to a value-based model, data will play a pivotal role in the transition [1].

The healthcare industry deals with a lot of information. For example, the vast amount of information that is continuously generated from patient medical experience remains untapped. Today, data is generated daily by mobile phones, sensors, patients, hospitals, researchers, organizations, pharmacies, medical centers, medical records, commerce, and organizations. Data has always been king, but handling and analyzing huge amount of data is a challenging task. In today's digital society, it is necessary that this data should be digitized. This huge, heterogeneous, and digitized data is known as big data (BD). Big data (BD) has opened up enormous opportunities for a wide range of industries, include the healthcare sector. Its management solutions will provide insightful information, which can help healthcare organizations make right decisions at the right time [2].

Although the healthcare industry has lagged behind other industries due to issues of patient privacy, confidentiality, and data security, the exploration of big data in healthcare is increasing at an unprecedented rate due to advanced technologies. Technological advances enable huge volumes of data to be analyzed through faster, more efficient, and cheaper computing devices.

This chapter provides an introduction to big data analysis in the healthcare sector. It begins by discussing the importance and characteristics of big data in healthcare. It presents big data analytics and big data ethics. It discusses several applications of big data in healthcare. It addresses the benefits and challenges of big data in healthcare. The last section provides some concluding thoughts.

7.2 WHY BIG DATA IN HEALTHCARE

"Big data" is a big all-too-common buzzword these days. The concept refers to massive amount of data generated through digitization of all sorts of information, including health records. It has rapidly made its way into a wide range of industries and it has changed the way we manage and analyze data. It is a major challenge for industries such as defense, transportation, agriculture, and banking. For healthcare industry, it is even more formidable due to the highly sensitive and highly dynamic nature of the data. In healthcare, big data comes from numerous sources including data from electronic health records, mobile applications, genomics, clinical reports, doctor's notes, wearable body sensors, medical devices, hospital admission notes, pharmacies, insurance companies, medical imaging, laboratories, ehealth, mhealth, social media, genomic sequencing, to name a few [3]. Some of these sources are illustrated in Figure 7.1 [4]. These include structured (such as from electronic health records (EHRs)), semi-structured (physician-to-patient and patient-to-patient communication through email, social media, and web), and unstructured (such as clinical notes and claims) data [5].

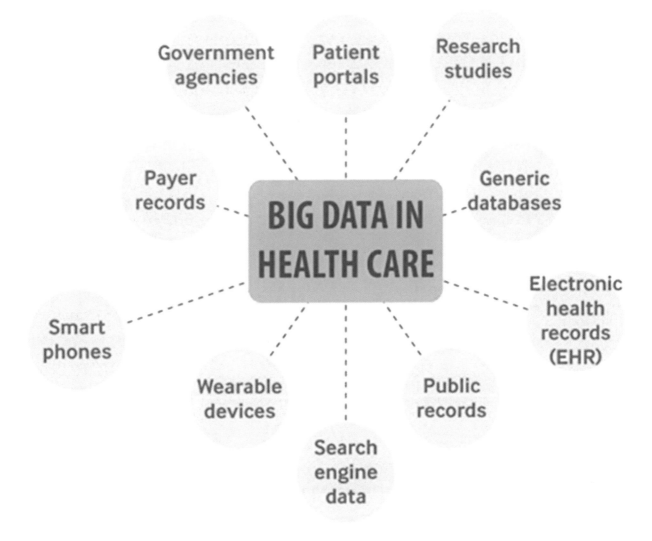

Figure 7.1 Sources of big data in healthcare [4].

The rise of healthcare big data is due to the rapid digitization across healthcare, the rise of value-based care, and the rise in healthcare cost in nations like the United States. Big data (BD) is essentially about gathering information from disparate sources and analyzing it to reveal trends that can directly improve patients' well-being. Healthcare is one of the most promising areas where big data can be applied to make a change. BD is a revolutionary, powerful tool in the healthcare industry; it is now becoming vital in current patient-centric care.

The era of big data has opened up new opportunities in personalized medicine, preventive care, chronic disease management, telemonitoring, and managing of patients with implanted devices. Data-driven healthcare enables autonomous decision-making [6].

7.3 BIG DATA CHARACTERISTICS

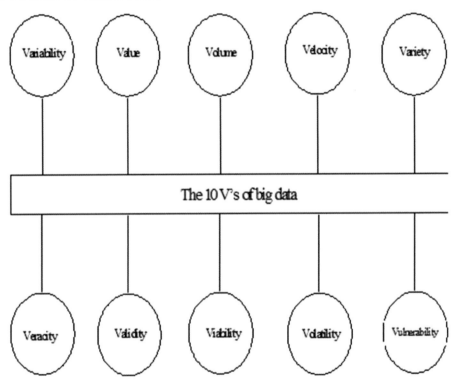

Figure 7.2 Big data's 10Vs [7].

As shown in Figure 7.2, big data are often described with the five "Vs": volume, velocity, variety, veracity, and value [7,8].

- *Volume*: This refers to the size of the data being generated from both inside and outside organizations, and is increasing annually. Some regard big data as data over one petabyte in volume. The volume of medical data are of the order of terabytes and petabytes.
- *Velocity*: This depicts the unprecedented speed at which data are generated by Internet users, mobile users, social media, etc. Data are generated and processed in a fast way to extract useful, relevant information. Big data could be analyzed in real time, and it has movement and velocity.

- *Variety*: This refers to the data types since big data may originate from heterogeneous sources and is in different formats (e.g., videos, images, audio, text, logs). BD comprises of structured, semi-structured or unstructured data.
- *Veracity*: By this, we mean the truthfulness of data, i.e. whether the data comes from a reputable, trustworthy, authentic, and accountable source. It suggests the inconsistency in the quality of different sources of big data. The data may not be 100% correct.
- *Value*: This is the most important aspect of the big data. It is the desired outcome of big data processing. It refers to the process of discovering hidden values from large datasets. It denotes the value derived from the analysis of the existing data. If one cannot extract some business value from the data, there is no use managing and storing it.

On this basis, small data can be regarded as having low volume, low velocity, low variety, low veracity, and low value. Additional five Vs has been added [9]:

- *Validity:* This refers to the accuracy and correctness of data. It also indicates how up to date is.
- *Viability:* This identifies the relevancy of data for each use case. Relevancy of data is required to maintain the desired and accurate outcome through analytical and predictive measures.
- *Volatility:* Since healthcare data are generated and change at a rapid rate, volatility determines how quickly data change.
- *Vulnerability:* The vulnerability of data is essential because privacy and security are of utmost importance for healthcare data.
- *Visualization:* Healthcare data need to be presented unambiguously and attractively to the user. Proper visualization of large and complex clinical reports helps in finding valuable insights.

Instead of the 5V's above, some suggest the following 5V's: Venue, Variability, Vocabulary, Vagueness, and Validity) [10].

Healthcare is a good example of how the five V's of big data are an innate aspect of the data it produces. Considered this way, healthcare has become one of the key emerging users of big data. Combining healthcare with big data can lead to improved decision making process and obtaining better solutions to curing diseases. Big data in health is concerned with structured and unstructured datasets that are too big, too fast, and too complex for healthcare providers to process and interpret with existing tools. Big data promises to connect physicians of different specialties, nurses, laboratory technologists, researchers, pharmaceutical, and healthcare companies to personalized patient experiences everywhere.

7.4 BIG DATA ANALYTICS

Tools for analyzing big data are generally referred to as big data analytics (BDA). Typical BDAs include [11]: (1) Google Big Query, (2) MapReduce, (3) Jaql, (4) Hadoop. MapReduce is Google's solution for processing big data. The Hadoop is the popular implementation of the MapReduce model. The main objective of big data analytics is to help healthcare organizations in making better and more informed decisions. Big data analytics tools have the potential to transform healthcare in many different ways. In healthcare sector, BDA has shown advantages on improving healthcare efficiency because BDA can recognize individuals' healthcare conditions, identify risks for serious health problems, and provide personalized healthcare services [12]. Prominent big data analytics companies include Oracle, IBM, Sparx, and Verisk. These are the leading vendors in the healthcare data analytics market.

A cloud-enabled big data analytic platform is the best way to analyze the structured and unstructured healthcare data. Common BDA techniques include data mining, statistical analysis, visualization, natural language processing, machine learning, and cloud computing.

The role of big data analytics in healthcare is illustrated in Figure 7.3 [13]. The objective of healthcare data analytics is to use data-driven findings to predict and solve a problem before it is too late. Big data analytics enables organizations to analyze structured, semi-structured, and unstructured data which scales to terabytes, petabytes, and exabytes in search of valuable insights. In healthcare, analytics in healthcare carries many benefits, promises, and presents great potential for transforming healthcare. Healthcare organizations or providers use big data analytics to transform data into actionable information [14,15].

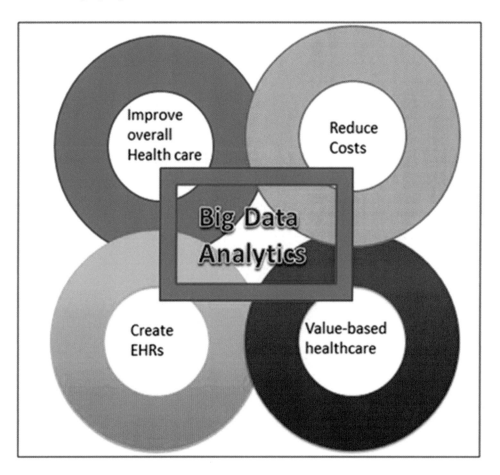

Figure 7.3 The role of big data analytics in healthcare [13].

7.5 BIG DATA ETHICS

Sharing data is an expectation of the human participants involved and thus a key part of ethical research. Data ethics is of increasing relevance as the quantity of data increases. Ethical questions may be considered in terms of accuracy, humane treatment, informed participants, and the necessity and applicability of the work. Ethics helps us to frame our ideas about what is right or wrong using rational argument. It can be applied in determining whether the use of big data is ethical [16].

Companies and professional organizations build codes of conduct and ethic. For example, professional organizations such as the Association for Computer Machinery (ACM), the Institute of Electrical and Electronics Engineers (IEEE), and the British Computer Society, have developed codes of ethics. Such professional codes of ethics set the standard for acceptable behavior within a profession and provide a signal to those that interact with the relevant group as to what to expect of the group members.

Ethics helps us to frame our ideas about what is right or wrong using rational argument. It can be applied in determining whether the use of big data is ethical. Five major ethical themes are identified [17]: (1) informed consent is taken for participating in a study, (2) privacy, which is the non-disclosure of personal information to the public, (3) ownership refers to rights regarding the modification of data, along with benefiting from intellectual property, (4) epistemology and objectivity, a number of sources reveal a connection between the ethics and epistemology of big data, and (5) big data divides between those who have or lack the necessary resources to analyze large datasets.

Big data ethics are integrated into a range of disciplines, such as computing, statistics, and data sciences, and user behavior using codes of conduct. Although data is ethically neutral, ethical considerations arise from the effort to align the organization actions with societal values. Big data will be useful to sustain and improve health care. Various forms of health sensitive information are being easily created, stored, and accessed. The risk that health information will be used inappropriately can never be fully eliminated, but it can be minimized. Patients whose data were used for research purposes have the right to initiate litigation.

7.6 APLICATIONS IN HEALTHCARE

Big data is generating a lot of attention in every industry including healthcare. It is capable of transforming business and clinical models for smart and efficient delivery of care. The important factors for implementing the usage of big data in healthcare include organizational analytics capability, data quality, data privacy and security, data standardization, and data experts. Big data analysis can better manage health records, generate new knowledge, care for the elderly, discover a remedy for illnesses, improve care, save patient's life, and lower healthcare cost. Healthcare professionals can apply big data analytics in the same way as other businesses, except that the stakes are higher. Data analytics in healthcare has the potential of transforming the ways healthcare organizations operate, both for business operations and health management. BD analytics in healthcare can be applied in the following areas [18-21].

- *Control Data for Public Health:* The healthcare industry is drowning in data. Without big data, those data are meaningless. Public health issues can be improved with data analytics approach. Large amount of data can help determine needs, offer required services, and predict and prevent the future crises.
- *Electronic Medical Record* (EMR): Currently, most hospitals have switched over to using EMR, which makes it easier for health care professionals to access data. An EMR contains

the standard medical data that can be evaluated with the data analytic approach to predict patients at risk and provide effective care.

- *Electronic Health Records* (EHRs): These are the most widespread application of big data in medicine. The digital record may include demographics, medical history, allergies, and laboratory test results. The widespread adoption of EHRs has created new opportunities for clinical investigation using big data techniques. Doctors sharing EHRs can aggregate and analyze data for trends and minimize duplicate tests.

- *Generating New Knowledge:* Integrating data about the patient might provide better predictions and help target interventions to the right patients. For example, the integrated system has improved outcomes in cardiovascular disease. The insights from big data have the potential to touch multiple aspects of healthcare.

- *Elderly Care:* A growing number of the elderly population wish to live an independent lifestyle. A big data solution uses wearable sensors capable of carrying out continuous monitoring of the elderly. The healthcare system connects with remote wrist sensors through mobile phones to monitor the elder's well-being. Such a big data system can provide rich information to healthcare providers about the elderly living conditions and environment [22].

- *Discovering a Remedy for Illnesses*: Analyzing big data can be used in identifying hidden associations and unrevealed patterns. Big data can learn about human genomes and discover the appropriate remedy or pills for cancer. With the genome information, a connection can be established between DNA and a specific illness [23].

- *Fraud Reduction:* The cost of fraud, waste, and abuse in the healthcare industry is a major contributor to spiraling healthcare costs in the United States, but big data analytics can be used to prevent fraud and security threats. Identifying, predicting, and minimizing fraud can be implemented using advanced analytic tools. This approach helps analyze greater number of claim requests to curtail fraud cases. An effective analysis can help reduce fraud, waste, and abuse. Medical insurers are using big data analytics to detect medical fraud and identity theft.

- *Monitoring of Patients:* Healthcare organizations are looking for ways to provide more proactive care to their patients by constantly monitoring patient vital signs. New wearables can track specific health trends and relay them back to the cloud where they can be monitored by physicians. Data analytics can be used to analyze real time large volumes of data in hospitals. The approach may help in monitoring patients.

- *Preventing Medication Errors:* Medication errors are a major concern in healthcare industry. Patients often end up with the wrong medication or dosage—which could cause harm or even death. Big data can help reduce these medication error rates dramatically by analyzing the patient's records with all medications prescribed, and flagging anything that seems out of place.

- *Identifying High-Risk Patients*: One major issue in healthcare on identifying high-risk patients is lack of data. Using predictive analytics, some hospitals have been able to reduce the number of emergency room visits by identifying high-risk patients and offering customized care.

- *Precision Medicine*: This can be regarded as an approach to provide the right treatments to the right patients at the right time. It replaces the imprecise one-size-fits-all medicine. Precision medicine allows individually tailored medicine and enables patients to receive care best matched to their specific health condition. It combines comprehensive data collected about an individual's genetics, environment, and lifestyle (such as smoking and heart disease), to advance disease understanding, aid drug discovery, and ensure delivery of appropriate therapies. Combining big data and personalized or precision medicine holds great promise for the future of medicine. Big data holds promise to transform clinical decision making toward precision medicine. Precision medicine powered by big data will also reduce costs [24,25]. With healthcare data analytics, prevention is better than cure.

- *Cardiovascular Care*: Cardiovascular diseases are well known to be heterogeneous in nature. Applying big data analytic to cardiovascular care will translate into better care at a lower cost. Although there are several risk models related to cardiovascular conditions, big data analytics may yield more powerful prediction of outcomes ranging from mortality to patient-reported outcomes [26]. Big data has tremendous potential to improve cardiovascular quality and outcomes of care.

- *Biomedical Research*: Big data is radically transforming biomedical research. The main issue in biomedical research is how to extract knowledge from big data. In the era of digital biomedicine, biomedical scientists are confronting with dealing with ever larger sets of data. Big data in biomedicine has tremendous potential to transform biomedicine, healthcare, drug discovery, and development [27]. It is also expediting biomedical discovery. In view of the complexity of biomedical big data, there is an urgent need to produce bioinformatics professionals who are capable of processing, analyzing, and interpreting big data.

- *Psychiatry:* The growth of big data in psychiatry will provide unprecedented opportunities for exploration. Psychiatrists will increasingly have to evaluate results from research studies and commercial analytical products that are based on big data. Big data from clinical, administrative, and imaging will increase understanding of existing and new questions in psychiatry [28].

- *Telemedicine:* This is used for primary consultations, real time remote patient monitoring, and medical education for healthcare practitioners. Clinicians use telemedicine to provide personalized treatment plans and prevent hospitalization. Such use of healthcare data analytics allows clinicians to predict acute medical events in advance and prevent deterioration of patient's conditions [29]. It is sometimes necessary to deliver telehealth services using mobile technology.

Some of these applications are depicted in Figure 7.4. These are just few areas where big data has been applied in healthcare industry. Other areas include diagnostics, cost reduction, prevention medicine, precision medicine, diabetes management, bioinformatics, patient profile analysis, genomic analytics, obesity, hospitals, medical image processing, clinical informatics, imaging informatics, and public health informatics.

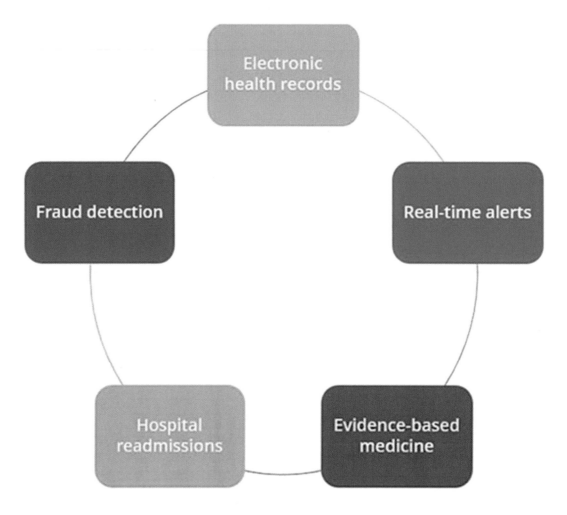

Figure 7.4 Some applications of big data in healthcare.

BENEFITS

The big data revolution holds great promise in the healthcare industry. It has the potential to provide unparalleled opportunities to answer questions that cannot be answered by clinical trials. Big data in healthcare allows providers to deliver more precise and personalized care. The more data is available to physicians, the easier it is to identify trends and identify bottlenecks in patient care. Big data is helping to solve healthcare problems in hospitals around the world, leading to reduced waiting times for patients and better quality of care. Today, big data allows for early identification of individual patient's illnesses. Healthcare analytics are on the rise. The benefits derived from big data analytics can be classified into five categories: IT infrastructure benefits, operational benefits, organizational benefits, managerial benefits, and strategic benefits [30].

The benefits of BD in healthcare industry include cost reduction, disease prediction, increase in operational efficiency, reduction in preventable mistakes, appropriate treatment, patient care improvement, more efficient healthcare system, improved patient outcomes, public health surveillance, early disease detection, fraud detection and prevention, and better healthcare quality [31]. It has led to the improvement of patients care at a lower cost and increased patient satisfaction. It can also benefit healthcare through data management, electronic medical records, and data analysis. Using BD in healthcare allows for strategic planning. BD can unify all patient related data to get a total view of the patient. It can improve clinical practices, new drug development, and health care financing process [32]. Big data will enable healthcare providers to deliver much more precise and personalized care. The opportunities for using big data in healthcare are endless.

Other benefits include the following [33]:

- *Change:* Big data analytics has the potential to drive real change in clinical practice, from personalized therapy to electronic health record mining.
- *Intelligence*: Big data has the ability to combine data from numerous sources and provide "intelligence" not derived from any single data source. It allows the prediction of patterns, trends, and outcomes.
- *Reduced Costs:* By using predictive analysis, healthcare expenses can be reduced. The greater insight that medical data gives physicians translates to better patient care, shorter hospital stays, fewer admissions, and cost reduction..
- *Eliminating Human Errors:* Making mistakes is inevitable and human. For example, medical professionals can prescribe the wrong medicine. Big Data can dramatically decrease the likelihood of errors.
- *Visualization:* This plays a crucial role in helping nurses and other healthcare professionals. It only proves to be a valuable tool if the data quality is assured.

CHALLENGES

While the adoption of big data technologies in healthcare industry offers limitless opportunities and benefits for patients and healthcare professionals, it also faces some challenges. Big data for healthcare may cause more problems than solutions. Big data analytics in healthcare faces huge challenges and barriers including data collection and analysis, data complexity, security and privacy of the information stored, ethical and legal issues, visualization, interoperability, portability, authenticity, implementation costs, transportability, complexity, accuracy, consistency, performance, management, storage, standards, governance, integration of data, data integrity, data quality, data accommodation, data classification, and incorporation of technology. Some of these challenges are computationally and storage intensive in nature and are further complicated by an increasing emphasis on fault tolerance, redundancy, and scalability.

Although data protection is everybody's duty, it is important that there is the right balance between data protection rights and the need to support public health [34]. Lack of skilled healthcare workers to work with big data toolsets is another big challenge. Cost is always a concern in many applications of BD, but the cost cannot be closely predicted.

Other challenges include [35,36].

- *Ethics and privacy:* The main issues in big data in medicine are security and privacy of the patients as well as ownership, stewardship, and governance of data due to the sensitive nature of health care data. These issues are important when gathering and accessing data in health care. The use of big data for medical research poses unprecedented ethical challenges. These information privacy laws are a major hurdle that prevents comprehensive data to be used in medicine. Big data projects are often distributed across nations with different laws, making issues of privacy, and consent complicated solving challenges associated with data privacy and security.

- *Collaboration:* Every step in the acquisition, processing, cleaning, analysis, and interpretation of big data is difficult because projects require the active collaboration of people with a wide range of expertise such as physicians, statisticians, biologists, software engineers, mechanical engineers, network security experts, and project managers.

- *Risks:* Different risks should to be carefully considered and monitored when looking at new sources of big data.

- *Fragmented Systems and Databases:* Healthcare data is often fragmented into institution-centered silos. Medical data is spread across many sources governed by different states, hospitals, and administrative departments. Healthcare providers often have no incentive to share patient information with one another, which has made it difficult to apply the power of big data.

- *Integration:* Inadequate integration of healthcare systems is a major challenge. To fully benefit from BD analytics, patient databases from different institutions such as hospitals, universities, and nonprofit organizations need to be linked up. This may be difficult to achieve due to incompatible data systems, patient confidentiality issues, and lack of willingness to share with others [37]. The integration of data is necessary to drive potential benefit in the care of patients. Integration of data sources would require developing a new infrastructure where all data providers collaborate with each other.

- *Standardization:* Healthcare data is rarely standardized, often generated with incompatible formats. Lack of standards creates interoperability challenges. There is need for standardization of data content, format, and clinical definitions. Standardization of samples allows for data generated from one individual to be used in other related studies.

- *Intellectual Property* (IP): IP protection, mainly provided by copyrights and patents, is the pillar of national research policies. It helps in effectively translating innovation by commercialization. In the absence of such protection, companies will be unwilling to invest in the development of diagnostic tests or treatments. However, the operation of the IP system is being fundamentally changed by new data driven techniques.

- *Noise*: Handling noisiness and incompleteness of EHRs are still challenging. More data often means more noise in which any true signals drown.

Some of these challenges are illustrated in Figure 7.5 [38]. These challenges must be properly addressed by healthcare organizations to achieve their data-driven clinical and financial goals. This may take time, commitment, funding, but doing so will ease the burdens of everyone.

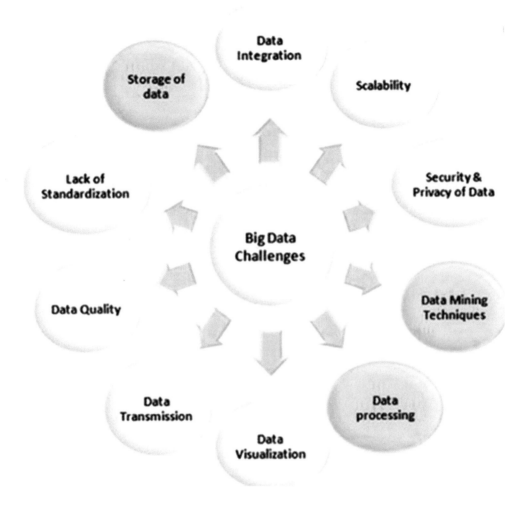

Figure 7.5 Big data challenges [38].

CONCLUSION

Whatever can be done to help physicians and healthcare workers with carrying out their jobs effectively should be encouraged. The key role of big data in addressing the needs of the healthcare system all over the world has been noticed by government, private, and academic sectors. Big data analytics has offered a new way to healthcare industry to develop actionable insights, boost up the outcomes, and help enhance the decision making capability of the healthcare leaders.

Big data is now a booming industry. It has started to revolutionize healthcare and move the industry forward on many fronts. The growing rate of data in healthcare organizations has necessitated the adoption of big data techniques so as to improve the quality of healthcare delivery. The applications of big data in healthcare are still in their formative stages and the future is bright. Although the healthcare industry is yet to fully grasp the potential benefits of big data analytics, it has increased its overall value by adopting big data techniques to analyze and understand its data from various sources. However, some organizations are simply not ready to invest in big data. There are some roadblocks to widespread adoption of BD analytics in healthcare.

Big data is already here. It has many implications for all healthcare constituents – patients, care providers, students, researchers, and health insurance companies. To survive, in this digital age, healthcare organizations must become data-driven. Healthcare organizations such as government agencies, medical schools, and research institutes will benefit from big data.

Since big data is poised to revolutionize healthcare industry and health professional education, nursing and medical students should be involved in the effort to increase big data literacy [39]. Training in data science will need to become a part of medical and nursing curricula so that healthcare practitioner will be more comfortable with the result that is generated by the new tools. Healthcare leaders must understand the value of big data science and how it affects their profession, as they aim to provide the best possible care to patients [40]. Big data is poised to have enormous impact on healthcare, especially on personalized medicine. The future of healthcare will definitely be enabled by big data. More information about the use of big data in healthcare can be found in books in [41-45] and the following related journals:

- *Journal of Big Data*
- *Big Data Research*
- *Journal of Healthcare Communications*

REFERENCES

[1] H. K. Patil and R. Seshadri, "Big data security and privacy issues in healthcare," *Proceedings of IEEE International Congress on Big Data*, 2014, pp. 762-765.

[2] M. N. O. Sadiku, K. G. Eze, and S. M. Musa, "Big data in healthcare," *International Journal of Trend in Research and Development*, vol. 7, no. 2, March-April 2020, pp. 189-190.

[3] M. N. O. Sadiku, E. Dada, K. B. Olarenwaju, and S. M. Musa, "Big data in healthcare," *International Journal for Research & Engineering Technology*, vol. 7, no. 9, September 2019, pp. 1165-1168.

[4] "Healthcare big data and the promise of value-based care," https://catalyst.nejm.org/doi/full/10.1056/CAT.18.0290

[5] M. S. Hossain and G. Muhammad, "Healthcare big data voice pathology assessment framework," *IEEE Access*, vol. 4, 2016.

[6] M. Grossglauser and H. Saner, "Data-driven healthcare: From patterns to actions," *European Journal of Preventive Cardiology*, vol. 21, 2014, pp.14–17.

[7] B. Ristevski and M. Chen,"Big data analytics in medicine and healthcare," *Journal of Integrative Bioinformatics, 2018.*

[8] M. N.O. Sadiku, M. Tembely, and S.M. Musa, "Big data: An introduction for engineers," *Journal of Scientific and Engineering Research*, vol. 3, no. 2, 2016, pp. 106-108.

[9] P/ K. D. Pramanik S. Pal, and M. Mukhopadhyay, "Healthcare big data: A comprehensive overview," in N. Bouchemal (ed.), *Intelligent Systems for Healthcare Management and Delivery.* IGI Global, chapter 4, 2019, pp. 72-100.

[10] J. Moorthy et al., "Big data: Prospects and challenges," *The Journal for Decision Makers*, vol. 40, no. 1, 2015, pp. 74–96.

[11] I. Olaronke and O. Oluwaseun, "Big data in healthcare: Prospects, challenges and Resolutions," *Proceedings of Future Technologies Conference*, San Francisco, US, December 2016, pp. 1152-1157.

[12] J. Wu, "Adoption of big data and analytics in mobile healthcare market: An economic perspective," *Electronic Commerce Research and Applications*, vol. 22, 2017, pp. 24–41.

[13] A. Pandey, "Big Data Analytics and augmented patient care," July 2019, https://blogs. mastechinfotrellis.com/big-data-analytics-augmented-patient-care

[14] M. N. O. Sadiku, J. Foreman, and S. M. Musa, "Big data analytics: A primer," *International Journal of Technologies and Management Research,* vol. 5, no. 9, September 2018, pp. 44-49.

[15] S. Rao, S. N. Suma, and M. Sunitha, "Security solutions for big data analytics in healthcare," *Second International Conference on Advances in Computing and Communication Engineering,* 2015, pp. 510-514.

[16] M. N. O. Sadiku, C. M. Kotteti, and S. M. Musa, "Big data ethics," *International Journals of Advanced Research in Computer Science and Software Engineering,* vol. 8, no. 12, December 2018, pp. 15-17.

[17] B. D. Mittelstadt and L. Floridi, "The ethics of big data: Current and foreseeable issues in biomedical contexts," *Science and Engineering Ethics,* vol 22, no. 2, April 2016, pp. 303–341.

[18] T. Hardy, "Significant benefits of big data analytics in healthcare industry," January 2016, https:// www.builtinla.com/blog/significant-benefits-big-data-analytics-healthcare-industry

[19]. M. N. O. Sadiku, K. B. Olanrewaju, and S M. Musa, "Examining big data in medicine: Applications, challenges and benefits," *European Scientific Journal,* vol. 16, no. 6, 2020, pp.1-11.

[20] R. Ayers, "5 ways the healthcare industry could use big data – and why it's not," August 2017, http://dataconomy.com/2017/08/5-ways-healthcare-big-data/

[21] M. Lebied, "12 Examples of big data analytics in healthcare that can save people," July 2018, https://www.datapine.com/blog/big-data-examples-in-healthcare/

[22] P. Jian et al., "An intelligent information forwarder for healthcare big data systems with distributed wearable sensors," *IEEE Systems Journal,* vol. 10, no. 3, September 2016, pp. 1147-1159.

[23] A. G. Alexandru, I. M. Radu, and M. L. Bizo, "Big data in healthcare - Opportunities and challenges," *Informatica Economică,* vol.22, no. 2, 2018, pp. 43-54.

[24] W. J. Hopp, J. Li, and G. Wang, "Big data and the precision medicine revolution," *Production and Operations Management,* vol. 27, no. 9, September 2018, pp. 1647-1664.

[25] B. E Huang, W. Mulyasasmita, and G. Rajagopal, "The path from big data to precision medicine," *Expert Review of Precision Medicine and Drug Development,* vol. 1, no. 2, 2016, pp. 129-143.

[26] R. U. Shah and J. S. Rumsfeld, "Big data in cardiology," *European Heart Journal,* vol. 38, no. 24, June 2017, pp. 1865–1867.

[27] F. F. Costa, "Big data in biomedicine," *Drug Discovery Today,* vol. 19, no. 4, April 2014, pp. 433-440.

[28] S. Monteith et al., "Big data are coming to psychiatry: A general introduction," *International Journal of Bipolar Disorders,* vol. 3, no. 21, 2015.

[29] "Big data use cases in the healthcare industry," https://www.allerin.com/blog/big-data-cases

[30] Y. Wang, L. A. Kung, and T. A. Byrd, "Big data analytics: Understanding its capabilities and potential benefits for healthcare organizations," *Technological Forecasting and Social Change,* vol. 126, January 2018, pp. 3-13.

[31] Q. K. Fatt and A. Ramadas, "The usefulness and challenges of big data in healthcare," *Journal of Healthcare Communications,* vol. 3, no. 2, 2018.

[32] L. Wang and C. A. Alexander, "Big data in medical applications and health care," *Current Research in Medicine,* vol. 6, no. 1, 2015.

[33] R. Ijaz, "5 ways big data is transforming the medical field," July 2018, https://www.smartdatacollective.com/5-ways-big-data-is-transforming-the-medical-field

[34] G. Roesems-Kerremans, "Big data in healthcare," *Journal of Healthcare Communications*, vol. 1, no.4, 2016.

[35] M. Bauer, "Big data, technology, and the changing future of medicine," https://www.medicographia.com/2018/02/big-data-technology-and-the-changing-future-of-medicine/

[36] T. Hulsen et al., " From big data to precision medicine," *Frontiers In Medicine*, vol. 6, March 2019.

[37] M. Lebied, "9 examples of big data analytics in healthcare that can save people," *Business Intelligence*, May 2017, https://www.datapine.com/blog/big-data-examples-in-healthcare/

[38] P. S. Mathew and A. S. Pillai, "Big data challenges and solutions in healthcare: A survey," in H. Sharma et al. (eds.), *Advances in Intelligent Systems and Computing,* Springer, 2020.

[39] C. Vaitsis, G. Nilsson, and N. Zary, "Visual analytics in healthcare education: Exploring novel ways to analyze and represent big data in undergraduate medical education," *PeerJ*, vol. 2, November 2014.

[40] M. N. O. Sadiku, K. G. Eze, and S. M. Musa, "Big data in nursing," *International Journal of Trend in Research and Development,* vol. 6, no. 4, July-Aug. 2019, pp.16-17.

[41] M. D. Lytras and P. Papadopoulou (eds.), *Applying Big Data Analytics in Bioinformatics and Medicine.* IGI Global, 2018.

[42] B. Wang, R. Li, and W. Perrizo, *Big Data Analytics in Bioinformatics and Healthcare.* IGI Gblobal, 2015.

[43] R. Suganya, S. Rajaram, and A. S. Abdullah, *Big Data in Medical Image Processing.* Boca Raton, FL: CRC Press. 2018.

[44] A. J. Kulkarni et al. (eds.), *Big Data Analytics in Healthcare.* Springer, 2020.

[45] Various Authors, *Big Data Analytics in Healthcare: Promise and Potential.* Amazon, 2015.

CHAPTER 8

ARTIFICIAL INTELLIGENCE IN HEALTHCARE

"Kind words can be short and easy to speak, but their
echos are truly endless." —Mother Teresa

8.1 INTRODUCTION

Recently, we have witnessed a wave of emerging technologies, from Internet of things and blockchain to artificial intelligence (AI), demonstrate significant potential to transform and disrupt multiple sectors, including healthcare. Healthcare is shifting from traditional hospital-centric care to a more virtual care that leverages the latest technologies around artificial intelligence, deep learning, big data, genomics, robotics, increased access to data, additive manufacturing, and wearable and implanted devices [1].

Artificial intelligence (AI), the core of the fourth revolution of science and technology, is the use of computer science to develop machine that can be trained to learn, reason, communicate, and make humanlike decisions. It is basically the intelligence of machines, as opposed to the intelligence of humans. AI is a technology that is rapidly being adopted in many industries to improve performance, precision, time efficiency, and cost reduction. The use of artificial intelligence in healthcare is an emerging scientific area that aims to generate healthcare intelligence by analyzing health data. AI is becoming increasingly attractive in healthcare industry and changing the landscape of healthcare and biomedical research.

Today, artificial intelligence (AI) is shorthand for any task a machine can perform just as well as, if not better than, humans. AI represents the hopes and fears of an industry seeking more intelligent solutions. AI is an interdisciplinary field covering numerous areas such as computer science, psychology, linguistics, philosophy, and neurosciences. The central objectives of AI research include reasoning, knowledge, planning, learning, natural language processing, perception, and the ability to move and manipulate objects [2].

Although AI is a branch of computer science, there is hardly any field which is unaffected by this technology. Common areas of applications include agriculture, business, law enforcement, oil and gas, banking and finance, education, transportation, healthcare, automobiles, entertainment, manufacturing, speech and text recognition, facial analysis, and telecommunications [3]. In healthcare, AI can help manage and analyze data. AI can have a significant impact in making healthcare more accessible, especially in developing countries, where shortages of healthcare practitioners are most severe. There are many cases in which AI can perform healthcare tasks as well or better than humans.

This chapter provides an introduction on a broad range of applications of AI in healthcare. It begins by providing an overview on AI. It covers some applications of AI in healthcare. It addresses the global policy developments and investments in AI. It highlights the benefits and challenges of AI in healthcare. The last sections concludes with some comments.

8.2 OVERVIEW ON ARTIFICIAL INTELLIGENCE

The term "artificial intelligence" (AI) was coined in 1956 by John McCarthy during a conference held on this subject. AI is the branch of computer science that deals with designing intelligent computer systems that mimic human intelligence. The ability of machines to process natural language, to learn, to plan makes it possible for new tasks to be performed by intelligent systems. The main purpose of AI is to mimic the cognitive function of human beings and perform activities that would typically be performed by a human being. AI is stand-alone independent electronic entity that functions much like human healthcare expert. Today, AI is integrated into our daily lives in several forms, such as personal assistants, automated mass transportation, aviation, computer gaming, facial recognition at passport control, voice recognition on virtual assistants, driverless cars, companion robots, etc. [4]. AI technologies are performing better and better at analyzing health data, thereby helping doctors better understand the future needs of their patients.

An important feature of AI technology is that is can be added to existing technologies. AI has benefited many areas such chemistry and medicine, where routine diagnoses can be initiated by AI-aided computers. It embraces a wide range of disciplines such as computer science, engineering, machine learning, chemistry, biology, physics, astronomy, neuroscience, and social sciences.

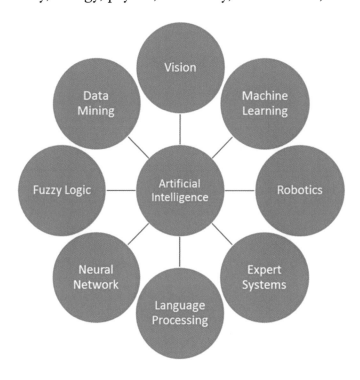

Figure 8.1 Branches of artificial intelligence [5].

AI is not a single technology but a range of computational models and algorithms. As illustrated in Figure 8.1, the major disciplines in AI include expert systems, fuzzy logic, and artificial neural networks (ANNs), machine learning, deep learning, natural language processing, computer vision, and robotics. The various computer-based tools or technologies that have been used to achieve AI's goals are the following [5-7]:

- *Expert Systems*: An expert system (ES) (or knowledge-based system) enables computers to make decisions by interpreting data and selecting between alternatives just as a human expert would do. It uses a technique known as rule-based inference in which rules are used to process data. Complex expert systems such as MYCIN, ONCOCIN, and INTERNIST gave the impression that AI technology would have a significant impact on the everyday practice of medicine.

- *Neural Networks*: These computer programs identify objects or recognize patterns after having been trained. Artificial neural networks (ANNs) are parallel distributed systems consisting of processing units (neurons) that calculate some mathematical functions. The ANN model represents nonlinear relationships which are directly learned from the data being modeled. Neural networks are being explored for healthcare applications in imaging and diagnoses, risk analysis, lifestyle management and monitoring, health information management, and virtual health assistance.

- *Natural Language Processors*: Computer programs that translate or interpret language as it is spoken by normal people. NLP techniques extract information from unstructured data such as clinical notes to supplement and enrich structured medical data. NLP targets at extracting useful information from the narrative text to assist clinical decision making. NLP includes applications such as speech recognition, text analysis, translation and other goals related to language. There are two basic approaches to NLP: statistical and semantic. Healthcare is the biggest user of the NLP tools. NLP has been used in the clinical setting for capturing, representing, and utilizing clinical information [8].

- *Robots*: Computer-based programmable machines that have physical manipulators and sensors. The introduction of intelligent robots in the healthcare domain enhances patients' satisfaction, accuracy of diagnosis, and operational efficiency of hospitals. Medical robots can help with surgical operations, rehabilitation, social interaction, assisted living, etc. Robotic-guidance is becoming common in spine surgery. The popularity of robot-assisted surgery is skyrocketing. Figure 8.2 shows AI and robotics [9].

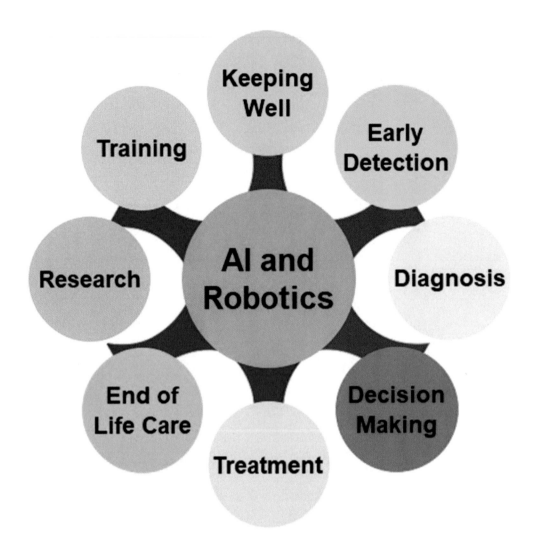

Figure 8.2 AI and robotics [9].

- *Fuzzy Logic:* Reasoning based on imprecise or incomplete information in terms of a range of values rather than point estimates. Fuzzy logic deals with uncertainty in knowledge that simulates human reasoning in incomplete or fuzzy data. The fuzzy model is robust to parameter changes and tolerant to impression.
- *Machine Learning:* Since intelligence is defined as learning and reasoning. Learning is an essential component in AI and is realized through machine learning (ML). ML refers to algorithms to make predictions and interpret data and "learn", without static program instructions. ML is a statistical technique for fitting models to data and training models with data. ML extracts features from input data by constructing analytical data algorithms and examines the features to create predictive models. The most common ML algorithms are supervised learning, unsupervised learning, reinforcement learning, and deep learning. The most common application of ML is precision medicine. Many hospitals have started using ML for predictive analytics for hospital management purposes. ML algorithms are capable of identifying suicide risk factors.

- *Deep Learning*: A subset of machine learning built on a deep hierarchy of layers, with each layer solving different pieces of a complex problem. It aims at increasing the capacity of supervised and unsupervised learning algorithms for solving complex real-world problems by adding multiple processing layers. An illustration of deep learning with two hidden layers is in Figure 8.3 [10]. As shown in Figure 8.4, artificial Intelligence is a broader umbrella under which machine learning (ML) and deep learning (DL) come [11].

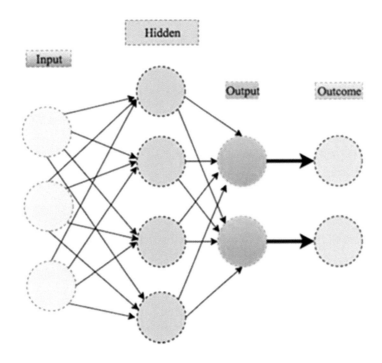

Figure 8.3 An illustration of deep learning with two hidden layers [10].

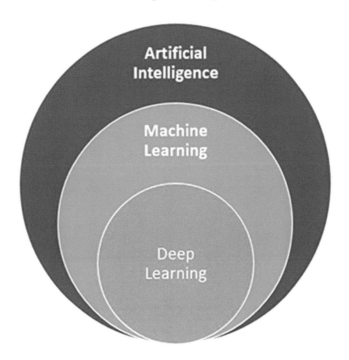

Figure 8.4 Artificial intelligence, machine learning, and deep learning [11].

- *Data Mining:* This deals with the discovery of hidden patterns and new knowledge from large databases. Data mining exhibits a variety of algorithmic tools such as statistics, regression models, neural networks, fuzzy sets, and evolutionary models.
- *Computer Vision:* With the progress in deep learning and neural networks, we have made great inroads in the field of computer vision. AI and computer vision have made eye tracking more efficient and affordable.
- *Computer Emotion:* The recent developments in human-computer interaction have emphasized user-centered rather than computer-centered approach. This led to design of intelligent and affective interfaces. Important discoveries in neuroscience and psychology have contributed to an interest in the scientific study of emotion. Without the ability to process such affect or emotion information, computers cannot be expected to communicate with humans in a natural way. The ability of machines to recognize, interpret, and respond according to human emotions is known as adaptive or affective computing. It is computing that relates to emotion or other affective phenomena. It involves the study and development of systems and devices that can recognize and express human affects or emotions. It uses both hardware and software technology to detect the affective state of a person [12].

Each AI tool has its own advantages. Using a combination of these models, rather than a single model, is recommended. AI technologies are drastically influencing the retail industry and customer experience.

8.3 APPLICATIONS IN HEALTHCARE

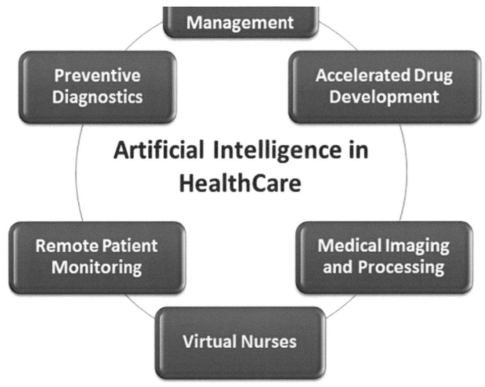

Figure 8.5 AI in healthcare [13].

AI techniques are now actively being applied in healthcare, as shown in Figure 8.5 [13]. The primary aim of AI applications in the health domain is to analyze relationships between prevention or treatment techniques and patient outcomes. The applications of AI in healthcare are countless. They fall into three categories [14]: patient-oriented AI, clinician-oriented AI, and administrative- and operational-oriented AI. Various AI applications have been developed to solve some of the most pressing problems that currently face healthcare industry. The following specialties in medicine have shown an increase in research regarding AI [6, 10,15,16].

- *Radiology*: This is the widest application of AI in medicine, but providers are just beginning to tap into the potential of what AI technology has to offer. The ability to interpret imaging results with radiology may aid clinicians in detecting a minute change in an image that a clinician might not notice otherwise. A radiologist is a medical doctor who is skilled in interpreting medical images such CT scans, MRI, digital radiographs, and ultrasounds. Today, radiologists are overwhelmed by the amount of imaging data they must review. AI technology, working alongside the radiologist, has the potential to improve accuracy, safety, efficiency, and productivity. The practice of radiology relies primarily on imaging for diagnosis and is very amenable to deep-learning techniques. As AI continues to expand in its ability to interpret radiology, it may be able to diagnose more people with the need for less doctors as there is a shortage in many nations. In radiology, machine learning algorithms are being used to detect breast cancer, colonic polyps, and pulmonary nodules. The emergence of AI technology in radiology is perceived as a threat by some specialists [17].

- *Disease diagnosis:* There are many types of diseases and there are many ways AI can be used to efficiently and accurately diagnose them. AI can predict and diagnose disease at a faster rate than medical professionals. It can now diagnose skin cancer more accurately, more efficiently, and faster than a board-certified dermatologist. The marriage of AI and data is helping to provide the right treatment to the right patients at the right time [15]. Since AI can collect and keep patient's data in a single place, the physicians can utilize this information on disease to make an accurate diagnosis. The role AI in the early diagnosis of diseases is invaluable in saving lives and avoiding premature deaths. For example, early detection of breast cancer through mammography can save lives.

- *Disease management*: AI and robots can help develop a comprehensive plan for disease management. This will help patients get the most effective, efficient care. Robots can be used in providing physical therapy, disease rehabilitation, and conducting repetitive tasks [18].

- *Oncology/Cancer*: Breast cancer is one of the leading causes of death among women. The penetration of AI into cancer treatment affects treatment capabilities and safety. AI could be useful for head/neck cancers, prostate cancer, colorectal cancers, breast cancer, and cervical cancer. In breast cancer diagnosis and the detection of lung cancer, AI algorithms have been shown to be better and more effective than a human. It has been demonstrated that the IBM Watson for oncology would be a reliable AI system for assisting the diagnosis of cancer. AI-based diagnostic algorithms applied to mammograms are helping in the detection of breast cancer. Machine learning algorithms include computer-aided detection applications that are used in mammography for the early diagnosis of breast cancer. AI will be part of the future of oncology [19].

- *Neurosciences:* The application of AI in neurosciences presupposes a good understanding of the intelligent functioning of the biological brain. Deployment of AI in neurosciences is slowly becoming a reality. Neurosurgeons and neurologists need to be prepared to use AI in their practice [20].

- *Diabetes Care*: Diabetes affects over 29 million Americans. Application of AI to diabetes, a global healthcare burden, can reform the diagnosis and management of this chronic condition. AI has changed the way diabetes is prevented, detected, treated, and managed. It allows a continuous remote monitoring of the patient's symptoms and blood sugar levels. It also allows patients with diabetes to be informed and empowered so that they can take daily decisions for diet and activity. The American Diabetes Association (ADA) supports the use of AI in diabetes care [21].

- *Dentistry:* The possibilities of combinations of robotics, artificial intelligence, machine learning, and dentistry are many. Smart robots can be used in dental offices as assistants to the dentist. Robotic implantology is also proposed to enable drilling of complex forms of dental implants. Human safety is a critical aspect in a human–robot co-working scenario. Changes in modern robot technology, ML, and AI that may contribute to the development of novel methodologies in dentistry are yet to be fully implemented [22]

- *Medical imaging:* The number of imaging performed annually has skyrocketed over the last two decades. Medical imaging data provides a rich source of information about patients. AI can support radiologists and pathologists as they use medical imaging to diagnose a wide range of conditions, accelerate their productivity, and improve their accuracy. For example, when a patient complains about shortness of breath, the chest radiograph is likely the first imaging study to be conducted. AI could help improve accuracy and efficiency of polyp detection at CT colonography (CTC). AI-based computer-aided detection is routinely used in breast cancer screening programs [23].

- *Aging:* AI can be used in aging and longevity research. Aging is a gradual, time-dependent process leading to the loss of function, biological and physical damage. It is a universal unifying feature possessed by all living organisms, tissues, and cells. Modern deep learning techniques can be used to develop age predictors. Most of the advances in deep learning in the context of aging research are in the area of biomarker development [24].

- *Telemedicine:* Telemedicine (also known as telehealth or ehealth) may be regarded as the transmission of medical images between healthcare centers for diagnosis across distance. It allows healthcare practitioners to diagnose, treat, and monitor patients at a distance using telecommunications technology. Telemedicine is used in a variety of specialties including radiology, neurology, and pathology. The ability to monitor patients using AI may allow for the communication of information to physicians if possible disease activity may have occurred [25,26].

- *Electronic Health Records:* Electronic health records are crucial to the digitalization and information spread of the healthcare industry. They contain the clinical history of patients and could be used to identify the individual risk of developing cardiovascular diseases, diabetes, and other chronic conditions. Using an AI tool to scan EHR data can accurately predict the course of disease in a patient.

- *Mobile Health:* Mobile health (or mHealth) refers to the practice of medicine via mobile devices such as mobile phones, tablet computers, personal digital assistants (PDAs), and wearable devices. It has emerged as the creative use of emerging mobile devices to deliver and improve healthcare practices. It integrates mobile technology with the health delivery with the premise of promoting a better health and improving efficiency. mHealth benefits immensely from AI. AI algorithms, sensor technology, and advanced data are helping transform smartphones into full health-management platforms. The evolution of mHealth can be seen in the improved availability of healthcare services, increased efficiency in the treatment process, reduced costs, and the creation unprecedented opportunities for preventive care. mHealth assistants will become a popular alternative in developed countries, where doctors are very busy [27,28].

- *Medical Research*: AI can be used to analyze and identify patterns in large and complex datasets. It can also be used to search the scientific literature for relevant articles. AI systems used in healthcare could also be valuable for medical research by helping to match suitable patients to clinical studies. AI can aid early detection of infectious disease outbreaks and sources of epidemics. AI has also been used to predict adverse drug reactions [29]. (not sure how the last 2 sentences have to do with medical research)

- *Virtual Assistants:* This application is designed to guide patients with medication reminders. AI is increasingly becoming sophisticated and capable of doing what humans do, but more efficiently, more quickly, and at a lower cost. For an example, robots can assist therapy for recovering stroke patients [30]. Machines are now capable of reminding or informing of things that we might otherwise forget or miss. An AI system can also assist clinicians by providing current medical information from journals, conference proceedings, textbooks, and clinical practices to improve patient care.

AI can also be used in neurology, cardiology, stroke, health surveillance health, health monitoring, hospital inpatient care, healthcare management, urban healthcare system, suicide risk prediction, emergence medicine, detection of disease, delivery of health services, and drug discovery. The scope of possible applications of AI in healthcare is almost limitless. The current and future applications of AI technologies can impact the healthcare industry. Future uses for AI include Brain-computer Interfaces (BCI) which will help those with trouble moving or speaking.

Medical institutions, such as The Mayo Clinic, Massachusetts General Hospital, Memorial Sloan Kettering Cancer Center, and National Health Service, have developed AI algorithms for their departments. Major technology companies such as IBM, Intel, Microsoft, and Google have also developed AI algorithms for healthcare [15].

8.4 INTERNATIONAL TRENDS

Artificial Intelligence has arrived in healthcare. The AI technology now moves towards globalization and it becomes necessary to track both government initiatives as well as regulatory changes around the world. There is global policy developments and investments in AI. Figure 8.6 shows the world map of AI startups in healthcare [31]. AI has been a strategic priority for governments around the world. The following are typical examples of international trends [32].

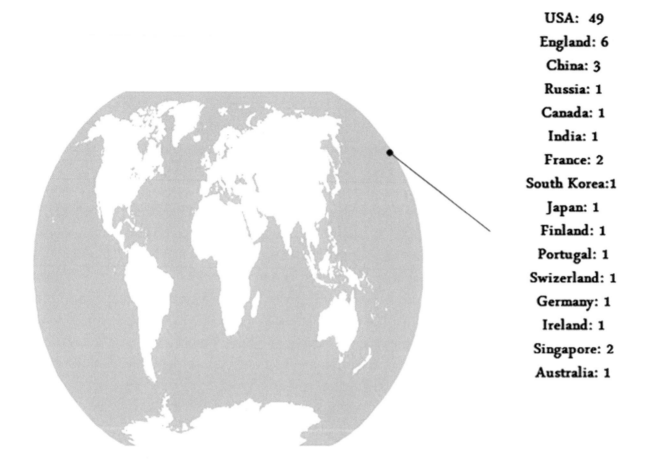

USA: 49
England: 6
China: 3
Russia: 1
Canada: 1
India: 1
France: 2
South Korea:1
Japan: 1
Finland: 1
Portugal: 1
Swizerland: 1
Germany: 1
Ireland: 1
Singapore: 2
Australia: 1

Figure 8.6 The world map of AI startups in healthcare [31].

- *Canada:* Canada has a unique and time-limited opportunity to be world leaders in system design using AI technology. It has established itself as a world leader in AI technology-related research. Its main cities, Montreal, Toronto, and Vancouver, have become hubs for AI research and development, attracting companies like Google, Facebook, Uber, Microsoft, and Samsung. Canada aims at establishing responsible development of human-centric AI and facilitate international scientific collaboration [33].

- *United Kingdom:* The British Government has announced its ambition to make the UK a world leader in AI and data technologies. The UK government has launched the *Centre for Data Ethics and Innovation*, as part of the UK's initiative to lead global governance on AI ethics.

- *France:* The government plans to establish France as leader in AI research. Its key initiatives include: (1) developing an open data policy to drive the adoption and application of AI in sectors like healthcare, (2) establishing a regulatory and financial framework to support the development of domestic "AI champions," and (3) putting in place regulation to ensure that AI developments remain transparent, explainable, and non-discriminatory.

- *China:* The government plans to develop intelligent and networked products such as vehicles, service robots, and identification systems. It announces investment in industry training resources, standard testing, and cybersecurity.

- *India*: India's AI strategy aims at promoting AI inclusion, an approach called *"AI for All."* India is also attempting to establish itself as an "AI Garage", which allows the AI technology developed in India to be useable to the rest of world. India is rich in data due to the volume of patients. Artificial intelligence (AI) and machine learning (ML) are witnessing increasing adoption in the Indian healthcare setting. However, India is fraught with several problems like aging population, lack of adequate infrastructure, limited access to healthcare facilities, adherence to treatment, and availability of care providers [34].

AI solutions could improve access, quality, and efficacy of global health systems. A common trend is the international focus on the development of transparent and responsible AI policy.

8.5 BENEFITS

AI has the potential to impact almost every aspect of healthcare, from prevention to detection and prediction. AI has unimaginable potential, and its benefits are enormous when implemented strategically. It may allow for better prevention, detection, diagnosis, and treatment of diseases. AI-enabled care is safe and effective. AI is ideally equipped to handle challenges that humans are naturally not able to tackle, such as collecting raw data from multiple sources into a single source for treating a hospitalized patient. Other benefits include the following [35].

- *Better Patient Care:* The use of AI will deliver major improvements in quality and safety of patient care. It will decrease medical costs as there will be more accuracy in diagnosis and better predictions in the treatment plan. AI is destined to drastically change clinicians' roles and everyday practices.
- *Efficiency:* While a healthcare practitioner can treat one patient at a time, automated AI-powered health assistants can serve millions of patients simultaneously, thereby multiplying productivity. AI has already begun making progress in healthcare by simplifying tedious and expensive procedures, guarding against human error, and promising to usher in a new era of patient care.
- *Cost Reduction:* AI algorithms can save time and costs. AI algorithms are more cost-efficient than conventional methods. It reduces unnecessary hospital visits. It can lower the cost of chronic disease management. Human-safe robots can work directly with human co-workers and relieve them of tedious and laborious tasks.
- *Forecasting and Prediction:* Artificial Intelligence (AI) is able to perform as humans and surpass human's performances in some tasks. Virtual assistants such as Apple's Siri and Google Assistant have illustrated the current and future potential of AI. Medicine has shifted toward prevention, personalization, prediction, and precision. In this shift, AI is the key technology that can bring this opportunity to everyday practice.

8.6 CHALLENGES

There are challenges hindering the successful AI technology adoption. There is lack of regulations specifically for the use of AI in healthcare. Medical costs are skyrocketing at an unsustainable rate. Failure of hospitals to use AI prevents both the use of potentially life-saving technology and potential cost savings. Other challenges include:

- *Complexity:* While AI has achieved widespread adoption in certain sectors, the complexities of healthcare have resulted in slower adoption. Clinical data can be messy, incomplete, complex, and potentially biased. Integration of healthcare data is complex, which can result in missing and disparate data.

- *Privacy and Security:* Healthcare providers must recognize that patient privacy and security must remain paramount. Therefore, AI companies should utilize valuable medical data while remaining compliant with laws governing the protection of patient information and data ownership. If a patient suffers harm due to an AI-based technology, who should be held responsible or accountable?

- *Fear:* There is a misconception that AI will replace human clinicians. As technology is increasingly implemented in workplaces, some fear that their jobs will be replaced by machines. Doctors and nurses still have a number of unique and important advantages over AI. They can do a lot of things (performing physical examinations, accessing patients well being, interpret non-verbal cues, take a blood test, show compassion, alleviate anxiety, communicate well, learn thoroughly about patients needs and their disease processes, etc.) that an AI assistant cannot do, because they are human traits that are difficult to model mathematically.
To eliminate fear, there is an urgent need for education and training of healthcare professionals to enhance AI literacy so that appropriate technologies can be rapidly adopted. This will also help healthcare professionals have the capabilities required to navigate the complex world of AI [36].

- *Shortage In Healthcare Professionals:* Due to shortages of doctors and nurses (especially in developing nations), care cannot be delivered to everyone. With increase consumer demands, increased life expectancy, and more complex disease processes, AI is expected to bridge the gap for this expected shortage. It is believed that AI can help streamline time consuming routine tasks [37].

- *Ethical Risks:* There are several ethical implications in the use of AI in healthcare. The social and ethical use of AI in healthcare presents significant challenges as some question about the ethical appropriateness of the use of AI. There is a need to minimize ethical risks of AI implementation, which can include threats to patient privacy, confidentiality, informed consent, and autonomy [38].

- *Automation complacency:* This is the tendencies for health professionals to trust AI tools implicitly, assuming all predictions are correct and failing to cross-check or consider alternatives. Errors and imperfect decision-making are inevitable in the world of healthcare, with or without AI.

- *Change is Difficult:* Despite its potential to unlock new insights and streamline the way providers interact with patients, some see AI as causing privacy problems, ethics concerns, and medical errors. The health care community is yet to be fully committed to adopt AI in healthcare practice.

Other significant challenges and issues include data preprocessing, consolidation, ubiquitous information, knowledge extraction, interpretability, and the need to ensure that the way AI is developed and used is transparent, accountable, and compatible with public interest [29].

8.7 CONCLUSION

Artificial Intelligence reflects the intelligence exhibited by machines and software. The use of artificial intelligence in healthcare is evolving at a rapid rate. It is already having a great impact on healthcare and medicine and the future looks exciting. AI is penetrating into every aspect of global healthcare. It has the potential to disrupt the healthcare industry. AI presents unprecedented opportunities in healthcare and major challenges for the patients, developers, providers, and regulators. Through our collective effort, AI can achieve all its lofty expectations to improve healthcare for patients across the world.

The current popularization of the Internet, universal existence of sensors, emergence of big data, and other emerging technologies have caused rapid advancement in AI, leading to a new Artificial Intelligence 2.0 [39].

Medicine is undergoing an evolutionary change with greatly priority being paid to "cost-effective" delivery of care. Medical education is also changing, with or without AI [40]. It is unlikely that machines will replace human doctors, but those in the medical profession must be willing to adapt, learn, and work alongside technological advancements. However, AI-based technologies are still quite controversial because they are not yet commonly used. In the near future, healthcare will be delivered as a seamless continuum of care and with a greater focus on prevention and early intervention. For more information about AI in healthcare, one should consult books in [41-54] and the following related journals:

- *Artificial Intelligence in Medicine*
- *Journal of Medical Artificial Intelligence.*
- *Artificial Intelligence*
- *Applied Artificial Intelligence*
- *Future Healthcare Journal*

REFERENCES

[1] M. Wehde, "Healthcare 4.0," *IEEE Engineering Management Review*, vol. 47, no. 3, Third Quarter, September 2019, pp. 24-28.

[2] I. Sniecinskia and J. Seghatchianb, "Artificial intelligence: A joint narrative on potential use in pediatric stem and immune cell therapies and regenerative medicine," *Transfusion and Apheresis Science*, vol. 57, 2018, pp. 422-424.

[3] M. N. O. Sadiku, "Artificial intelligence", *IEEE Potentials*, May 1989, pp. 35- 39.

[4] Y. Mintz and R. Brodie, "Introduction to artificial intelligence in medicine," *Minimally Invasive Therapy & Allied Technologies*, vol. 28, no. 2, 2019, pp. 73-81.

[5] "Artificial intelligence technologies and their categories," https://www.auraportal.com/artificial-intelligence-technologies-and-their-categories/

[6] R. O. Mason, "Ethical issues in artificial intelligence," *Encyclopedia of Information Systems,* vol 2, 2003, pp. 239-258.

[7] A. N. Rames et al., "Artificial intelligence in medicine," *Annals of the Royal College of Surgeons of England*, vol. 86, 2004, pp. 334–338.

[8] M. N. O. Sadiku, Y. Zhou, and S. M. Musa, "Natural language processing in healthcare," *International Journal of Advanced Research in Computer Science and Software Engineering*, vol. 8, no. 5, May 2018, pp. 39-42.

[9] "No longer science fiction, AI and robotics are transforming healthcare," https://www.pwc.com/gx/en/industries/healthcare/publications/ai-robotics-new-health/transforming-healthcare.html

[10] F. Jiang et al., "Artificial intelligence in healthcare: Past, present and future," *Stroke and Vascular Neurology*, 2017.

[11] "Basic concepts of artificial intelligence, machine learning, deep learning," https://noveltybilisim.com.tr/deep-learning/basic-concepts-of-artificial-intelligence-machine-learning-deep-learning/

[12] M. N. O. Sadiku, A. E. Shadare, and S. M. Musa, "Affective computing," *International Journal of Trend in Research and Development*, vol. 5, no. 6, November-December 2018, pp. 144-145.

[13] D. Naik, "AI in the healthcare world," August 2017, https://medium.com/@humansforai/ai-in-the-healthcare-world-88d13a815f35

[14] A. Kaushal et al., "The future of artificial intelligence in health care," December 2019, https://www.modernhealthcare.com/technology/future-artificial-intelligence-health-care

[15] "Artificial intelligence in healthcare," *Wikipedia*, the free encyclopedia https://en.wikipedia.org/wiki/Artificial_intelligence_in_healthcare

[16] M. N. O. Sadiku, T. J. Ashaolu, and S. M. Musa, "Artificial intelligence in medicine: A primer," *International Journal of Trend in Research and Development*, vol. 6, no. 1, Jan.-Feb. 2019, pp. 270-272.

[17] T. Nawrocki et al., "Artificial intelligence and radiology: Have rumors of the radiologist's demise been greatly exaggerated?" *Academic Radiology*, vol. 25, no. 8, February 2018, pp. 967–972.

[18] A. Karam, "Artificial intelligence in health care," August 2017, http://azikar24.com/tag/artificial-intelligence

[19] R. F. Thompson et al., "The future of artificial intelligence in radiation oncology," *International Journal of Radiation Oncology, Biology, and Physics*, vol. 102, no. 2, 2018, pp. 247-248.

[20] K. Ganapathy, S. S., Abdul, and A. A. Nursetyo, "Artificial intelligence in neurosciences: A clinician's perspective," *Neurology India*, vol. 66, no. 4, 2018, pp. 934-939.

[21] S. Ellahham, "Artificial intelligence in diabetes care," *The American Journal of Medicine*, 2020.

[22] J. Grischke et al., "Dentronics: Towards robotics and artificial intelligence in dentistry," *Dental Materials*, vol. 36, no. 6, June 2020, pp. 765-778.

[23] M. I. Faza et al., "The past, present and future role of artificial intelligence in imaging," *European Journal of Radiology*, vol. 105, 2018, pp. 246-250.

[24] A. Zhavoronko et al., "Artificial intelligence for aging and longevity research: Recent advances and perspectives," *Ageing Research Reviews*, vol. 49, 2019, pp. 49-66.

[25] M. N. O. Sadiku, M. Tembely, and S.M. Musa, "Telemedicine: A primer (Part 1)," *International Journal of Advanced Research in Computer Science and Software Engineering*, vol. 9, no. 6, June 2019, pp.43-46.

[26] M. N. O. Sadiku, M. Tembely, and S.M. Musa, "Telemedicine: Teleeverything phenomena (Part 2)," *International Journal of Advanced Research in Computer Science and Software Engineering*, vol. 9, no. 6, June 2019, pp.35-38.

[27] M. N. O. Sadiku, A. E. Shadare, and S.M. Musa, "Mobile health," *International Journal of Engineering Research*, vol. 6, no. 11, Oct. 2017, pp. 450-452.

[28] B. Dickson, "How artificial intelligence is revolutionizing the mhealth industry," https://www.magzter.com/articles/1642/241037/59c9590a889f7

[29] Nuffield Council on Bioethics, "Artificial intelligence (AI) in healthcare and research" http://nuffieldbioethics.org/wp-content/uploads/Artificial-Intelligence-AI-in-healthcare-and-research.pdf

[30] K. Joy, "Artificial intelligence in healthcare: Why transparency matters," March 2020, https://healthtechmagazine.net/article/2020/03/artificial-intelligence-healthcare-why-transparency-matters-perfcon

[31] O. Iliashenko, Z. Bikkulova, and A. Dubgorn, "Opportunities and challenges of artificial intelligence in healthcare," *E3S Web of Conferences*, vol. 110, 2019.

[32] S. E. Davies, "Artificial intelligence in global health," Ethics & International Affairs, vol. 33, no. 2, Summer 2019.

[33] A. Kassam and N. Kassam, " Artificial intelligence in healthcare: A Canadian context," *Healthcare Management Forum*, 2019, pp. 1-5.

[34] R. Mabiyan, "How artificial intelligence can help transform Indian healthcare," ETHealthWorld, May 2018, https://health.economictimes.indiatimes.com/news/health-it/how-artificial-intelligence-can-help-transform-indian-healthcare/64285489

[35] "AI in healthcare: Keys to a smarter future," https://www.gehealthcare.com/-/media/b3a5e32538454cf4a61a4c58bd775415.pdf

[36] D. Wiljer and Z. Hakim, "Developing an artificial intelligence–enabled health care practice: Rewiring health care professions for better care," *Journal of Medical Imaging and Radiation Sciences*, vol. 50, no. 4, December 2019, pp. S8-S14.

[37] J. Bennett, "Artificial intelligence in healthcare: Is it beneficial?" *Journal of Vascular Nursing*, vol. 37, no. 3, September 2019, p. 159.

[38] M. J. Rigby,"Ethical dimensions of using artificial intelligence in health care," *AMA Journal of Ethic*, February 2019.

[39] Y. Pan, "Heading toward Artificial Intelligence 2.0," Engineering, vol. 2, 2016, pp. 409–413.

[40] V. K. Sondak and N. E. Sondak, "New directions for medical artificial intelligence," *Computers & Mathematics with Applications*, vol. 20, no. 4-6, 1990. pp. 313-319.

[41] P. Vasant (ed.), *Handbook of Research on Artificial Intelligence Techniques and Algorithms*. Information Science Reference, 2015.

[42] D. D. Luxton, *Artificial Intelligence in Behavioral and Mental Health Care*. San Diego, CA: Elsevier, 2016.

[43] A. Panesar, *Machine Learning and AI for Healthcare: Big Data for Improved Health Outcomes*. Apress, 2019.

[44] C., Gunnar and, F. X Campion, *Machine Intelligence for Healthcare*. CreateSpace Independent Publishing, 2017.

[45]A. Agah, *Medical Applications of Artificial Intelligence*. Boca Raton, FL: CRC Press, 2017.

[46] S. M. Richins, *Emerging Technologies in Healthcare*. Boca Raton, FL: CRC Press, 2015.

[47] S. Russell and P. Norvig, *Artificial Intelligence: A Modern Approach*. Upper Saddle River, NJ: Prentice Hall, 3rd edition, 2009.

[48] M. Fieshi (translated by D. Cramp), *Artificial Intelligence in Medicine: Expert Systems.* Paris, Springer Science, 1990.

[49] A. Agah, *Medical Applications of Artificial Intelligence.* Boca Raton, FL: CRC Press, 2017.

[50] P. Szolovits, *Artificial Intelligence in Medicine.* Westview Press, 1982.

[51] E. Topol, *Deep Medicine: How Artificial Intelligence Can Make Healthcare Human Again.* New York: Hachette Book Group, 2019.

[52] P. S. Mahajan, *Artificial Intelligence in Healthcare.* Parag Suresh Mahajan, 2nd edition, 2019.

[53] A. Bohr and K. Memarzadeh, *Artificial Intelligence in Healthcare.* Academic Press, 2020.

[54] M. Chang, *Artificial Intelligence for Drug Development, Precision Medicine, and Healthcare.* Chapman and Hall/CRC, 2020.

CHAPTER 9

MACHINE LEARNING IN HEALTHCARE

"The closest thing to being cared for is to care for someone else." - Anonymous

9.1 INTRODUCTION

In today's information era, an organization should deduct meaningful information from their data in order to be able to compete. Like other fields, healthcare sector is going through data revolution. With the emergence big data, the explosion in data available for analysis is as evident in healthcare as anywhere else. Clinical medicine has always required doctors to handle enormous amounts of data. Diagnostic and imaging techniques generate such an incredible amount of data. Machine learning techniques emerged as an objective tool to assist practitioners to diagnose certain conditions and make clinical decisions [1].

Most computer-based algorithms in healthcare are "expert systems." Expert systems work the way an ideal medical student would: they take general medical principles and apply them to patients. Machine learning handles problems as a doctor progressing through residency might: by learning rules from data. It is a branch in computer science that employs knowledge from artificial intelligence, optimization, and statistics to develop algorithms. It focuses on how computers learn from data. Such an algorithmic method allows data to speak for themselves.

Machine learning is a branch of artificial intelligence which is based on the notion that systems can learn from data, identify patterns, and make decisions with minimal human intervention. Today, machine learning is playing an integral role in the healthcare industry. This is due to its ability to process huge datasets beyond the scope of human capability, and then convert the data analyzed into clinical insights that aid physicians in providing care. Machine learning is a powerful, relatively easy to implement tool with numerous possibilities to enhance medical practice. The applications of machine learning in medicine are advancing medicine into a new realm. Therefore, educating the next generation of medical professionals with machine learning is essential.

Although machine learning (ML) is widely used in other industries, such as retail and banking, it is not routine in healthcare because of the complexity and limited availability of data. In healthcare, the bottom line is to use machine learning to augment patient care, save more lives, improve more care, while saving money at the same time. ML can automate the manual processes carried out by practitioners, which are usually time-consuming and subjective. Thus, using ML can save time for practitioners and provide unbiased, repeatable results.

This chapter provides an introduction to applying machine learning in healthcare. It begins by giving an overview on what machine learning is all about. It also covers extreme machine learning. Then it applies ML to various areas in healthcare. It addresses the benefits and challenges of ML. The last section concludes with comments.

9.2 OVERVIEW ON MACHINE LEARNING

Machine learning (ML) is the discipline that gives computers the ability to learn without being explicitly programmed. The term "machine learning" (ML) was initially coined in 1959 by Arthur Samuel, a computer scientist. Machine learning (or statistical learning) is part of artificial intelligence. It assists computers in estimating future events and modelling based on experiences gained from previous information. Machine learning focuses on how computers "learn" from data and it is a major domain within predictive analytics [2]. It allows computers to learn from past examples and to detect hard-to-discern patterns from large data sets. An example of how a machine learner is trained is shown in Figure 9.1 [3]. It describes a class of algorithms which learn model parameters from a set of training data with the purpose of accurately predicting outcomes for previously unseen data. ML is a marriage between statistics and computer science [4,5].

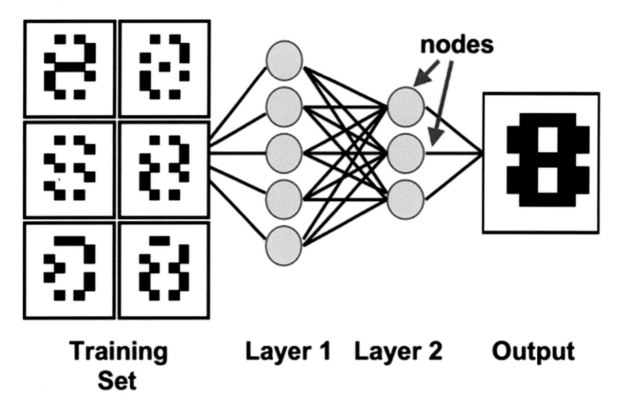

Figure 9.1 An example of how a machine learner is trained [3].

Machine learning is the study of tools and methods for identifying patterns in data. ML algorithms can be supervised or unsupervised. As illustrated in Figure 9.2, the algorithms may be classified as follows [6]:

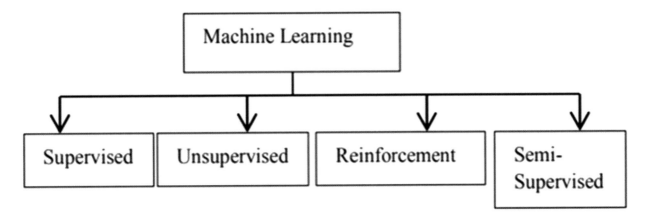

Figure 9.2 Classification of machine learning techniques [6].

- *Supervised ML:* The program is "trained" on a pre-defined set of "training examples" from a "teacher," which then facilitate its ability to reach an accurate conclusion when given new data. In this case, the data comes with additional attributes that we want to predict. A common case of supervised learning is to use historical data to predict statistically likely future events. Under supervised ML, we have regression ML and classification ML. Supervised learning focuses on classification and prediction. It involves building a statistical model for predicting or estimating an outcome based on one or more inputs. It is often used to estimate risk. Supervised ML is where algorithms are given training data. Learning from data is used when there is no theoretical or prior knowledge solution, but data is available to construct an empirical solution. Supervised ML is increasingly being used in medicine such as in cardiac electrophysiology.
- *Unsupervised ML:* This is used against data that has no historical labels and the system is not told the "right answer." Unsupervised algorithms do not need to be trained with desired outcome data. The program is given a bunch of data and must find patterns and relationships therein. A typical goal of unsupervised learning may be as straightforward as discovering hidden patterns within a dataset. Without being told a "correct" answer, unsupervised learning methods can look at complex data and organize it in potentially meaningful ways. Unsupervised learning algorithms are used for more complex processing tasks than supervised learning systems. In unsupervised learning, we are interested in finding naturally occurring patterns within the data. Unlike supervised learning, there is no predicted outcome. Unsupervised learning looks for internal structure in the data [7]. Unsupervised learning algorithms are common in neural network models. A common application of such a process is to explore interrelationships between genetics, biochemistry, histology, and disease states.
- *Classification ML*: This involves seeking a yes-or-no prediction, such as "Does this product meet our quality standard?" We want to learn from already labeled data how to predict the class of unlabeled data. An example of classification problem would be the handwritten digit recognition.

- *Regression ML*: If the desired output consists of one or more continuous variables, then the task is called regression. In this case, the value being predicted falls somewhere on a spectrum. An example of a regression problem would be the prediction of the length of a salmon as a function of its age and weight.

In addition, we also have "reinforcement" ML, which is often used for robotics, gaming, navigation, and network routing. Reinforcement learning is a technique that allows an agent to modify its behavior by interacting with its environment.

The most commonly used ML algorithms include neural networks, support vector machines, and decision trees. Other ML techniques include classification, regression, and clustering. There are some software packages that do some form of machine learning [8].

There is significant interest in the use of ML in healthcare. ML techniques can 'learn' from the vast amount of medical data and assist clinical decision making. They are often suitable for detecting complex patterns in large and noisy data sets.

For a ML system to be useful in solving medical diagnostic tasks, the following features are desired: good performance, the ability to appropriately deal with missing data, the transparency of diagnostic knowledge, the ability to explain decisions, and the ability of the algorithm to reduce the number of tests necessary to obtain reliable diagnosis [9]. However, success in using ML is not always guaranteed. Like any technique, an appreciation of the limitations of ML algorithms is crucial.

Machine learning is applied in various fields such as healthcare, manufacturing, transportation, financial services, face recognition, object recognition, speech recognition, self-driving cars, natural language processing (NLP), optical character recognition, affective computing, Internet fraud, medical diagnosis, IoT, marketing, stock market prediction, economics, automotive, defense and security, government, insurance, utilities, oil and gas, advertisement, email spam detection, drug recognition, robotics, education, social science, linguistics, management, computer vision, materials science, smart city, and remote sensing, and communication networks such wireless sensor networks and mobile ad-hoc networks (MANETs).

9.3 EXTREME LEARNING MACHINE

The extreme learning machine (ELM) is an emerging learning technique due to its faster learning speed, ease of implementation, least human intervention, and simplicity. Traditional machine learning techniques (such as deep neural networks, support vector machines, and back-propagation algorithm) face some challenging issues such as: intensive human intervention, slow learning speed, overfitting problems, and poor learning/computational scalability. To overcome these challenges, extreme learning machine (ELM) was introduced in 2006 by Huang, Zhu, and Siew at Singapore [10]. ELM is a new algorithm for single-hidden layer feed-forward artificial neural network. The two basic characteristics of ELM are universal approximation capability with random hidden layer and various learning techniques that can be easily implemented [11]. Figure 9.3 shows the architecture of ELM model [12].

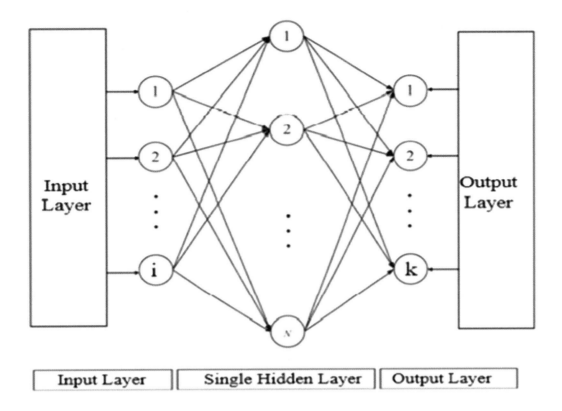

| Input Layer | Single Hidden Layer | Output Layer |

Figure 9.3 Architecture of ELM model [12]

An extreme learning machine (ELM) is basically a modified version of an artificial neural network. We get an extreme learning machine when you subtract propagation from a classic feed-forward neural network with one hidden layer. ELM is a single-hidden layer feedforward neural network, in which the parameters connecting the input layer and the hidden layer are generated randomly. It is basically the idea of a random projection followed by linear regression. Various variants or extensions of the original ELM have been proposed in the literature to improve its stability, sparsity, and accuracy under specific conditions or applications. Such variants include incremental ELM, evolutionary ELM, online sequential ELM, voting-based ELM, ordinal ELM, pruned ELM, memetic ELM, manifold regularized ELM, self-adaptive ELM, weighted or unweighted ELM, two-dimensional ELM, orthogonal ELM, and symmetric ELM [13]

Extreme learning machines (ELMs) are primarily applied to supervised learning problems. Only a few existing studies on ELMs have dealt with unsupervised learning. In practical applications, ELM has slow response speed and low generalization ability for unknown test data. Applications of ELM include medical diagnosis, human robot, electric power systems, credit scoring, economics signal processing, and automatic control [14]

9.4 APPLICATIONS OF ML IN HEALTHCARE

Machine learning techniques were first applied to medicine with the use of electronic health records. They emerged in the medical sciences as clinical decision-support techniques to improve sensitivity, disease detection, and monitoring. Machine learning has virtually endless applications in the healthcare industry. Both supervised and unsupervised can be applied to clinical data sets for the purpose of developing robust risk models and redefining patient classes. Some selected applications of machine learning include the following [15-18]:

- *Radiology:* This is one of the most sought-after applications of machine learning in healthcare. Medical image analysis has many discrete variables. Since ML-based algorithms learn from the multitude of different samples available on-hand, it becomes easier to diagnose and find the variables. One of the most popular uses of machine learning in medical image analysis, is the classification of objects. Machine learning can be trained to examine images and identify areas that need attention. ML is transforming radiology from a subjective perceptual skill to an objective science.

- *Oncology:* This is a branch of the medicine that deals with the prevention, diagnosis, and treatment of cancer. Almost all works in this field apply machine learning techniques, which perform deep statistical analysis of a set of clinical cases supported by gene expression data. Researchers are using deep learning to train algorithms to recognize cancerous cells at a level comparable to trained physicians. Google has developed a machine learning algorithm to help identify cancerous tumors on mammograms. Stanford is using a deep learning algorithm to identify skin cancer. IBM Watson Oncology is at the forefront of this movement by leveraging patient medical history to help generate multiple treatment options [3].

- *Pathology:* This is the medical specialty that is concerned with the causes and effects of a disease or injury. It involves examining specimens (organs, tissues, fluids, etc) on a gross, microscopic, chemical, immunologic or molecular level. Machine vision and other machine learning technologies can enhance the efforts traditionally left only to pathologists with microscopes. ML algorithms can provide the speedy and more accurate way of diagnosis.

- *Genomic Medicine*: One of the goals of genomic medicine is to determine how variations in the DNA of individuals can affect the risk of different diseases. Machine learning can help to model the relationship between DNA and the quantities of key molecules in the cell [19].

- *Disease Prediction:* Prediction of a disease can be a challenge, but it can help practitioners make data-informed timely decisions about patient's health and treatment. Accurate prediction is essential in finding out the risk of the disease in a patient. There are several machine learning techniques that are used to perform predictive analytics. Machine learning can help hospital systems identify patients with a chronic disease, predict the likelihood that patients will develop a chronic disease, and present patient-specific prevention interventions. For example, ML approaches have significant potential in predicting acute exacerbations in asthma patients [20].

- *Personalized Medicine:* This is individualization, recognition of the micro-variables within a patient that may cause them to be different from their peers. ML for personalized medicine is a growing area. It involves the ability to draw on large data sets and predictive models, which allows for clinicians to confidently diagnose, predict and treat their patients.

- *Reduce Readmissions*: Machine learning can reduce readmissions. Clinicians can receive daily guidance as to which patients are most likely to be readmitted and how they might be able to reduce that risk.

- *Clinical Decision*: In conjunction with data and personnel, machine learning can advance clinical decision support and help providers deliver optimal care. ML and clinical decision support tools can analyze large volumes of data and suggest steps for treatment [21].

- *Smart Health Records:* Keeping and maintaining up-to-date health records is an exhaustive process and a majority of the processes take a lot of time to complete. It is safe to say there are still many manual processes involved. The main task of machine learning in record keeping is to ease processes to save time, effort, and money. This will to help with diagnosis, clinical treatment suggestions, etc. Machine learning applied to electronic health records (EHRs) will produce actionable insights. A machine remembers and stores all data, preparing it for global research.

- *Pharmacy:* There are various uses of machine learning in pharmacy. They are broadly classified into [22]: (1) Disease Identification/Diagnosis, (2) Personalized Treatment/Behavioral Modification, (3) Drug Discovery/Manufacturing, (4) Clinical Trial Research, (5) Radiology and Radiotherapy, (6) Smart Electronic Health Records. AI and ML techniques are increasingly being chosen by big names in the pharma industry to solve the complex problem of successful drug discovery. They will play a major role in understanding how a drug is performing in real-time.

These advances would have been unimaginable without machine learning. Some are illustrated in Figure 9.4. Other areas include surgery, emergency medicine, psychiatry, and ophthalmology. ML provides methods, techniques, and tools that can help solve diagnostic and prognostic problems in various medical domains. Machine learning techniques have been successfully applied to different branches of healthcare as a tool to help diagnose diseases. ML algorithms have immense potential to enhance diagnostic and intervention research in smoking, depression, asthma, and chronic obstructive pulmonary disease (COPD). ML is also being used for data analysis and interpretation of continuous data used in the Intensive Care Unit. With time, the healthcare environment will become more and more reliant on computer technology and ML capabilities will reach into all aspects of healthcare [23,24].

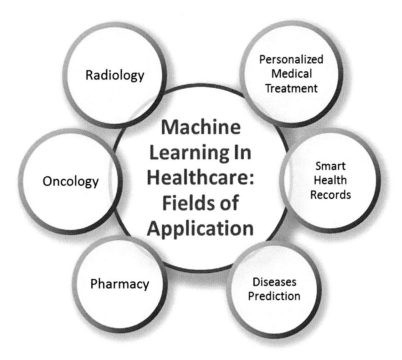

Figure 9.4 Applications of machine learning in healthcare [23].

9.5 BENEFITS

It can be helpful in alerting a physician or a patient's family when things begin to go wrong. It has the potential to positively change the role of physicians in patient care. By analyzing thousands of bits of information to make decisions, ML algorithms go far beyond anything a human analyst can do. Application of ML models could improve patient safety, improve quality of care, and reduce healthcare costs. Other benefits include [25]:

- *Reduce Readmissions:* Machine learning can reduce readmissions in a targeted, efficient, and patient-centered manner.
- *Reduce Hospital Length-of-Stay* (LOS): Health systems can reduce LOS and improve other outcomes like patient satisfaction.
- *Predict Chronic Disease:.* Machine learning can help hospital systems identify patients with undiagnosed or misdiagnosed chronic disease. Machine learning is helping to create many new clinical prediction tools. The tools can predict future patients' probability of having specific diseases based on certain risk factors and help foster early screening parameters and encourage annual physical exams.
- *Machine accuracy:* Machine accuracy will soon exceed that of humans. ML can lead to more accurate diagnostic algorithms and individualize patient treatment. It provides accurate data to help evaluate images of breast cancer.
- *Improved Healthcare Delivery:* Machine learning in healthcare changes the way healthcare practitioners practice and enhances their current role.
- *Self-trained systems:* They can follow supervised and unsupervised learning, facilitating early detection and diagnosis greatly.
- *Analysis of fraud:* Fraud in the healthcare system is a major problem. Healthcare fraud is committed in different ways at different levels. ML techniques can be used to provide sophisticated tools for the analysis of fraudulent patterns in these vast health insurance databases.

9.6 CHALLENGES

While ML has the potential to significantly help medical practice, some negative consequences that may arise from using ML decision support in healthcare. Machine learning algorithms often require thousands of observations to reach acceptable performance levels. How doctors handle these challenges will create winners and losers in medicine.Critical voices have emerged warning of potential problems surrounding the use of ML. Some challenges include the following 26-28]:

- *Privacy:* Personal health information must be handled in a privacy-preserving manner. Patients should be fully informed about using their data for data processing. Data used to train algorithms should have the necessary user' consent and authorizations, but determining which data uses are permitted for a given purpose is easy.
- *Ethics:* Ethical and regulatory concerns about health data have expressed for long. ML algorithms use data that are subject to privacy protections, requiring that their developers pay close attention to ethical and regulatory restrictions.
- *Fear:* Some fear that machine learning is the beginning of a process that could replace healthcare practitioners. People are understandably hesitant when they learn that healthcare

professionals are being replaced by algorithms. Although ML applications can perform some of what doctors do today, but they will not replace doctors because patients will always need the human touch and the caring relationship with care givers.

- *Reproducibility:* ML tools present unique challenges and obstacles to reproducibility. Reproducibility is the ability of researchers to get or reproduce the same results as the original study. Many sub-fields such as machine learning are experiencing a reproducibility crisis.

Some of these challenges are depicted in Figure 9.5. To advance the translation of machine learning into clinical care, healthcare leaders must address these challenges.

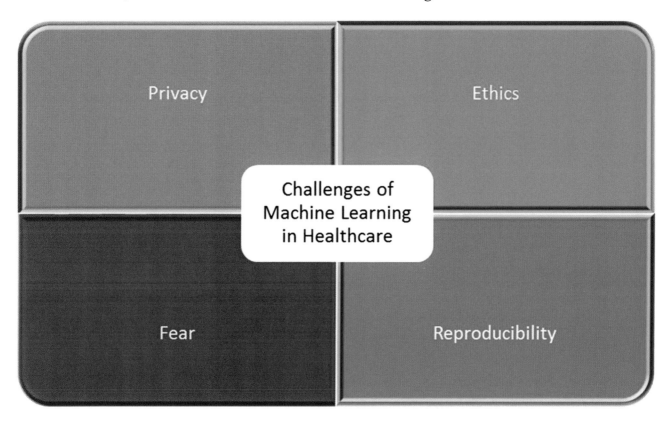

Figure 9.5 Some of the challenges of ML in healthcare [28].

9.7 CONCLUSION

Machine learning is the process of teaching computers to automatically recognize patterns of interest in data. It is an incredibly powerful tool that is used in a wide range of compelling application domains because it is applicable to many real-life problems. It is regarded as one of the disruptive technologies of our time. Much of machine learning will initially come from businesses and organization with big datasets.

Machine learning should no longer be regarded as a futuristic concept but a real-world tool that can be deployed today. Machine learning is critical for anyone practicing healthcare in the 21st century. Today, ML techniques are suited for analyzing medical data and serving as tools for medical diagnosis in a variety of medical domains. They will become indispensable tools for clinicians who truly seek to understand their patients.

In today's highly competitive global market, winning requires near-perfect quality and high productivity. The healthcare industry is turning to machine learning to improve the performance of its operations. If technology is to improve medicine in the future, the data provided to doctors needs to be enhanced by the power of analytics and machine learning. This will help them make better decisions about patient diagnoses and treatment option. Machine learning represents the next wave in advancing modern healthcare. The next generation of medical professionals should be equipped with the right ML techniques that will enable them to become part of this emerging revolutionary technology [29]. Machine learning is set to be a pillar of our future civilization. Additional information on ML application in healthcare is available in the books in [30-38] and the following related journals:

- *International Journal of Machine Learning and Cybernetics*
- *Applied Artificial Intelligence.*

REFERENCES

[1] A. Consejo, T. Melcer, and J. J. Rozema, "Introduction to machine learning for ophthalmologists, seminars in ophthalmology," November 2018.

[2] H. Saber et al., "Predictive analytics and machine learning in stroke and neurovascular medicine," *Neurological Research,* vol. 41, no. 8, 2019, pp. 681-690.

[3] J. A. Cruz and D. S. Wishart, "Applications of machine learning in cancer prediction and prognosis," *Cancer Informatics*, vol. 2, 2006, pp. 59–78.

[4] Z. Obermeyer and E. J. Emanuel, "Predicting the future — Big data, machine learning, and clinical medicine," *New England Journal of Medicine*, vol. 375, no. 13, September 2016, pp. 1216–1219.

[5] M. N. O. Sadiku, S. M. Musa, and O. S. Musa, "Machine learning, " *International Research Journal of Advanced Engineering and Science*, vol. 2, no. 4, 2017, pp. 79-81.

[6] K. Shailaja, B. Seetharamulu, and M. A. Jabbar, "Machine learning in healthcare: A review," *Proceedings of the 2nd International conference on Electronics, Communication and Aerospace Technology*, May 2018, pp. 910-914.

[7] R. C. Deo, "Machine learning in medicine," *Circulation*, vol. 132, no. 20, November 2015, pp. 1920–1930.

[8] A. K. Waljee and P. D. R. Higgins, "Machine learning in medicine: A primer for physicians," *The American Journal of Gastroenterology*, vol. 105, June 2010, pp. 1224–1226.

[9] I. Kononenko, "Machine learning for medical diagnosis: History, state of the art and perspective," *Artificial Intelligence in Medicine*, vol. 23, no. 1, August 2001, pp. 89-109.

[10] G. B.Huang, Q. Y. Zhu, and C. K. Siew, "Extreme learning machine: theory and applications," *Neurocomputing*, vol. 70, no. 1-3, 2006, pp. 489–501.

[11] G. B. Huang, D. H. Wang, and Y. Lan, "Extreme learning machines: A survey," *International Journal of Machine Learning and Cybernetics*, vol. 2, 2011, pp. 107-122.

[12] J.. Lei and Q. Liu, "Three-dimensional temperature distribution reconstruction using the extreme learning machine, " *IET Signal Processing*, vol. 4, no. 11, 2017, pp. 406-414.

[13] S. Ding, X. Xu, and R. Nie, "Extreme learning machine and its applications," *Neural Computing & Applications*, vol. 25, 2014, pp. 549–556.

[14] M. N. O. Sadiku, J. Foreman, and S. M. Musa, "Extreme learning machines: A primer," *International Journal of Scientific Engineering and Technology*, vol. 7, no. 8, August 2018, pp. 76-77.

[15] K. Sennaar, "Machine learning for medical diagnostics – 4 current applications," December 12, 2018, https://emerj.com/ai-sector-overviews/machine-learning-medical-diagnostics-4-current-applications/

[16] G. S. Handelman, "eDoctor: Machine learning and the future of medicine," *Journal of Internal Medicine*, vol. 284, no. 6, December 2018, pp. 603-619.

[17] M. N. O. Sadiku, S. M. Musa, and A. Omotoso, "Machine learning in medicine: A primer," *International Journal of Trend in Scientific Research and Development*, vol. 3, no. 2, Jan.-Feb. 2019, pp. 98-100.

[18] "Top 10 applications of machine learning in healthcare," https://www.flatworldsolutions.com/healthcare/articles/top-10-applications-of-machine-learning-in-healthcare.php

[19] M. K. K. Leung et al., "Machine learning in genomic medicine: A review of computational problems and data set," *Proceedings of the IEEE*, vol. 104, no. 1, January 2016, pp. 176-197.

[20] J. Finkelstein1 and I. C. Jeong, "Machine learning approaches to personalize early prediction of asthma exacerbations," *Annals of the New York Academy of Sciences*, vol. 1387, 2017, pp. 153–165.

[21] "How machine learning is transforming clinical decision support tools," https://healthitanalytics.com/features/how-machine-learning-is-transforming-clinical-decision-support-tools

[22] M. A.Jabbar, S. Samreen, and R. Aluvalu, "The future of health care: Machine learning," *International Journal of Engineering & Technology*, vol. 7, no. 4.6, 2018, pp. 23-25.

[23] "Machine learning in healthcare to enhance your solution," January 2020, https://innovecs.com/blog/machine-learning-in-healthcare/

[24] G. D. Magoulas and A. Prentza, "Machine learning in medical applications," chapter in G. Paliouras, V. Karkaletsis, and C.D. Spyropoulos (eds.): *Advanced Course on Artificial Intelligence*, 1999, Springer, pp. 300-307.

[25] E. Corbett, "The real-world benefits of machine learning in healthcare," August 2017, https://www.healthcatalyst.com/clinical-applications-of-machine-learning-in-healthcare

[26] L. McDonald et al., "Unintended consequences of machine learning in medicine?" *F1000Research*, vol. 6, 2017.

[27] E. Vayena, A. Blasimme, and I. G. Cohen, "Machine learning in medicine: Addressing ethical challenges," *PLoS Medicine*, vol. 15, no. 11, 2018.

[28] A. Ray, "What's holding back machine learning in healthcare," https://amitray.com/what-holding-back-machine-learning-in-healthcare/

[29] V. B. Kolachalama and P. S. Garg. "Machine learning and medical education," *npj Digital Medicine*, vol. 54, September 2018.

[30] T. J. Cleophas and A. H. Zwinderman, *Machine Learning in Medicine, Part 2*. Springer, 2018.

[31] V. Jain and J. M. Chatterjee (eds.), *Machine Learning with Health Care Perspective: Machine Learning and Healthcare*. Springer, 2020.

[32] S. Dua, U. R. Acharya, and P. Dua (eds.), *Machine Learning in Healthcare Informatics*. Springer, 2014.

[33] Y. W. Chen and L. C. Jain (eds.), *Deep Learning in Healthcare: Paradigms and Applications*. Springer, 2019.

[34] P. Natarajan, J. C. Frenzel, and D. H. Smaltz, *Demystifying Big Data and Machine Learning for Healthcare*. Boca Raton, FL: CRC Press, 2017.

[35] D. A. Clifton, *Machine Learning for Healthcare Technologies*. The Institution of Engineering and Technology, 2016.

[36] N. Dey et al. (eds.), *Machine Learning in Bio-Signal Analysis and Diagnostic Imaging*. Academic Press, 2018

[37] A. Subasi, *Practical Guide for Biomedical Signals Analysis Using Machine Learning Techniques*. Academic Press, 2019.

[38] Eduonix Learning Solutions, *Machine Learning for Healthcare Analytics Projects: Build smart AI Applications Using Neural Network Methodologies Across the Healthcare Vertical Market*. Packt Publishing, 2018.

CHAPTER 10

NATURAL LANGUAGE PROCESSING IN HEALTHCARE

"One of the deep secrets of life is that all that is really worth doing is what we do for others." - Anonymous

10.1 INTRODUCTION

Although globalization has opened borders for exchange, users may find sensitive data in foreign websites in foreign languages. Language is crucial around the world in communication, entertainment, media, culture, drama, movie, and economy. There is the need for the establishment of language processing systems. Also, there is explosion of clinical data in the healthcare industry and the data is represented in structured or unstructured non-standardized formats in electronic health records (EHR). There is a need to extract what is relevant so that clinicians can make the best decisions for their patients. It is expected that natural language processing (NLP) tools should be able to bridge the gap between the mountain of data generated daily and the limited cognitive capacity of the human mind [1].

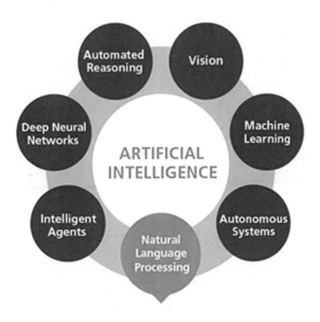

Figure 10.1 Natural language processing is a branch of artificial intelligence [2].

As shown in Figure 10.1, natural language processing (NLP) is a branch of artificial intelligence and it is used for extracting the elements of concerns from raw plain text information [2]. NLP lies at the intersection of artificial intelligence and linguistics. Its goal is to create intelligent agents than understand and manipulate human languages. It deals with how to program computers to fruitfully process large amounts of natural language data. It can be broadly described as utilizing computer algorithms to process and extract meaning from the natural language like speech or written text. Healthcare is the biggest user of the NLP tools. NLP has been used in the clinical setting for capturing, representing, and utilizing clinical information.

NLP is a discipline of computer science and is also known as computational linguistics. It involves using computer system for processing natural (human) languages such as English, Arabic, Chinese, Japanese, Spanish, Italian, German, Yoruba, and French [3]. It is a multidisciplinary field that is related to linguistics, cognitive science, psychology, philosophy and logic.

This paper provides an introduction on the use of NLP in healthcare. It begins by discussing NLP basics and different aspects of NLP. It covers some applications of NLP in healthcare. It addresses global healthcare NLP. It highlights some benefits and challenges of NLP in healthcare. The last section concludes with some comments.

10.2 NLP BASICS

NLP (also known as computational linguistics or "text mining") is a interdisciplinary field involving computer science, linguistics, logic, and psychology. NLP as an area of research and application began in the 1950s as the intersection of artificial intelligence (AI) and linguistics. Since then, NLP research has been focusing on tasks such as machine translation, information retrieval, text summarization, question-answering, information extraction, and opinion mining [4]. The late 1980s witnessed a revolution in NLP with the introduction of machine learning algorithms and statistical techniques for language processing. Machine learning approaches extract statistical information from large amounts of documents and learn the rules of language without explicitly listing them.

Natural language processing (NLP) refers to the application of computational techniques to the understanding and generation of human language. It is the field of study that focuses on the interactions between human language and computers. It is a computational approach to text analysis. It is the application of a wide range of computational techniques for the understanding, automatic analysis, and representation of human language

NLP is a technique where machine can become more human and thereby making humans to communicate with the machine easily. It involves the study of mathematical and computational modeling of various aspects of language. It implies the development of a wide range of systems such as spoken language systems that integrate speech and natural language, multilingual interfaces, and machine translation. NLP seeks to make software intelligent enough to process a natural language as humans. For example, imagine a machine that takes instructions by voice. NLP systems perform useful roles, such as correcting grammar, converting speech to text, and automatically translating between languages.

10.3 DIFFERENT ASPECTS OF NLP

Human language is inherently complex and diverse. We express ourselves in many ways, both verbally and in writing. There are hundreds of languages (English, Spanish, Chinese, etc.) and dialects, each with a unique set of grammar and syntax rules, accent, and slang [5]. We share meaning in several ways: texts, gestures, sign languages, and face expressions.

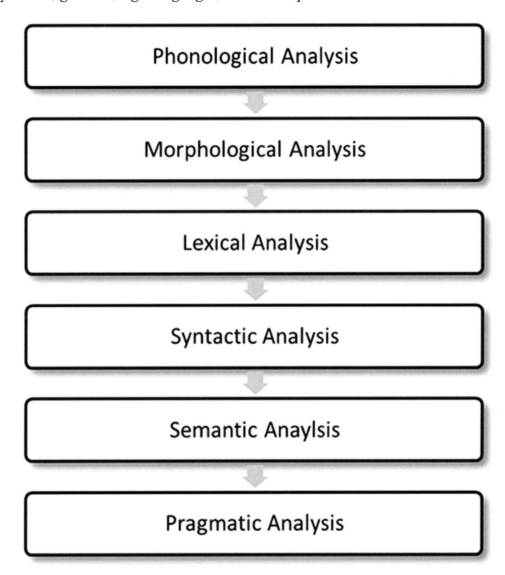

Figure 10.2 Levels of NLP in Healthcare [3].

NLP analysis generally consists of the following five levels (in a hierarchy) [6-10], shown in Figure 10.2,

- *Phonetics*, the level that deals with pronunciation or sounds to the words. It analyzes the phonetic composition of a word. Three rules used in phonological analysis are: (1) for sounds within words, (2) for variations of pronunciation when words are spoken together, and (3) for fluctuation in stress and intonation across a sentence.
- *Morphology*, the study which relates to word construction from basic units called morphemes. In other words, morphology is the study of word composition from *morphemes*, i.e. word stem/

root and affixes. It determines the relation between a word, its roots, and derived forms. Computational morphology is the study of the computational analysis of word forms for eventual use in NLP applications.

- *Syntax,* the study of sentence structure. Syntax deals with the formation of a sentence from individual words. Syntax alone suggests the proper interpretation of "Jimmy loves Lucy."
- *Semantics,* the study of context-independent meaning. This derives the meaning of a sentence based on the meanings of the words/phrases. For example, semantics determines whether the word "bank" refers to a river bank or to a financial institution.
- *Pragmatics,* the study of context-dependent meaning. Pragmatics deals with how meaning changes in the presence of a specific context and how the contexts affect the meaning of the sentences. This level is concerned with the purposeful use of language in situations

Specific tasks for NLP systems include summarizing lengthy blocks of narrative text (e.g. clinical note), mapping data elements present in unstructured text to structured fields in an electronic health record, converting data from machine-readable formats into natural language, answering unique free-text queries, optical character recognition, and conducting speech recognition [11].

Applications for processing large amounts of texts require NLP expertise. These include classifying text into categories, indexing, automatic translation, speech understanding, information extraction, automatic summarization, knowledge acquisition, games, opinion mining, spell-checking, context-based thesaurus, and genre-based word prediction, and text generations [8]. Some of NLP applications involve generation as well as analysis of the language. Over the years, a significant number of NLP software have been developed; some of these are available freely, while others are available commercially.

10.4 APPLICATIONS IN HEALHCARE

Natural language processing may be regarded as the automatic processing of the natural human language by a machine. NLP has great potential in healthcare, mobile technology, cloud computing, virtual reality, election, social work, and social networking. It has many potential applications in healthcare. It is a major factor that is driving big data analytics in healthcare. It converts providers' notes and narratives into structured formats. It is being used to extract the facts needed to enable many kinds of clinical decisions [12]. NLP in healthcare may be segmented into four categories: NLP for physicians, NLP for researchers, NLP for patients, and NLP for clinical operators. NLP approaches can also be divided into either symbolic or statistical techniques.

The following include typical applications of NLP in healthcare.

- *Radiology*: Radiology report generates large quantities of digital content within the electronic health record. NLP supports the extraction of important data from pathology reports to create patient profiles. It provides techniques that aid the conversion of text into a structured representation, and thus enables computers to derive meaning from human input (i.e. natural language). NLP techniques enable automatic identification and extraction of information that are used in radiology reports [13]. The need for application expertise in natural NLP is increasing in radiology

- *Mental Health:* The field of mental health has seen a drastic increase in the use of NLP strategies and methods, partly because most clinical documentation is in free-text [14].
- *Clinical Decision Support:* Natural language processing may be the key to effective clinical decision support. There is all sorts of data in the healthcare industry and the industry must decide the best ways to extract relevant data to help clinicians make the best decisions. Natural language processing extract and structure text-based clinical information, making clinical data available for use in healthcare delivery. NLP technology improves clinical outcomes and simplify data entry. It enables many voice-to-text technologies to simplify clinical documentation. NLP is also being used to aid physicians in checking symptoms and making better decision [15].
- *Electronic Health Records* (EHRs): An EHR is a computerized medical record for documenting patient information. It was conceived to alleviate limitations of the paper-based medical record and to improve its organization. EHRs offer portability of large volumes of information and faster access to patient information. They capture "real-world" disease and care processes. Although EHRs were intended to promote clinician efficiency, they have increased physician documentation time. NLP can be used to analyze and process large sets of unstructured data, namely spoken or written communication. It can enhance the accuracy of electronic health records by translating free text into standardized data [16]. NLP has almost unlimited potential to turn EHR from burden to boon.
- *Clinical Data:* The amount of data in healthcare is massive and growing. Clinical data is represented in structured and unstructured form. Structured data is created through constrained choices in the form of data entry devices. The unstructured clinical record contains a wealth of insight into patients that is not available in the structured record. Unstructured text records are usually significantly larger that structured records. NLP is essential because it can transform relevant information locked in text into structured data that can be used by computer processes. It plays a crucial role in extracting valuable information that can benefit decision making, administration reporting, and research. Figure 10.3 shows how NLP classifies, extracts, and summarizes unstructured text [17].

Electronic Medical Records

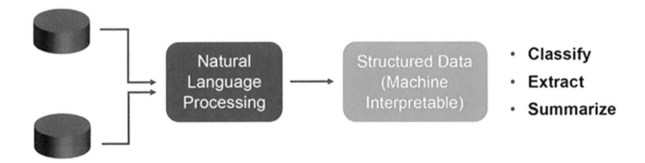

MEDLINE Articles / Abstracts

Figure 10.3 NLP classifies, extracts, and summarizes unstructured text [17].

- *Computer-Aided Coding* (CAC): CAC extracts information about procedures and therapies to capture every possible code to maximize claims. Although CAC may have improved the speed of coding, it has not improved accuracy. NLP-driven CAC systems are in use at several healthcare facilities across the country for hospital coding. They promise to improve coder accuracy. NLP is being used in professional coding as well.
- *Speech Recognition:* Speech offers unique distinction. Today, NLP technology is used as the basis for speech recognition in clinical documentation. NLP uses speech recognition by allowing clinicians to transcribe notes for useful EHR data entry.
- *Prior Authorization:* Before treating the patient, the physicians need to know whether payers will agree and authorize reimbursement. Payer prior authorization requirements on physicians are on the rise. IBM Watson Health and Anthem are working on an NLP module used by the payer's network of providers to rapidly determine prior authorization quickly.
- *Patient Safety*: This is a major concern in healthcare. Errors are inevitable in an age when long clinical hours are increasingly becoming standard operating practice. The possible consequences of errors and patient safety issues remain ominous. NLP workflows can help reduce the likelihood of error and improve patient safety.

Some of these applications are shown in Figure 10.4. In addition to the above applications, healthcare NLP systems specifically can help coping with the following tasks [18]:

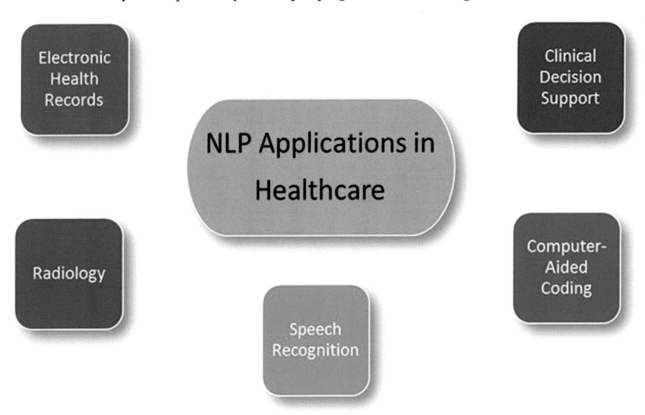

Figure 10.4 Applications of NLP in healthcare.

- Locating, extracting, and summarizing key concepts or phrases from blocks of narrative texts (e.g. clinical notes or a patient's account).
- Converting data from machine-readable formats into natural language (speech or written text).
- Doing speech recognition tasks that will allow users to dictate notes that can be instantly turned into text with high accuracy.
- Implementing EHR NLP can improve risk management for patients with chronic diseases. Using NLP with an EHR greatly improves postoperative complication identification.
- Generating a set of predictive words that detect medical nonadherence and predicting patient nonadherence in the ICU setting.
- Detecting the presence of an indwelling urinary catheter and urinary symptoms in hospitalized patients [19].
- Extracting information on healthcare-associated pneumonia (an infectious disease) in infants using NLP of radiology reports [20].
- Using of NLP software to improve the accuracy of estimating infusion dates and doses, especially when combined with Healthcare Common Procedure Coding System (HCPCS) codes [21].
- Aiding in clinical decision support for protocoling and prioritization of magnetic resonance imaging (MRI) brain examinations [22].
- Applying NLP tools to develop a task-specific EMR interface for timely stroke thrombolysis [23].
- Assessing hospital readmissions for patients with COPD [24].
- Adapting existing NLP resources for cardiovascular risk factors identification in clinical notes [25].
- Automatically identifying heart failure patients with ineffective self-management status in the domains of diet, physical activity, and medication adherence [26].

Other applications include colonoscopy reports, identification of critical limb ischemia, standardizing unstructured clinical information, and extracting mammographic findings. The potential applications of NLP seem endless.

10.5 GLOBAL HEALTHCARE NLP

Currently, the adoption of the NLP technology is growing in the global healthcare industry. It is garnering more and more attention across the nations. Both private and public healthcare service providers are implementing NLP technology for clinical applications to improve their patient engagement and overall decision making capabilities. Several organizations worldwide have been exploring the potential of natural language processing for risk stratification, population health management, and decision support. Currently, North America and Europe are leading the global healthcare natural language processing (NLP) market and the United States is the most significant revenue contributor to the global NLP in Healthcare. NLP holds the promise of enhancing the availability, quality, and utility of clinical information with the goal of improving documentation and efficiency of the healthcare system in the United States. NLP can efficiently use the data resources that have been relatively unavailable for meaningful clinical or research use until now [27].

Efforts are being made to apply natural language processing to human languages other than English. Multilingual NLP, whether it concerns analysis or generation of sentences, requires a sound language-independent representation. The major growth in the NLP in healthcare is caused by the growing demand for improving electronic health records (EHRs) data usability to better patient care. Electronic medical information systems are now used worldwide, replacing traditional handwritten medical reports. The international movement toward the broad implementation of EHRs implies that more clinical data will be captured and stored electronically. It is necessary to extract and structure the data by natural language processing.

For an example, colorectal cancer is the third most common cancer occurring in men and women and has been the cause of deaths of many people in the USA. In Germany, colorectal cancer is the second most common cancer in women and the third most common in men. An NLP-based algorithm for entity recognition was developed for the German language and used for processing German clinical notes of colorectal cancer [28].

10.6 BENEFITS

NLP tools are designed to assist machines in understanding the language used by humans to communicate both reading and writing. NLP is important to healthcare. The benefits of using NLP in healthcare include easy implementation, ease of use, portability between languages, robustness towards poorly written documentation, computer assisted coding, clinical decision support, and interoperability. There is also NLP-based approach to extract information from patient records [6].

Other benefits of NLP in healthcare include the following:

- *Transforming Care:* Natural language processing is transforming healthcare. NLP along with machine learning can be used to flag patients with heart disease. *NLP techniques have been used to review EHR documents for indications of PTSD, depression, and potential suicidal patients.* NLP-based computer programs have been developed. For example, NLP enables assessment of smoking-cessation care delivery. (what does this last sentence mean?)

- *Clinical Decision Support:* NLP clinical systems can be used to represent clinical knowledge and clinical decision support interventions in standardized formats. They have been developed to process unstructured text and transform it into a desired coded form to support several healthcare-related activities. Such systems require a higher degree of accuracy as results are incorporated into critical decisions related to patient care. NLP often works in the background and makes everyday work easier for doctors.

- *Improve Patient Care:* Clinical NLP can improve patient care, improve medical record coding productivity and consistency, and boost doctors' efficiency. Using NLP, the computer can read, interpret and organize important health data that is buried in unstructured free-text fields, such as physicians' notes.

- *Liberate Clinicians:* A bot (cognitive agent) could ask questions via NLP and help the clinician-spend more time looking after their patients and less time searching through EMR menu screens. It could help reduce the mundane aspects of their work and liberate time to do what they were trained for.

10.7 CHALLENGES

NLP is not without its challenges. Although NLP is the key to effective clinical decision support, there are some challenges that need to be addressed before the healthcare industry can make good on NLP's promises. Some challenges in clinical NLP have little to do with NLP. In spite of the advances in NLP techniques, building models is often expensive, time-consuming, and slow to develop. Training and refining algorithms for NLP is a time-consuming task. Other challenges include the following.

- *Unstructured Data:* Unstructured clinical notes and narrative text are still a major challenge for NLP because the notes often use acronyms and abbreviations making them highly ambiguous. For example, the abbreviation "qhs" means nightly at bedtime but can be mistaken as "qhr" which means every hour, which can be a detrimental mistake during medication administration.
- *Languages are Complex:* In the clinical care setting, misuse or misinterpretation of a word or gesture could mean life or death. Interpretation of an expression can be uncertain or ambiguous. Some medical reports are compact and omit information that can be assumed by experts.
- *Garbage In, Garbage Out:* This old saying applies to NLP. As an algorithm, NLP depends on the input it gets from its users. NLP has the ability for a computer to accept input, spoken or typed, in a conversational manner - even using slang or shorthand.

These challenges must be addressed to drive the usefulness of NLP in the healthcare industry. The grand challenge for future research is to develop an NLP-based system for better clinical NLP that can meaningfully communicate with humans. Many miles remain in our journey toward overcoming this challenge.

10.8 CONCLUSION

Natural language processing (NLP) refers to the process of using computer algorithms to identify key elements in everyday language and extract meaning from unstructured spoken or written communication. It involves utilizing computer algorithms to process and extract meaning from the natural language like speech or written text. The explosive growth in healthcare industry is the main market driver of NLP. With the increase in EHR systems, NLP techniques will be needed to create decision support systems. NLP products for radiology and emergency medicine are now commercially available the mainstream market. NLP algorithms will become more accurate and capable of performing more advanced functions in the following years. If properly executed, NLP enables a more natural transition between healthcare practitioners and database. More information about NLP can be found in the books in [29-34].

REFERENCES

[1] M. N. O. Sadiku, Y. Zhou, and S. M. Musa, "Natural language processing," *International Journal of Advances in Scientific Research and Engineering,* vol. 4, no. 5, May 2018, pp. 68-70.

[2] "Natural language processing," https://www.optum.com/resources/library/nlp-ai-roi.html

[3] O. G. Iroju and J. O. Olaleke, "A systematic review of natural language processing in healthcare", *International Journal of Information Technology and Computer Science*, vol.7, no.8, 2015, pp.44-50.

[4] E. Cambria and B. White, "Jumping NLP curves: A review of natural language processing research," *IEEE Computational Intelligence Magazine*, May 2014, pp. 48-57.

[5] "Natural-language processing," *Wikipedia*, the free encyclopedia, https://en.wikipedia.org/wiki/Natural-language_processing

[6] C. Friedman, T. C. Rindflesch, and M. Corn, "Natural language processing: State of the art and prospects for significant progress, a workshop sponsored by the National Library of Medicine," *Journal of Biomedical Informatics*, vol. 46, 2013, pp. 765–773.

[7] J. Hirschberg, B. W. Ballard, and D. Hindle, "Natural language processing," *AT&T Technical Journal*, Jan./Feb. 1988, vol. 67, no. 1, 1988.

[8] S. M. Chandhana, "Natural language processing future," *Proceedings of International Conference on Optical Imaging Sensor and Security*, Tamil Nadu, India, July 2-3, 2013.

[9] J. P. Zagal, N. Tomuro, and A. Shepitsen, "Natural language processing in game studies research: An overview," *Simulation & Gaming*, vol. 43, no. 3, 2012, pp. 356–373.

[10] E. D. Liddy, "Natural language processing," https://surface.syr.edu/cnlp/11/

[11] "What is the role of natural language processing in healthcare?" https://healthitanalytics.com/features/what-is-the-role-of-natural-language-processing-in-healthcare

[12] M. N. O. Sadiku, Y. Zhou, and S. M. Musa, "Natural language processing in healthcare," *International Journal of Advanced Research in Computer Science and Software Engineering*, vol. 8, no. 5, May 2018, pp. 39-42.

[13] E. Pons et al., "Natural language processing in radiology: A systematic review," *Radiology*, vol. 279, no. 2, May 2016, pp. 329-343.

[14] S. Velupillai et al., "Using clinical natural language processing for health outcomes research: Overview and actionable suggestions for future advances," *Journal of Biomedical Informatics*, vol 88, December 2018, pp. 11-19.

[15] D. Demner-Fushman, W. W. Chapman, and C. J. McDonald, "What can natural language processing do for clinical decision support?" *Journal of Biomedical Informatics*, vol. 42, 2009, pp. 760–772.

[16] R. Attrey and A. Levit, "The promise of natural language processing in healthcare," March 2019, https://www.researchgate.net/publication/331718974_The_promise_of_natural_language_processing_in_healthcare

[17] "Healthcare NLP: The secret to unstructured data's full potential," April 2019, https://www.healthcatalyst.com/insights/how-healthcare-nlp-taps-unstructured-datas-potential

[18] "Natural language processing in healthcare: Is it worth implementing?" https://www.romexsoft.com/blog/nlp-in-healthcare/

[19] A. V. Gundlapalli et al., " Detecting the presence of an indwelling urinary catheter and urinary symptoms in hospitalized patients using natural language processing," *Journal of Biomedical Informatics*, vol. 71, 2017, pp. S39–S45.

[20] E. A. Mendonc et al., "Extracting information on pneumonia in infants using natural language processing of radiology reports," *Journal of Biomedical Informatics*, vol.38, 2005, pp. 314–321.

[21] S. D. Nelson et al., "The use of natural language processing of infusion notes to identify outpatient infusions," *Pharmacoepidemiology and Drug Safety*, vol. 24, 2015, pp. 86–92.

[22] A. D. Brown and T. R. Marotta, "A natural language processing-based model to automate MRI brain protocol selection and prioritization," *Academic Radiology*, vol 24, no 2, February 2017, pp. 160-166.

[23] S. F. Sung, "Applying natural language processing techniques to develop a task-specific EMR interface for timely stroke thrombolysis: A feasibility study," *International Journal of Medical Informatics*, vol. 112, 2018, pp. 149–157.

[24] A. Agarwal et al., "A natural language processing framework for assessing hospital readmissions for patients with COPD," *IEEE Journal of Biomedical and Health Informatics*, vol. 22, no. 2, March 2018, pp. 588-596.

[25] A. Khalifa and S. Meystre, "Adapting existing natural language processing resources for cardiovascular risk factors identification in clinical notes," *Journal of Biomedical Informatics*, vol. 58, 2015, pp. S128–S132

[26] M. Topaz et al., " Studying associations between heart failure self-management and rehospitalizations using natural language processing," *Western Journal of Nursing Research*, 2017, vol. 39, no. 1, 2017, pp. 147–165.

[27] A. M. Rassinoux et al., "Tuning up conceptual graph representation for multilingual natural language processing in medicine," *International Conference on Conceptual Structures*, 1998, pp 390-397.

[28] M. Becker et al., "Natural language processing of German clinical colorectal cancer notes for guideline-based treatment evaluation," *International Journal of Medical Informatics*, vol. 127, July 2019, pp. 141-146.

[29] S. Bird, E. Klein, and E. Loper, *Natural Language Processing with Python*. O'Reilly Media, 2009.

[30] J. Olive, C. Christianson, and J. McCary (eds.), *Handbook of Natural Language Processing and Machine Translation: DARPA Global Autonomous Language Exploitation*. Springer, 2011.

[31] C. D. Manning and H. Schutze, *Foundations of Statistical Natural Language Processing*. Cambridge, MA: The MIT Press, 1999.

[32] D. Jurafsky and J. H. Martin, *Speech and Language Processing*. Englewood Cliffs, NJ: Prentice Hall, 2000.

[33] K. B. Cohen and D. Demner-Fushman, *Biomedical Natural Language Processing*. Philadelphia, PA: John Benjamins Publishing Co., 2014.

[34] M. Farhangfar, H. Keshvari, and S. Tofighi, *Natural Language Processing in Hospital Beds* (Persian Edition). CreateSpace Independent Publishing Platform, 2015.

CHAPTER 11

HEALTHCARE CHATBOTS

"A prudent person foresees danger and takes precautions. The simpleton goes blindly on and suffers the consequences." — Proverbs 27:12, NLT

11.1 INTRODUCTION

Technology has transformed our modern society, pushing new boundaries every day. Virtually anything can be accessed via a computer or phone app. The development of conversational system as a medium of conversation between humans and a computer has made a great stride. Healthcare providers are now offering telemedicine options like chatbots. The idea of visiting a physician in person has tremendously increased, especially during the 2020 Covid-19 Pandemic [1].

Healthcare is important for living a good life. In the US, healthcare is a highly rapidly developing field. The healthcare industry has seen a wave of emerging technologies such as AI, Internet of things, and 3D printing with significant potential to alter and disrupt the sector. It is moving toward personalized care, where patients are expected to take more control of their own health. This is something that can be accomplished with machine learning technology.

Chatbots (also known as a talkbots or chatterbots) are artificial intelligence (AI) programs designed to simulate human conversation via text or speech. They are also known as conversational agents, interactive agents, virtual agents, virtual humans, or virtual assistants [2]. Chatbots are becoming more prevalent in our daily lives. They can be used in various fields like education, healthcare, route assistance, business, market, stock, banking, customer care, counselling, recommendation systems, support system, entertainment, brokering, journalism, online food and accessory shopping, telecom, travel, and many more [3]. Chatbots are gradually being adopted into the healthcare industry. Chatbots are effective tools in healthcare due to their simplicity in interaction.

This chapter provides an introduction on the uses of healthcare chatbots. It begins by discussing the concept of chatbots. It presents many applications of chatbots in healthcare. It discusses some benefits and challenges of chatbots in healthcare. The last section concludes with comments.

11.2 CONCEPT OF CHATBOTS

Chatbots are also known as conversational agents, interactive agents, virtual agents, virtual humans, or virtual assistants. Chatbots, as part of AI devices, are computer programs designed to carry on a dialogue with users using natural languages. Healthcare has become an attractive market for chatbot applications. The main purpose of healthcare chatbots is to help patients in less time and for less money than it would take to visit a medical professional. Healthcare chatbots have great potential, but they still have a long way to go to win over consumers.

The first chatbot (Eliza) was developed in 1966 by Joseph Weizenbaum for psychiatric patients. Since then, Chatbots have gained popularity in all the domains such as banking, e-commerce, healthcare, education, and smart homes [4]. A chatbot describes a computer system or the situation in which human is chatting with the robot (computer).

Chatbots may be regarded as mimic systems which imitate the conversations between two individuals. They employ different degrees of human-like appearance and behavior, such as facial expressions, compassion, humor, and tone of voice. Thus, chatbots are computer programs with a conversational user interface capable of emulating natural, conversational interpersonal exchange. Fueled by artificial intelligence (AI), chatbots are becoming a viable option for human–machine interaction.

Healthcare chatbot can diagnose the disease and provide basic details about the disease before consulting a doctor. It is designed to reduce the healthcare costs and improve accessibility to medical knowledge. The healthcare chatbot is an entity which imitates human discussion using AI. Healthcare chatbots depend on natural language processing (NLP) that helps users to submit their health problem [5]. Figure 11.1 illustrates a chatbot based on three key structures in AI.

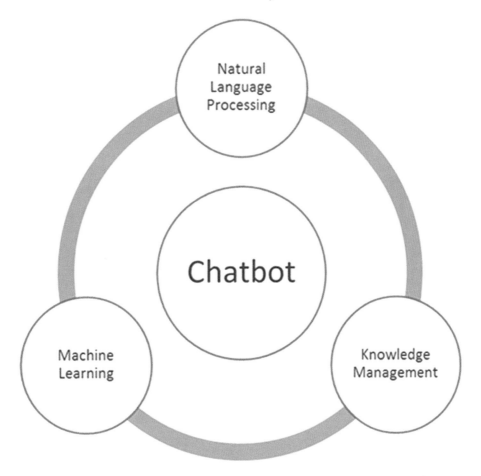

Figure 11.1 A chatbot based on three key structures in AI [5].

There are essentially two types of chatbots: (1) Fixed chatbots: These are programs with fixed information and hence offer limited help; (2) AI-based: These chatbots thrive on dynamic learning and constantly update themselves using various customer interactions. An AI-based chatbot has three domains: databases, natural language processing (NLP), and machine learning (ML). Mostly chatbots are some kind of computer programs that use natural language processing (NLP) for interpreting the user input and generating the corresponding response. In other words, NLP helps users to submit their problem about the health. The aim of the system is to replicate a person's discussion. Chatbots interact with users using natural languages. Chatbot may ask a review of symptoms and relevant information such past medical or surgical history. It provides response by use of an efficient Graphical User Interface (GUI). The GUI is an artificial creation invented to enable interactions between human and computers. The chatbot system helps users to freely submit their complaints and queries regarding health by voice since customer satisfaction is the major concern for developing this system [6,7].

One may also regard a chatbot as a software system that allows you to simulate real conversations between devices and users by means of a conversational interface [8]. Chatbots use three types of conversation styles [9]: static, semi-automated, and fully-automated conversation dialogue. The static conversation style is rule-based and it is easy to build. Automated refers to the generative-based model, which uses deep learning models to build interaction. This is very complex and requires a lot of training data. The semi-automated automates some parts while the rest is handled by a human.

11.3 APPLICATIONS IN HEALTHCARE

Chatbots are generally used for the intelligent assistant applications. They can act as automated conversational agents, capable of promoting health, providing education, and potentially prompting behavior change. They have been applied in health education, diagnostics, and mental health. The chatbots can handle several healthcare needs, such as personalized medical follow-up, communication and transmission of test results, dissemination of information, advice patients, and provide patients with more information about the medications they use. They can be used by clinicians to easily retrieve information about drug interactions and side effects and streamline the interaction with electronic health records. For patients, chatbots perform customer service tasks such as booking appointments [10]. It is endless what chatbots may provide healthcare. Figure 11.2 shows some examples of what chatbots can do [11]. A typical healthcare chatbot is depicted in Figure 11.3 [12].

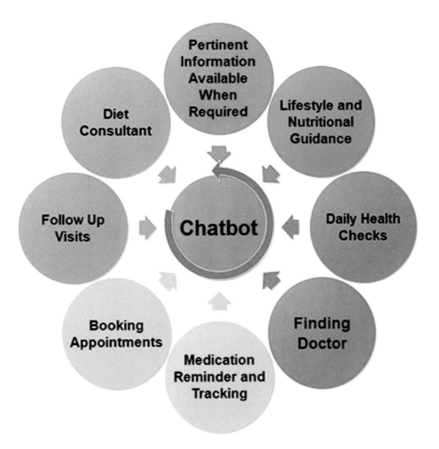

Figure 11.2 Typical examples of what chatbots can do [11].

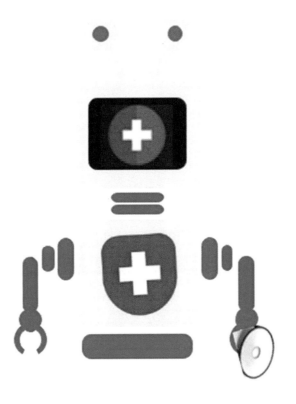

Figure 11.3 A typical healthcare chatbot [12].

Some of these applications are explained as follows.

- *Surgery*: Having surgery can be a traumatic experience. Some healthcare chatbots are for surgery for patients with cancer, mental health, dementia, phobic disorders, stress, and eating disorders. Special chatbots have been designed to aid surgery.

- *Mental Health:* Mental disorders is regarded as one of the most common causes of disability. There is a global shortage of mental health practitioners. This has prompted the utilization of newly emerging technology such as chatbots. Chatbots can be useful tools for individuals with mental disorders [13].

- *Cancer:* The cancer chatbot would help cancer patients to clarify their doubt regarding cancer. According to WHO, cancer is the second major cause of death. Chatbots can be leveraged in the field of radiation oncology: from cancer screening, diagnosis to patient information on treatment modalities and potential toxicities [14]. The number of cancer patients is increasing exponentially. Chatbots can be used to follow up with patients during their treatments and save time for health care providers.

- *Hospital Administrator:* A medical registrar at the hospital has to answer the same questions by phone several times a day. This repetitive activity can be easily performed by a chatbot [15]. Chatbot as a hospital administrator can schedule appointments, answer questions, collect user requests, and schedule doctor visits. A chatbot can be used for internal record-keeping and booking visits.

- *Healthcare Consultant:* Sometimes patients have concerns or inquiries about their health condition. It would be beneficial to have a chatbot on your hand held device as a healthcare consultant to answer your questions. The chatbot can play the role of a physical, mental, and social health consultant. If you have a question or need advice on nutrition, medications, medical diagnoses, or medical equipment, you can simply ask the chatbot and get an instant answer [15]. Chatbots provide real-time instructions and can recommend treatments based on patient symptoms. They can connect patients with suitable health care providers within the community. Although chatbots are not designed to offer diagnoses, as the physician has the final say, the chatbot can collect pertinent information and process it to make the job of the physician easier.

- *Patient Reminders:* Being human, patients can forget to take their medication at appropriate times or forget the appointment with their doctor. Patient compliance and medication adherence is an ongoing struggle for healthcare providers. Chatbots can update patient records and help with appointment reminders [16].

- *Elderly Care*: There is a need for systems that can interact with aging populations to gather information, monitor health condition, and provide support. A chatbot application can come in handy for the elderly patients and can function as an healthcare assistant. Chatbot application can monitor breathing and heart rate [17].

Other applications of healthcare chatbots include behavior change, personalized diagnosis, and patient-doctor interaction.

Today, chatbots are offered by Apple (Siri), Amazon (Alexa), Google (Assistant), Microsoft (Cortana) or Samsung (Bixby). Most of them are marketed without any specific use in mind. They can answer questions about knowledge stored in their data base place orders, play music, manage appointments, etc. Chatbots with a health focus include Florence, Molly, Lark, Babylon, Melody, Koko, and Dara. For example, Babylon has claimed that its chatbot perform as well as human doctors at providing patients with health advice [18]. Your.MD claims that it is uses artificial intelligence and machine learning to provide personalized health information and relevant products and services.

11.4 GLOBAL HEALTHCARE CHATBOTS

Chatbot is a computer program designed to help in carrying on a dialogue with humans. Chatbots are gradually being adopted into the healthcare industry and are generally in the early phases of implementation. Increasing internet connectivity, rapidly increasing adaptation of smart devices are the major factors driving the growth of the global healthcare chatbots market. The technological advances in voice recognition, natural language processing (NLP), and artificial intelligence (AI) have smoothened the interactions between computers and human. Geographically, the global healthcare chatbots market is segmented into four major regions such as Europe, North America, Asia Pacific, and the rest of the world.

- *United States:* In the United States, the use of chatbots is skyrocketing. Chatbots are now widely used in several forms as voice-based agents, such as Siri (Apple) Google Now (Google), Alexa (Amazon), Messenger (Facebook) or Cortana (Microsoft). Patients can now use chatbots to check for symptoms and to monitor their health. Healthcare chatbots can provide users with access to validated medical information on-demand. Applications of healthcare chatbots are very promising, particularly in the field of oncology.
- *United Kingdom*: The British chatbot, Babylon Health, is gradually gaining popularity among the citizens of London. Babylon Health was founded in 2013 and is now valued at more than $2 billion. The users inform the app about the symptoms of their illness. The chatbot checks them in a database of diseases using speech recognition and offers an appropriate action to take. The UK's National Health Service (NHS) started to use the chatbot for dispensing medical advice and plans to extend its service to other cities in the UK.
- *Germany:* In Germany, David Hawig developed Florence to remind patients about taking their prescriptions, a handy feature for older patients. The chatbot is essentially a "personal nurse assistant." Florence can track the user's health and find the nearest pharmacy or doctor's office. The German ADA chatbot asks personalized questions and connects the patient with a real doctor if necessary.
- *Africa:* This is the second largest continent in the world and the second most populous continent in the world. Some communicable diseases (such as malaria, tuberculosis, and HIV/AIDS) and non-communicable diseases (such as cancer, hypertension, diabetes) are still prevalent. An AI-based intelligent chatbot, named Likita (meaning "doctor" in an African language), interacts with patients and connects them to healthcare practitioners when necessary. Likita will revolutionize healthcare in Africa with respect to diagnosis and treatment of patients.. Likita's availability as a mobile app is very helpful since Africa has a very high mobile phone penetration [5].

11.5 BENEFITS

Chatbots bring several benefits: anonymity, asynchronicity, personalization, scalability, authentication, consumability, etc. [19]. The benefits of using chatbots in health include providing a personalized diagnoses based on symptoms, improving patient education and treatment compliance, increasing access to healthcare, improving doctor–patient and clinic–patient communication, reducing healthcare costs, and improving accessibility to healthcare information. Other benefits include the following [20]:

- *Personalized Care:* Chatbot is the perfect way to deliver personalized patient care. Chatbots are being used for various personal matters such reminding one to take medication, follow diets, aiding in scheduling appointments, preparation for a colonoscopy, notify nurses of problems, etc. It can improve patient experience with their doctors, so they can become more involved in their care and make well informed decisions regarding their health. Healthcare chatbots can help with diagnostic decision support as well.
- *Reduced Costs:* Without using chatbots, you incur a recurring expense of paying your customer support team every month. Chatbots eliminate the requirement of any manpower during online interaction. They can handle as many queries as required at once. They can also be used to market your latest products and send out updates to your customers.
- *24-7 availability:* Unlike humans, chatbots once installed can operate and attend queries at any time of the day. They can provide support to customers around the clock. Healthcare chatbots can advise you at any time of the day. Chatbots are useful programs that help you save a lot of manpower by ensuring the all-time availability and serving to several clients simultaneously.

There are countless cases where a healthcare chatbot could help physicians, nurses, and patients.

11.6 CHALLENGES

There are some issues to be resolved about the uses of chatbot technology. Chatbots suffer from performance issue due to limitations with their programming and training. Some have suggested that chatbot technology should be used in less complicated roles such as administrative and organizational tasks. Other challenges are as follows [2].

- *Fears:* Fears have been expressed that chatbots could eventually replace the physician or interfere with the patient-physician relationship. While chatbots can handle many simple or repetitive tasks, robots and chatbots will never replace humans. They cannot do the physical observation or manual work as a healthcare provider.
- *Privacy:* User privacy is important when working with chatbots since nobody wants their personal information to be disclosed. The users may be reluctant to share their personal information with your chatbot.
- *Data security:* Security and personality are crucial elements for building user confidence in the chatbot. Building natural language interaction with a chatbot is still complicated.
- *Trust:* Trust is the willingness of users to provide confidential information, accept the recommendations, and follow the suggestions. Reliability, transparency, and explainability affect the trust-building process. Patients must be able to trust chatbot regarding their privacy and security. Chatbots are highly prone to cybercrime, and the patient's data can be at risk.

Chatbot developers also must be very careful when providing information that is crucial in healthcare.

- *Conservation*: While other industries, such e-commerce, hospitality, and the food industry, have embraced chatbot technology, healthcare industry lags behind, resiss change, and still lean towards the traditional way of operation.
- *Maintenance:* Chatbots require ongoing maintenance and updating in terms of their knowledge base and the way they communicate with your customers. One would need to train the chatbot to respond to frequently-asked questions and improve customer satisfaction.

These challenges with healthcare chatbots should be addressed before the technology is widely endorsed in the healthcare community.

11.7 CONCLUSION

The advancement in artificial intelligence and machine learning has led to the rise of chatbots. Chatbots are used in many fields to reduce or eliminate the amount of tedious, repetitive tasks. They are efficient when their work is complemented by a healthcare professional. Chatbots are becoming increasingly popular as a human-computer interface as well as smart healthcare tools. Chatbots in healthcare industry are still in early stage of implementation. Most chatbots are implemented in stand-alone software. Their future will largely depend on how they are perceived by healthcare professionals and patients. Future chatbots will reliably, accurately, and cheaply help diagnose patients, recommend medication and treatment plans for the patient. Chatbots are here to stay.

More information on healthcare chatbots can be found in the book in [21] and in *Chatbots Magazine.*

REFERENCE

[1] "Healthcare chatbot diagnosis: Will consumers trust them with their health?" https://info.usertesting. com/rs/709-WMS-542/images/usertesting-healthcare-chatbot-diagnosis-benchmark-report.pdf

[2] A. Palanica et al., "Physicians' perceptions of chatbots in health care: Cross-sectional web-based survey," *Journal of Medical Internet Research*, vol. 21, no. 4, April 2019.

[3] N. Bhirud et al., "A literature review on chatbots in healthcare domain," *International Journal of Scientific & Technology Research*, vol. 8, no.7, July 2019, pp. 225-231.

[4] R. V. Belfin et al., "A graph based chatbot for cancer patients," *Proceedings of the 5th International Conference on Advanced Computing & Communication Systems*, 2019, pp. 717-721.

[5] M. N. O. Sadiku, P. O. Adebo, A. Ajayi-Majebi, and S. M. Musa, "Chatbots in healthcare," *International Journal of Trend in Research and Development*, vol. 7, no. 3, May-June 2020, pp. 91-93.

[6] R. Dharwadkar and N. A. Deshpande, "A medical chatBot," *International Journal of Computer Trends and Technology*. vol. 60, no. 1, June 2018, pp. 41-45.

[7] S. Divya et al., "A self-diagnosis medical chatbot using artificial intelligence," *Journal of Web Development and Web Designing*, vol. 3, no. 1, 2018.

[8] S. Valtolina, B. R. Barricelli, and S. D. Gaetano (2019): "Communicability of traditional interfaces VS chatbots in healthcare and smart home domains," *Behaviour & Information Technology*, 2019.

[9] A. Fadhil and G. Schiavo, "Designing for health chatbots," https://arxiv.org/ftp/arxiv/papers/1902/1902.09022.pdf

[10] M. Bates, "Health care chatbots are here to help," *IEEE Pulse*, vol. 10, no. 3, May-June 2019, pp.12-14.

[11] "The best free chatbot platform," September 2019, https://in.pinterest.com/pin/346988346289381600/

[12] S. Loeb,"Chatbots to save healthcare industry $3.6B in 2022," October 2017, https://vator.tv/news/2017-10-13-chatbots-to-save-healthcare-industry-36b-in-2022

[13] A. A.. Abd-alrazaqa et al., "An overview of the features of chatbots in mental health: A scoping review," *International Journal of Medical Informatics*, vol. 132, December 2019,

[14] J. E. Bibaulta et al., "Healthcare ex Machina: Are conversational agents ready for prime time in oncology?" *Clinical and Translational Radiation Oncology*, vol. 16, May 2019, pp. 55-59.

[15] M. Savonin, "Chatbots in healthcare: Advantages and disadvantages," September 2019, https://chatbotslife.com/chatbots-in-healthcare-advantages-and-disadvantages-346448ed634c

[16] "Personalized care: Virtual assistants trigger innovation in healthcare," Unknown source.

[17] A. Fadhil, "Beyond patient monitoring: Conversational agents role in telemedicine & healthcare support for home-living elderly individuals," https://arxiv.org/ftp/arxiv/papers/1803/1803.06000.pdf

[18] "The top 12 health chatbots," *The Medical Futurist*, May 2018, https://medicalfuturist.com/top-12-health-chatbots/

[19] J. Pereira1 and Ó. Díaz, "Using health chatbots for behavior change: A mapping study," *Journal of Medical Systems*, vol. 43, 2019.

[20] M. Gupta, "Chatbots: boon or bane?" January 2018, https://blog.bluelupin.com/chatbot-advantages-and-disadvantages/

[21] S. Janarthanam, *Hands-on Chatbots and Conversation UI Development*. Birminghan, UK: Packet Publishing, 2017.

CHAPTER 12

HEALTHCARE ROBOTICS

"I'm just a robot. I have no fears. I lack emotion. And I shed no tears." - Anonymous

12.1 INTRODUCTION

Robots have moved from science fiction to your local hospital, where they are changing healthcare. Today, robots perform vital functions in homes, industries, outer space, hospitals, and on military instillations. Robots can support, assist, and extend the services of healthcare professionals. In jobs with repetitive and monotonous functions they might even completely replace humans. Robotics and autonomous systems is regarded as the fourth industrial revolution. Robotics is part of AI. Robots are rapidly becoming part of the modern healthcare landscape.

Given the successful performance of robotics in a wide range of industries, from vehicle manufacturing to space exploration, robots have been introduced to transform a healthcare procedure like a surgery into an assisted operation definitely safer and more convenient for both doctors and patients. All stakeholders (e.g. patients, doctors, hospitals, care institutions, health insurance companies, and authorities) must prepare for them.

With the development of human living standard, the importance of medical healthcare is on the increase and many countries are facing pressure on their healthcare systems due to the rapidly aging population. Robots have the potential to provide assistance to healthcare providers in daily caregiving tasks. Transport, telemedicine, and service robots in healthcare promise to create a new level of quality healthcare by providing experts to patients. Robots also bridge multiple hospitals together, democratizing them as well as empowering smaller hospitals. They have been used across a range of environments, including hospitals, clinics, homes, schools, and nursing homes [1,2]. Factors that affect widespread adoption of robots in healthcare are illustrated in Figure 12.1.

143

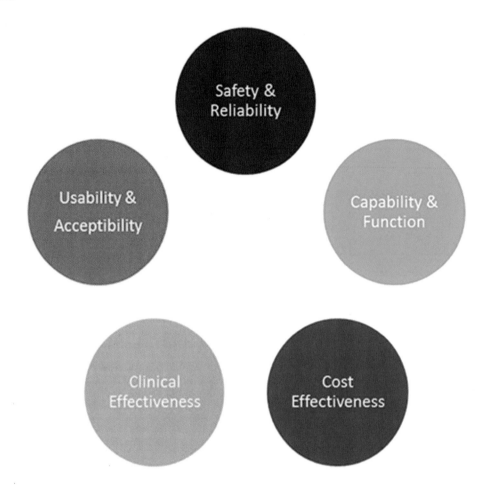

Figure 12.1 Factors that affect widespread adoption of robots in healthcare

This chapter provides a brief introduction to healthcare robots and their applications. It begins by discussing what robots are. It covers the various applications of robots in healthcare. It addresses global healthcare robotics. It highlights benefits and challenges facing robots in healthcare. The last section concludes with final remarks.

12.2 WHAT IS A ROBOT?

Robotics is a branch of engineering and computer science that involves the conception, design, manufacture, and operation of robots. It is an interdisciplinary discipline embracing mechanical engineering, electrical engineering, computer science, biotechnology, nanotechnology, information technology, and robot technology. It may be regarded as one of the technologies used to design and operate robots. The goal of robotics is to create intelligent machines (called robots) that behave and think like humans.

A robot is a mechanical intelligent device which can perform human tasks on its own or with guidance. It can sense, act, think, or process information. A robot functions as an intelligent machine, meaning that, it can be programmed to take actions or make choices based on input from sensors. It involves using electronics, computer science, artificial intelligence, mechatronics, and bioengineering.

A robot can also be regarded as a mechatronic device that is designed and programmed to perform some specific tasks. The word "robot" was first coined by the Czech playwright Karel Capek in 1921.

Isaac Asimov coined the term "robotics" in 1942 and came up with three rules to guide the behavior of robots [3]: (1) Robots must never harm human beings; (2) Robots must follow instructions from humans without violating rule 1, and (3) Robots must protect themselves without violating the other rules. There are several ways to classify robots: form, motion, application, or degree of agency of the robot. Programs are the core essence of a robot since they provide intelligence. There are three different types of robotic programs: remote control, artificial intelligence, and hybrid [4].

Early robots were simple mechanical automated machines. Modern robots employ microprocessors and computer technology. They can be programmed and "taught" to perform certain tasks. They are taking on more "human" traits such as sensing, dexterity, memory, and trainability.

Robots typically use sensor data to make decisions. Mobile robots share basic elements such as sensors, batteries, computer, drive motors, and case. The first known robot used in the healthcare industry was in 1985, when the robot PUMA (Programmable Universal Manipulation Arm) 560 placed a needle for a brain biopsy using CT guidance.

Robots are commonly used in dangerous environments where humans cannot survive such as manufacturing, defusing bombs, finding survivors in unstable ruins, welding, and exploring mines and shipwrecks. Today, robots perform important functions in homes, hospitals, industries, military institutions, education, entertainment, and outer space. Robots are applied in many fields including agriculture, education, manufacturing, entertainment, healthcare/medicine, industry, space exploration, undersea exploration, sex, power grid, agriculture, construction, meat processing, household, mining, aerospace, electronics, and automotive.

Robots have become increasingly important not only for industrial automation, but also for various human services in our daily life. Unlike industrial robots that assist in factories and have limited contact with humans, social robots are designed to interact with us. A social robot is an autonomous robot that interacts with people in a safe and comfortable manner. It must communicate and interact within the social rules attached to its task, which may be easy, moderate or complex [5]. A service robot is a robot which operates autonomously to perform useful services for humans. Service robots have been deployed in various indoor environments such as homes, hospitals, offices, and stores to provide services [6].

12.3 APPLICATIONS

A robot is a system that contains sensors, control systems, power supplies, and software all working together to perform a task. A healthcare robot is one used in healthcare. Robots play an important role in healthcare as they can improve diagnosis, lower the number of medical errors, and improve the overall quality and effectiveness of healthcare delivery. They hold the promise of addressing major healthcare issues in surgery, diagnostics, prosthetics, physical and mental therapy, monitoring, and support. With unmatched precision and the ability to work without fatigue, healthcare robots are definitely one of the most useful applications of robotic technology [7].

Robotics moves in all shapes and forms in healthcare. A wide range of robots is developed to serve different purposes within the healthcare environment. This results in various kinds of healthcare robots such as surgical robots, logistics robots, disinfectant robots, medication despensing robots, laboratory robots, rehabilitation/exoskeleton robots, nursing robots, care robots, eldercare robot, hospital robots, telepresence robots, therapy/ therapeutic robots, assistive robots, robotic prosthetic limbs, humanoid robots, mobile robots, diagnostics robots, nanorobots, space robots, military robots, and many other types.

The following applications are the top seven in the field of healthcare.

1. *Surgical Assistant*: Surgery is an unpleasant, daunting experience at best for most patients. It is the most commonly discussed application area for robots in healthcare. Robots assist surgeons increase precision during surgical procedures. Robots offer the following benefits in the surgical field [8]:
   - Repeatable tool position and trajectory
   - Steady motion
   - Ability to react rapidly to changes in force level
   - Remote operation
   - Ability to remain poised in a fixed position
   - Greater three-dimensional spatial accuracy
   - More reliable system design
   - Ability to achieve much greater precision

Robots can be used to disinfect operating rooms, reducing post operative infection for patients and reduce transmission to medical staff. Although robotics was commonly used to treat urologic oncologic conditions, it has also been widely adopted for gynecologic (i.e., myomectomy, hysterectomy), general (i.e., gastric, colorectal, hepato-biliary-pancreatic, bariatric), thoracic, and head and neck surgeries, neurosurgery and endocrine surgery [9][10].

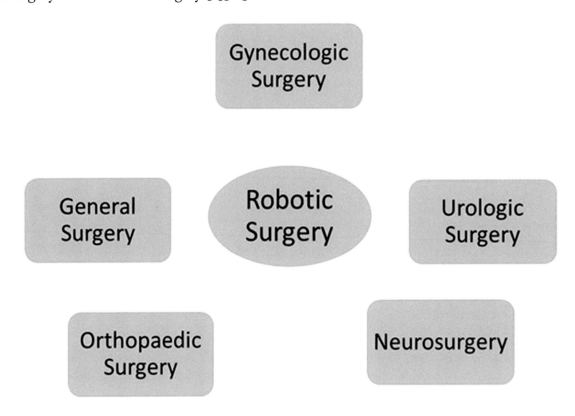

Figure 12.2 Different types of robotic surgery [11].

Because of these diverse uses, there are different types of robotic surgery, as illustrated in Figure 12.2 [11]. A specific application using the da Vinci robot for surgery is shown in Figure 12.3 [12].

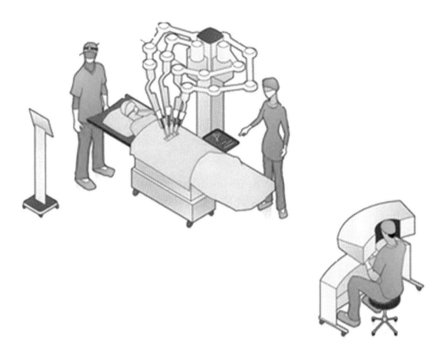

Figure 12.3 Using the da Vinci robot for surgery [12].

2. *Telepresence*: Telerobotics enables a doctor to perform a surgery at a distance. This way, physicians can use robots to examine and treat patients in rural or remote locations. A fundamental component for effective telesurgery is data transmission speed; latency in data transmission limits telemanipulation to a distance of a few hundred kilometers [13].

3. *Rehabilitation*: The most extensive use of robotic technology for healthcare applications has been in rehabilitation robotics, which traditionally includes assistive robots and therapeutic robots. Rehabilitation robotics is often regarded as robotic aids to assist people handicapped by a manipulative disability. Rehabilitation robots are used in the recovery of people with disabilities as well as the elderly population [14]. Virtual reality is being incorporated in these robots to improve balance, walking, etc.

4. *Nursing*: Nurses interact a lot with patients during a hospital stay. They draw blood, assess vital signs, administer medications, monitor patients' condition, etc. Robotic nurses can help carry these repetitive tasks. They can help a nurse to lift an elderly patient. They can monitor patient vital statistics and alert the nurses when there is a need for a human presence in the room. They will help administer care and support to people in hospitals, care facilities, and homes. They will have to make complicated decisions regarding patients on a daily basis [15]. Compared to humans, robot nurses are easy to train, cheaper to maintain, and able to do mundane and repetitive tasks.

5. *Pharmacies:* Pharmacists perform repetitive tasks that could be eliminated by utilizing the advancing robotics in healthcare. A robot could process information much faster and much more accurately than humans. Due to the potential hazards and high volumes, some hospitals

utilize robotics to dispense medication. Pharmaceutical robots reduce cost and provide flexibility and efficiency [16].

6. *Care:* Robots can be used to provide care and support to elderly and disabled patients living at home. As mentioned earlier, care robots can assist nurses with the various tasks they perform. Care robots can help older adults and chronically ill patients to remain independent. The robots can be provided with surveillance capability to monitor patients. Caregivers can also use robots to enhance telemedicine for those confined to their homes.

7. *Elderly care:* According to recent statistics, the number of people aged over 65 is predicted to triple between 2000 and 2050. The elderly population is straining healthcare services as there is a shortage in caregivers. By developing technologies to aid older people, they can become independent, healthier and improve their quality of life. Companion robots are appreciated for their ability to offer improved communication between patients and healthcare professionals and provide medical monitoring needs [17]. Figure 12.4 shows a typical robot for the elderly [18].

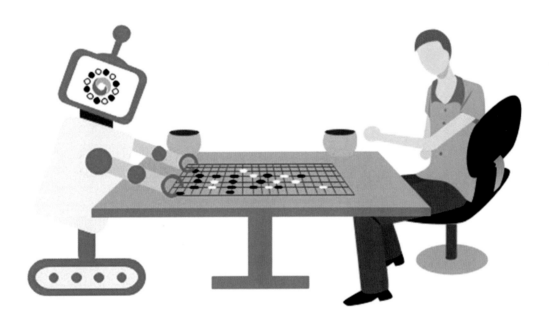

Figure 12.4 A robot for the elderly [18].

Other areas of applications include clinical training, ICUs, AI diagnostics, medical device packaging, lab automation, therapeutic massage, medical transportation, sanitation and disinfection robots, prostheses, endoscopy, autism, orthopedics, and training for healthcare workers

14.4 GLOBAL HEALTHCARE ROBOTICS

Robotics technologies are emerging technologies in the field of medicine and healthcare. They are advanced and affordable enough for broader experimentation and adoption. The healthcare robotics can benefit all stakeholders across nations. Robots can be a game changer in healthcare: improving health and well-being, filling care gaps, supporting care givers, and aiding health care workers. As the world population is aging, with an increasing shortage of healthcare professionals, robots will continue to grow in presence in the global healthcare. The global healthcare robotics market was valued at $5.40 billion in 2017 and is estimated to reach $11.44 billion by 2025. The countries with the highest number of patent claims on robots are US, Japan, China, and South Korea. We typically consider healthcare robots in some countries.

- *United States:* Robots are being introduced into the US healthcare system at a growing rate. Research and innovation in the area of healthcare robotics has seen a significant growth in recent years. Robots are intelligent and autonomous; they can take care of the elderly. Not only has healthcare been well established in hospitals or nursing facilities, but also in patient homes. In the US, all consumer in-the-body robots and many on-the-body robots must undergo regulatory approval before they can be marketed and sold. The approval is through the FDA, which requires evidence showing the effectiveness and safety of a medical robot [19]. The robotics industry has created millions of jobs since robot technology is being applied in several domains and incorporated into multiple daily activities. Typical examples of robot intervention include medication administration, assisting children with autism, telemedicine, lifting patients, and aiding in surgical procedures [20]

- *European Union:* Europe has world leading expertise in healthcare robotics. Robotics promises revolutionary changes in the EU health sector. Significant investments for the development of healthcare solutions are necessary, possibly through partnerships between the public and private sectors. The European Parliament is leading in establishing civil law rules applicable for robotics and fostering cooperation across the EU [21].

- *Japan:* In Japan, as well as in several other nations, people are living longer and fewer babies are being born. The issue of elderly care is becoming a serious issue in Japan. Although robotics applications may not be the final solution to the challenge of an aging society, they are worth considering. A more user-oriented, multi-disciplinary approach is needed. The importance of paying attention to safety, ethical, and privacy issues is commonly agreed on in Japan. Currently, there are no central rules on using caring healthcare robots for the elderly. In Japan, the law is made after a case has occurred and new issues are treated as they occur [22]. Effective law and regulation for robotics create trust: trust in brands, trust in functions, trust in privacy, trust in a fair market [23]. One robot developed in Japan named Robear helps patients get in or out of a bed or a wheelchair and help performs other tasks. The usage of such service robot has been recently growing in nursing or care homes in most advanced countries with Japan currently leading the world in advanced robotics.

- *Korea:* Robots are designed and manufactured to support different fields such as entertainment, health devices, and sport training systems. For example, the research on a healthcare service robot platform contains three types of robot platforms: ChairBot for relaxation, RideBot for exercising, and LifecareBot for human emotions. ChairBot is a robotic massage chair that uses the bioinformation of its human user for health monitoring. RideBot is a robotic riding machine for fitness. LifecareBot is a home service robot platform that can produce a positive mental and social effect on its users [24].

Key players in healthcare robotics include such companies as Accuray Incorporated, Corindus Vascular Robotics, Inc., Intuitive Surgical Inc., ReWalk Robotics Ltd., Smith & Nephew plc, Stereotaxis, Inc., Stryker Corporation, Zimmer Biomet, Medtronic plc, Fujifilm Holdings Corporation, Auris Health, Inc., Endomaster Pte Ld., Hocoma AG, Restorative Therapies, Think Surgical, and Tyromotion GmbH [25].

12.4 BENEFITS

Healthcare robotics is an emerging field that can greatly benefit the healthcare industry. Healthcare robots could take over administrative monotonous and repetitive tasks. While some are concerned about machines replacing people in the workforce, some see the benefits of healthcare robots.

- *Improve Patient Care:* Robots play an important role in healthcare as it can improve diagnosis, lower the number of medical errors, and improve the overall quality and effectiveness of healthcare delivery.They help hospitals save costs, reduce waste, and improve patient care.
- *Reduce Cost of Care*: Robots can reduce the cost of care, offload menial tasks from human personnel, improve the accuracy of repetitive tasks, and enable enhanced forms of therapy and rehabilitation. Robots assure a high level of productivity and efficiency at reduced costs compared with humans.
- *Precision and Repeatability:* A major advantage of robotic is performing heavy-duty jobs with accuracy, precision, and repeatability (you've repeated this sentence a lot). A machine does not need sleep or have prejudices as humans do. Robots eliminate human error in delicate, high-risk procedures. Surgical robots bring precision to meticulous procedures.

Other benefits of robots include remote treatment, precise diagnosis, supporting mental health. Despite these advantages, there are certain skills to which humans will be better suited than machines for some time to come. Humans have the advantages of creativity, decision-making, flexibility and adaptability. With the right expertise and technology, the benefits can outweigh the disadvantages.

14.5 CHALLENGES

As with all innovations in healthcare, robotics has faced numerous challenges, notably questions regarding efficacy, safety, and cost-effectiveness. Some see them as intrusive and controlling. They need regulation because of the new legal and ethical issues they raise. It is great to develop robots to solve practical healthcare problems, but it is important to do so with patient safety in mind. The ultimate question for robotics in healthcare is whether they will take jobs away from humans. Apart from cost, one of the key barriers to the successful translation of robotic advances into clinical practice has been the large and imposing nature of the system [26]. The task of building small robotic system (in the nanoscale) will likely present a new set of challenges. Other challenges include [27]:

- *Safety and Security Issues:* Security, safety and avoidance of harm should be of utmost importance in healthcare domain when using robots. This is incredibly important when robots and humans work in close proximity. Multidisciplinary teams are needed to develop the tools and methods required to ensure safe operation of robots. Another concern about security is how to protect robots from being hacked.

- *Cost-effectiveness:* This is the biggest challenge in adopting medical robots. When robots are being acquired in healthcare, their cost effectiveness should be considered beyond the purchase, maintenance, and training costs. In regular healthcare systems, where the cost of robotic instruments is passed directly to the patient, there has been limited adoption. Most hospitals simply cannot afford the technology. Also, space is required to set up robot technologies.
- *Societal Acceptance:* The problem with robots is not just an issue of technology, but also heavily depends on societal acceptance, safety, and reliability issues as well as regulations. Robots can be dangerous and absolute safety is not guaranteed with their use. "Safe robots" should be built that do not harm workers in case of an accident or collision
- *Ethical Concerns:* The legal and ethical barriers are high. Advances in robotic technology have social, legal, and ethical ramifications. Are robots primarily introduced to solve problems in healthcare or replace humans in order to save money? Will robots replace the nurses, leaving the sick and elderly in the hands of machines? Can robots deliver the same quality of care? What kind of tasks and decisions can be delegated to the machine? Robots lack the capacity of moral reasoning. Ethical issues such as personal moral responsibility, privacy, and accountability are emerging concerning the use of robots. This suggests the need for developing robot ethics and examining the laws and regulations governing its use [28,29].
- *Required Training*: Another block to success is that training is required in various uses of robots. A challenge exists when healthcare robots are to work effectively in homes. The people who interact with them may have little or no training in robotics, and so any interface will need to be extremely intuitive.

Other challenges include trust, deception, privacy and data protection, safety and avoidance of harm. Improvements in healthcare robotics must address these real problems, ultimately providing a clear improvement in quality of life when compared with the alternatives [30].

12.6 CONCLUSION

Robotics has benefited a wide range of industries, from car manufacturing to space exploration. And as much fun as robots are to play with, robots are even much more fun to design and construct. Automotive and electronics are the largest patent filers on robots.

Healthcare robotics is causing a major paradigm shift in therapy despite that the field is still in its infancy. Robots can be a game changer in healthcare: improving patient's health and well-being, supporting care givers, and aiding healthcare workers. Advancing the use of robotics in the healthcare requires integration across all stakeholders. Although robots are expensive, their use is changing healthcare. As the world's population ages and with an increasing shortage of healthcare professionals especially in developing nations, robots will become more relevant in the healthcare system. A robot may soon become a regular member of the healthcare professionals. The future of healthcare robot is bright and awe-inspiring.

The introduction of healthcare robots to the mass market depends on cost reduction. Robots as well as related sensors and software are becoming cheaper and more capable. Graduates with backgrounds in healthcare robotics and related areas are in short supply and high demand. It is imperative for medical students and nurses to acquire some basic knowledge about robotics while in school. More information about healthcare robotics can be found in the books in [31-38] and the following international journals devoted to robot-related issues:

- *Journal of Robotic Systems*
- *Advanced Robotics*
- *Journal of Robotics*
- *Journal of Robotic Surgery*
- *Journal of Intelligent & Robotic Systems*
- Intelligent Service Robotics
- *IEEE Journal on Robotics and Automation*
- *IEEE Robotics & Automation Magazine*
- *IEEE Transactions on Robotics*
- *International Journal of Medical Robotics and Computer Assisted Surgery*
- *International Journal of Robotics Research*
- *International Journal of Social Robotics*
- *International Journal of Humanoid Robotics*
- *Robotics and Autonomous Systems*

REFERENCES

[1] N. M. Su, L. S. Liu, and A. Lazar, "Mundanely miraculous: The robot in healthcare," *Proceedings of the 8th Nordic Conference on Human-Computer Interaction: Fun, Fast, Foundational*, October 2014, pp. 391-400.

[2] L. D. Riek, "Healthcare robotics," *Communications of the ACM*, vol 60, no. 11, November 2017, pp. 68-78.

[3] "Human–robot interaction," *Wikipedia*, the free encyclopedia https://en.wikipedia.org/wiki/Human–robot_interaction

[4] M. N. O. Sadiku, S. Alam, and S.M. Musa, "Intelligent robotics and applications," *International Journal of Trends in Research and Development*, vol. 5. No. 1, January-February 2018, pp. 101-103.

[5] M. N. O. Sadiku, M. Tembely, and S.M. Musa, "Social robots," *International Journal of Advanced Research in Computer Science and Software Engineering*, vol. 8, no. 10, October 2018, pp. 73-75.

[6] M. N. O. Sadiku, A. M. Oteniya, and S. M. Musa, "Service robots," *International Journal of Trend in Research and Development*, vol. 5, no. 4, July – Aug. 2018, pp. 555-556.

[7] M. N. O. Sadiku, Y. Wang, S. Cui, and S.M. Musa, "Healthcare robotics: A primer," *International Journal of Advanced Research in Computer Science and Software Engineering*, vol. 8, no. 2, Feb. 2018, pp. 26-29.

[8] L. Zamorano et al., "Robotics in neurosurgery: State of the art and future technological challenges," *International Journal of Medical Robotics and Computer Assisted Surgery*, vol. 1, no.1, 2004, pp. 7–22.

[9] H. Y. Yu, "The current status of robotic oncologic surgery," *A Cancer Journal for Clinicians*, vol. 63, no. 1, Jan./Feb. 2013, pp. 46-56.

[10] S. J. Baek and S. H. Kim, "Robotics in general surgery: An evidence-based review," *Asian Journal of Endoscopic Surgery*, vol. 7, 2014, pp. 117-123.

[11] R. Wason et al., "Smart robotics for smart healthcare," *Advances in Robotics & Mechanical Engineering*, January 2019, pp. 73-74.

[12] "Robotic surgery has come a long way in 10 years," May 2020, http://herald-citizen.com/stories/robotic-surgery-has-come-a-long-way-in-10-years,24144

[13] M. Diana and J. Marescaux, "Robotic surgery," *BJS*, vol. 102, 2015, pp. e15-e28.

[14] N. Tejima, "Rehabilitation robotics: A review," *Advanced Robotics*, vol. 14, no. 7, 2001, pp. 551-564.

[15] J. Borenstein and Y. Koren, "A mobile platform for nursing robots," *IEEE Transactions on Industrial Electronics*, vol. 32, no. 2, May 1985, pp. 158-165.

[16] P. Fiorini and D. Botturi, "Introducing service robotics to the pharmaceutical industry," *Intelligent Service Robotics*, vol. 1, no. 4, October 2008, pp. 267–280.

[17] H. Robinson, B. MacDonald, and E. Broadbent, "The role of healthcare robots for older people at home: Review," *International Journal of Social Robotics*, vol. 6, 2014, pp. 575–591.

[18] https://www.la-croix.com/Journal/Quand-robots-font-leur-entree-maisons-retraite-2017-12-05-1100897002

[19] L. D. Riek, "Healthcare robotics," *Communications of the ACM*, 2017

[20] K. Lorelei. "How have robotics impacted healthcare?" *The Review: A Journal of Undergraduate Student Research*, vol 12, 2010, pp. 6-8.

[21] "Robots in healthcare: A solution or a problem?" http://www.statewatch.org/news/2019/may/ep-analysis-robots-health.pdf

[22] Y. Yasuhara et al., "Potential legal issues when caring healthcare robot with communication in caring functions are used for older adult care," *Enfermería Clínica*, vol. 30, Supplement 1,February 2020, pp. 54-59.

[23] C. Holder et al., "Robotics and law: Key legal and regulatory implications of the robotics age (Part I of II)," *Computer Law & Security Review*, vol. 32, no. 3, June 2016, pp. 383-402.

[24] S. Yi et al., "Healthcare robot technology development," *Proceedings of the 17th World Congress, The International Federation of Automatic Control*, Seoul, Korea, July 2008, pp. 5318-5323.

[25] "Global healthcare robotics market to reach $11.44 billion by 2023," January 2019, https://www.prnewswire.com/news-releases/global-healthcare-robotics-market-to-reach-11-44-billion-by-2023-897457224.html

[26] A. Hussain et al., "The use of robotics in surgery: A review," *The International Journal of Clinical Practice,* vol. 68, no. 11, November 2014, pp. 1376-1382.

[27] B. C. Stahl and M. Coeckelbergh, "Ethics of healthcare robotics: Towards responsible research and innovation," *Robotics and Autonomous Systems,* vol. 86, December 2016, pp. 152-161.

[28] K. Kernaghan, "The rights and wrongs of robotics: Ethics and robots in public organizations," *Canadian Public Administration*, vol. 57, no. 4, December 2014, pp. 485-506.

[29] B. CarstenStahl and M. Coeckelbergh, "Ethics of healthcare robotics: Towards responsible research and innovation," *Robotics and Autonomous Systems*, vol. 86, December 2016, pp. 152-161.

[30] R. A. Beasley, "Medical robots: Current systems and research directions," *Journal of Robotics*, 2012.

[31] J. S. Sequeira (ed.), *Robotics in Healthcare: Field Examples and Challenges*. Springer, 2019.

[32] N. Wilkins, *Artificial Intelligence: The Ultimate Guide to AI, The Internet of Things, Machine Learning, Deep Learning + A Comprehensive Guide to Robotics*. Bravex Publications, 2019.

[33] N. Katevas (ed.), *Mobile Robotics in Healthcare*. Amsterdam, Netherlands: IOS Press, 2001.

[34] A. van Wynsberghe, *Healthcare Robots: Ethics, Design and Implementation.* Routledge,, 2016.

[35] M. Sood and S. W. Leichtle (eds.), *Essentials of Robotic Surgery.* Spry Publishing, 2013.

[36] F. Gharagozloo and F. Najam, *Robotic Surgery.* McGraw-Hill Education / Medical, 2008,

[36] A. Saxena, *A Practical Approach to Robotic Surgery.* Jaypee Brothers Medical Publishers, 2017.

[37] P. Gomes (ed.), *Medical Robotics: Minimally Invasive Surgery.* Woodhead Publishing, 2012.

[38] M. H. Abedin-Nasab, *Handbook of Robotic and Image-Guided Surgery.* Elsevier; 2019.

CHAPTER 13

HEALTHCARE DRONES

"Drones, with their agility and small size, seem perfect for search and rescue operations." – Grant Imahara

13.1 INTRODUCTION

Technological advances are changing the world around us. They have revolutionized the medical field and changed the way healthcare is delivered. Drones (otherwise known as Unmanned aerial vehicles) are the next wave of technological advance that can make a huge impact on healthcare. They are gradually becoming a recognizable facet of everyday life.

Drones are autonomous or remotely controlled multipurpose aerial vehicles driven by aerodynamic forces. They are devices which are capable of sustained flight and do not need a human on board. Typically, a drone consists of an air frame, propulsion system, communication system, and navigation system [1]. Common drone configurations include fixed-wing, rotary-wing, multirotor, and hybrid designs. Their obvious usage areas are transportation and package delivery. As illustrated in Figure 13.1, compared with other transport modes, drones are the fastest and the least expensive [2]. Since a drone can fly over an inaccessible road, organizations have begun to use drones for healthcare delivery. While governments and regulators may be cautious about allowing drones to roam the skies, healthcare deliveries have a compelling reason to go for it. Amazon announced its plan to use drones to deliver packages to customers.

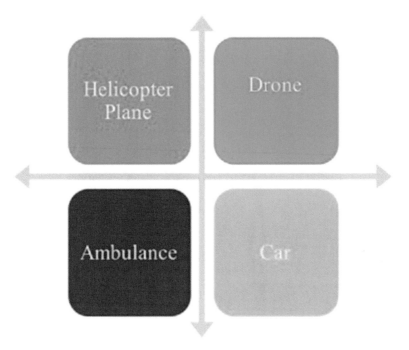

Figure 13.1 Drone is compared with other means of transportation [2].

Drones are increasingly being used as innovative tools for healthcare. Hospitals are experimenting with drones for numerous tasks that would often take twice as long for humans to do. The days are fast approaching when cars and trucks will be replaced by drones for moving things across hospital campuses.

This chapter discusses the use of drones in the field of healthcare. It begins by discussing the concept of drones. It provides some common applications of drones in healthcare. It covers the adoption of healthcare drone around the world. It discusses their benefits and challenges in healthcare. The last section concludes with comments.

13.2 CONCEPT OF DRONES

Drones are autonomous robots that fly in the sky. They may also be regarded as pilotless aircrafts that were initially used by the military, but are now used for scientific and commercial purposes. The word "drone" was coined due to the similarity of its sound to a male bee. Drones are pilotless aircraft and are formally known as either unmanned aerial vehicles (UAVs) or unmanned aircraft systems (UAS). Drones are also called "remotely piloted vehicle" or "unmanned aerial systems." Drones were first used in the 1990s by military organizations. The notion of drones began around 1918 when the US Navy commissioned Charles Kettering built a militarized unmanned aerial vehicle (UAV). Their original use was to take strategic pictures for the military. From the beginning of the 21st Century, civil activities of drones started to get more attention.

Drones are classified in different ways: size, weight, flight time, commercial or military, and cost. The US Federal Aviation Administration (FAA) defines consumer and commercial drones as those that weigh less < 1.0 lb (0.45kg) with approximately a maximum 500 m altitude and 2km range from the base operator. A drone is a pilotless aircraft that operates through a combination of technologies, including computer vision, artificial intelligence, object avoidance tech, automation, robotics, and miniaturization.

Drones in the medical field have been used for blood delivery, food delivery, and package delivery. They are now used in different fields including transportation, healthcare, news media, commerce, safety and security, disaster management, rescue operations, crop monitoring, weather tracking, environmental protection, intelligence gathering, surveillance, aerial photography, express shipping, recreation, agriculture, wildlife, military, law enforcement, home, cemetery management, power, infrastructure,, telecom sectors, marine, weather forecasting, sports, space, insurance, hotels, journalism/news coverage, and logistics [3,4]. Drones have been used by the military in combat and for humanitarian aid. Drones have emerged as interaction devices in home and research applications. A drone can be used as a companion, personal drone, agent, sensing tool, delivery tool, ambulance drone, etc. Drones are commonly used by hobbyists just for the fun of it. Healthcare is benefitting from this disruptive technology. Thus, we have different kinds of drones: military or armed drones, healthcare drones, medical drones, biomedical drones, smart drones, humanitarian drones, collaborative drone, ambulance drones, courier drones, nano or micro or mini drones, etc.

The technology involved in drone construction is impressive. Modern drones are empowered by sensor technology. Accelerometers are often used to determine position and orientation of the drone in flight. Inertial measurement units combined with global positioning systems (GPS) are critical for maintaining direction and flight paths [5]. Drones have to provide a reliable connection regarding tracking as well as remote control purposes and communicate this with users. They can maneuver unobtrusively above the ground towards a target without disturbing human movement on the ground.

Examples of drones used in healthcare include [6]:
- Seattle's Village Reach
- Flirtey
- Ehang
- ZipLine
- Tu Delft
- Google Drones
- Project Wing
- HiRO (Healthcare Integrated Rescue Operations)
- Vayu Drones

13.3 APLICATIONS

Some drone applications involve surveillance using an on board camera. Drones can also deliver small loads. They can gather real time data effectively. Drones have been used in different areas in healthcare including transfer of blood products, enhance search and rescue efforts, collection of different types of data, delivery of rural healthcare, offer remote telemedicine or patient care at home, transport samples and deliver blood, vaccines, medicines, organs, life-saving medical supplies (i.e., automated external defibrillators), and equipment. Healthcare drones are regarded as "medicine from the sky." Figure 13.2 shows some medical uses of drones [7].

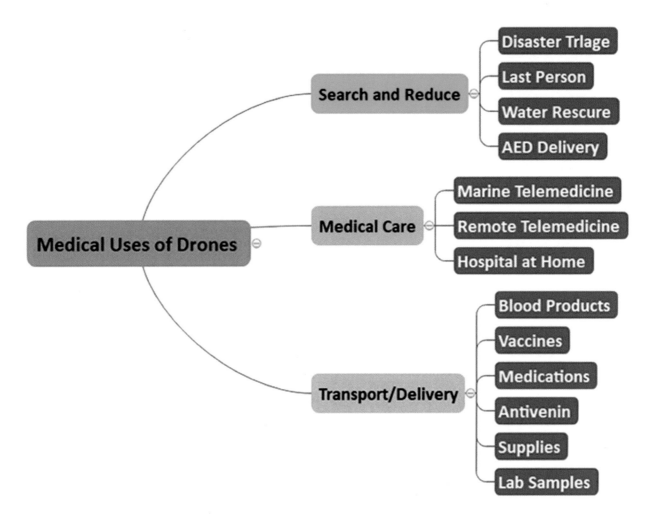

Figure 13.2 Medical uses of drones [7].

Some other potential uses of drones in healthcare include the following [8,9]:

- *Rural Healthcare:* This is perhaps the most popular use of healthcare drones. Patients often die due to lack of access to a basic medical product. Drones can be used to deliver blood, vaccines, birth control, and other medical supplies to rural areas or areas with mountains, deserts, or forests, roads are impassable and take long-distance travel. This could mean the difference between life and death. Health Wagon, a clinic based in Southwest Virginia, partnered with NASA researchers to fly the first drone approved by the Federal Aviation Administration (FAA) to deliver medication to rural Americans, particularly Native American populations. Zipline started transporting blood and vaccines to remote areas in Rwanda in harsh weather.
- *Care Delivery:* Drones can be used to transport blood, medical supplies, and water. This is a big step forward in saving time and lives. Drones can deliver supplies and medications from floor to floor or building to building. Drones can make it easier for clinicians to administer care to these patients in their homes by sending them necessary medications and other essentials for treatment. They are enabling healthcare delivery by providing faster response times, reduced transportation costs, and improved medical services to remote areas. Figure 13.3 shows a healthcare drone for delivery and pickup service in rural area [10].

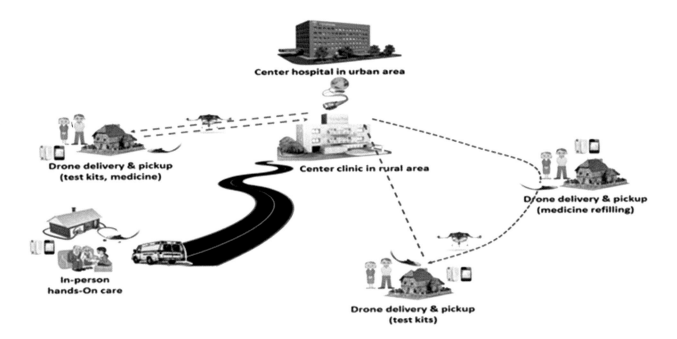

Figure 13.3 Healthcare drone for delivery and pickup services in rural area [10].

- *Bedside Medication Delivery:* Instead of nurses bringing medication to patients, drones could do the same job. Nurses and pharmacists can work more efficiently as supplies can be summoned to the bedside of a patient being cared for in the hospital or home.
- *Healthcare Transportation:* Drones are used as a means of transport. Drones can be used to transport urine, blood, sputum, and other samples from patients' rooms to hospital labs for testing. An example is the transportation of organs between two hospitals in the same city. Figure 13.4 illustrates typical medical drone transporting human organ [11].

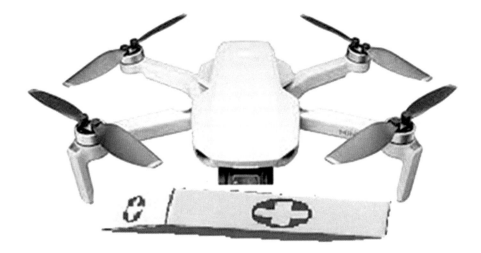

Figure 13.4 A typical medical drone transporting human organ [11].

- *Helping the Elderly:* Research is being done to use drones to benefit the growing senior population. Drones can be used to create ambient assisted living environments for the elderly. This is an efficient and cost-effective way of providing care for the elderly while extending their independent life. Drones can be used to deliver medication refills and pick up blood and urine tests [12].
- *Emergency:* Time is critical in emergency situations, especially when patients need blood, intravenous fluids or medications. For example, time is crucial in out-of-hospital cardiac arrest. Emergency medical services can sometimes have a long response time. Drones have been used to deliver supplies during an emergent lifesaving situation. A drone can serve as an ambulance during emergencies or be a viable alternative to ambulance response [13]. The drones always outperform the ambulances. Two hospitals in Switzerland started using drones to deliver blood samples.

Drones are used in other areas of healthcare including epidemiology, telemedicine, transfer units, humanitarian logistics, disaster relief, delivering aid packages, adverse weather conditions, and transporting medical goods over urban traffic jams.

13.4 GLOBAL HEALTHCARE DRONES

Drones are a rapidly developing technology with increasing worldwide applications. Healthcare drones are increasingly being used around the globe, especially in the following places:

- *Africa:* In spite of its poverty and poor infrastructure, subSaharan Africa has led the way in the adoption of mobile banking and healthcare, and now medical drones [14]. Necessity is the mother of invention; the rapid adoption of drone technology in sub-Saharan Africa is exemplary. The drone technology caught on so quickly in developing nations such as Rwanda, Tanzania, and Ghana with poor roads and lack of accessibility. These are among a group of early adopters of transport drones for healthcare systems in sub-Saharan Africa, with the first drone airport established in Rwanda. Figure 13.5 shows World Bank president, Jim Yong Kim, hailing Rwanda's use of drones in healthcare delivery [15]. The drone is operated by Zipline, a company based in San Francisco, California, focused on lifesaving medical supplies. Zipline argues that minimizing waste in the medical system will help the drones pay for themselves. Zipline plans to expand its operations to more African nations. The United Nations has used drones to drop condoms over rural parts of Ghana, where a fraction of women have access to contraceptives to prevent the transmission of sexual transmitted diseases. Threats of criminality, security breaches, and loss of privacy make drones too risky in developed countries. The World Economic Forum in partnership with Zipline and the World Bank has been raising awareness for using drones in Africa and beyond [16]. Tanzania is planning to have the largest drone healthcare delivery operation in the world. In spite of the fast adoption of drones in the continent, drones are manufactured elsewhere, e.g. USA and China.

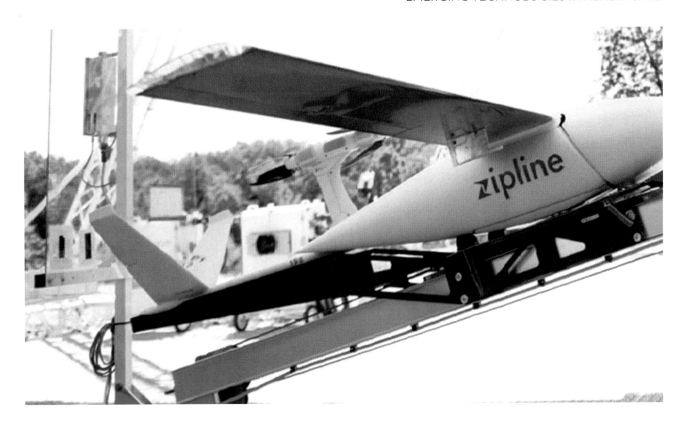

Figure 13.5 World Bank president hails Rwanda's use of drones in healthcare delivery [15].

- *United States*: Commercial use of drone in the US has been held back by regulations. The use of drones at hospitals in the US is relatively new. Some are of the opinion that deploying drones for public safety and humanitarian aid will be key to public acceptance in the United States. FAA defines consumer and commercial UAS as those that weigh less than 1.0 lb (0.45kg) with approximately a maximum 500 m altitude and 2km range from the base operator. FAA approved open drone fields (to indulge drone hobbyist) are dotted around the United States. The US Department of Defense is investigating drones as a battle space platform for medical logistics delivery. The National Aeronautics and Space Administration (NASA) recently tested a medical supply delivery (included medications for asthma, hypertension and diabetes) to a small clinic in rural Virginia using a drone.
- *India:* In India, there is a shortage of safe blood in hard-to-reach places. In rural India, the delay in diagnosing diseases due to lack of laboratory facilities nearby can be overcome by the use of drones. In December 2018, India's Ministry of Civil Aviation released a comprehensive framework for the operation of drones. In 2020, the government of Telangana (a state in India) in collaboration with the World Economic Forum has formalized the plan called "medicines from the sky." Telangana is known for using technology to improve the lives of the citizens. The National Disaster Management Authority (NDMA) has started using drones to handle disaster relief and rescue in India. Drones could be a gamechanger in states that are particularly geographically difficult to traverse.
- *China:* Consumer delivery was challenging in some areas in China. Drones sped the delivery of much-needed consumer goods replacing hours-long drives. The outbreak of coronavirus in

China has led to significant adoption of drones. China is known for building the most small drones.

- *Pakistan:* Consumers in Pakistan perceive privacy issues as a primary concern in relation to drone delivery, and unfortunately the Pakistani government does respect the rights of its citizens to privacy [17].. The typical Pakistani consumer now increasingly prefers variety, convenience, and ease. Drones can be used by businesses for making home delivery of packages in urban areas. They are also used for transporting medical supplies to remote areas that are hard to reach by road.

- *Singapore:* Tiny high-tech Singapore, with a population of 5.6 million, is ultra-modern, well-ordered and a tightly regulated nation. Drones are being used across the nation to deliver life-saving medical supplies. Its uses could include transporting blood samples, delivering emergency medical supplies, responding to security incidents, and in military operations. The drones would be operated remotely by pilots and be able to travel relatively long distances across the city-state [18].

13.4 BENEFITS

Drones are increasingly being used as innovative tools for healthcare. They address a specific niche application and provide an interesting non-traditional solution. They present a tremendous opportunity to address supply chain shortcomings in the healthcare sector. They can overcome the logistic challenges since they are not subjected to traffic delays. They have become a solution to transport challenges for medical products such as emergency blood supplies, vaccines, medicines, diagnostic samples, and organs. In Places like Rwanda, Ghana, and the Philippines, drones are already being used to transport lifesaving medical goods such as blood, drugs, and other critical medical supplies on a regular basis. The major benefit of using drones is that they decrease the travel time for diagnosis and treatment. Other benefits include the following [19].

- *Cost Advantages:* Drones have cost benefits. Drones have gained their popularity due to their affordability. Lightweight drones are probably less expensive than a car or motorcycle and faster. A lost drone is less expensive than a lost helicopter or airplane. Almost any hospital can use this modern healthcare technology to its advantage. The operating costs of drones can be reduced by working with drone battery manufacturers to create rechargeable batteries.

- *Better Mode of Transportation*: Compared to ground transportation, the benefits of drones include avoiding traffic in populous areas and circumventing dangerous fly zones in war-torn countries. Drones could also mitigate safety issues that arise with traditional modes of transport. Traffic conditions (such as icy roads, foggy skies, rush hour, mountains, canyons, or snow-covered ground) impose dangerous slowdowns in delivery. Drones could offer effective alternatives in those hazardous situations. Inaccessible roads no longer have to prevent healthcare delivery.

- *Can Save Lives:* Drones can also be used as lifesavers. For example, mountain rescuers use drones in hard to reach areas. They can also make it possible to identify victims in delicate situations.

- *Saves Time:* With just a push of a button, users can fly a drone and start recording moving images to its surroundings in a lesser time. Users will no longer have to wait for a photographer or digital artist to record images. Drone photography is a dynamic and fun new type of photography.
- *Easily Deployable:* Drones can be deployed and operated with relatively minimal experience. They are becoming accessible to a wide range of healthcare purposes. They can fly lower and in more directions, allowing them to reach traditionally hard-to-access areas.

Ground-to-drone communications must be protected to prevent hackers from using their data for evil purposes. Drones can carry defibrillators to heart attack victims faster than an ambulance. A drone that could bring medical aid to people in distress or rural areas. Drones can be useful during urgent and non-urgent medical disaster relief efforts.

Other benefits of using drone in healthcare delivery include [7]:
- Increased ability to reach victims who require immediate medical attention
- Increased ability to care for the elderly
- Increases the efficiency of providing care to patients in remote locations

13.5 CHALLENGES

The rise of drones in various fields, from using them for recreational use (i.e., play toys) to mass destruction weapons (i.e., military), brings its own challenges. Restrictions on drones have limited their use in healthcare:

- *Privacy and Safety Concern:* Privacy and safety are major issues with drones. Drones can invade an individual's privacy and gather sensitive data about the person. As a relatively new technology, there are no regulations regarding drone safety. Security is an important part of patient safety. Security refers to measures used to prevent health data from unauthorized access. Many things can go wrong when an autonomous flying vehicle flies across a busy road. The widespread adoption of drone in healthcare can create security concerns for healthcare practitioners: physicians, nurses, information technology, administrators, and healthcare management.
- *Regulatory Issues:* Healthcare drones raise some regulatory issues. A major hurdle in the use of healthcare drones is the need for permission from Aviation authorities. In the United States, the Federal Aviation Administration (FAA) provides license to fly drones, provided the drone meets certain requirements. In Europe, the European Aviation Safety Agency (EASA) is the legislative body with regulatory authority over drone usage. Regulations in some nations do not allow for a drone above certain size and weight.
- *Technical Limitations*: Drones cannot carry heavy loads or deliver goods long distance like commercial planes and helicopters. Weather and electromagnetic interference (EMI) can affect the performance of drones. Drones have limited carrying potential. They are unable to provide door-to-door services, which means the technology is limited to observation benefits only. Another major drawback is that a drone is powered by batteries and can exhausted after 15 minutes of flight.

- *Hacking:* Drones make it possible for unidentifiable individuals to spy on us from a distance. The vulnerability of mobile devices in the healthcare environment makes them an attractive target for hackers [20]. Ground-to-drone communications must be protected so that hackers do not hijack the drones.

Other challenges associated with using drone in healthcare delivery include [7]:
- Maintaining the integrity of specimens during delivery
- The need for special equipment (packaging)
- Payload capacity
- Limited battery life and weight carrying constraints
- Security for controlled substances
- Regulations on a local, state and federal level
- Consumer demand

These challenges have caused healthcare applications of drone technology to be slower to develop.

13.6 CONCLUSION

The age of drones has arrived and drones are here to stay. Autonomous flying is being applied in several industries ranging from transportation to law enforcement and defense. They are emerging as a new healthcare tool that can help mitigate logistical problems and make healthcare more accessible and save lives. They are increasingly being used for healthcare purposes around the world. They now let us do things we could not do before.

Drones could ultimately be a healthcare technology game-changer. In the not-too-distant future, drones could become an essential part of the hospital delivery healthcare services within the hospital and to your home. The future of drone deliveries of all kinds in America and elsewhere rests with regulators. More information about the use of drones can be found in the book in [21] and the following related journals:
- *Journal of Unmanned Vehicle Systems*
- *Journal of Intelligent Robot System*

REFERENCES

[1] P. Kardasz et al., "Drones and possibilities of their using," *Journal of Civil & Environmental Engineering,* vol. 6, no.3, 2016.

[2] "Drones and blood transportation: Will drone impact society?" https://mbamci.com/drones-and-blood-transportation/

[3] S. H. Alsamh et al., "Survey on collaborative smart drones and Internet of things for improving smartness of smart cities," *IEEE Access,* vol. 7, 2019, pp. 128125- 128152.

[4] M. N. O. Sadiku, O. D. Olaleye, P. Oyekanmi, and S. M. Musa, "Drones in healthcare: A primer," *International Journal of Trend in Research and Development,* vol. 8, no. 1, Jan.-Feb. 2021, pp. 39-41.

[5] C. Winkler, "Sensor solutions play critical roles in enabling innovation in drone," June 2016, https://www.designworldonline.com/sensor-solutions-play-critical-roles-in-enabling-innovation-in-drones/

[6] F. Scott, "Drones in healthcare: The rise of the machines," http://csohio.himsschapter.org/sites/himsschapter/files/ChapterContent/csohio/Drones%20in%20Healtcare%20Rise%20of%20the%20Machines.pdf

[7] "A role for drones in healthcare," https://www.dronesinhealthcare.com/

[8] J. White, "How drones could revolutionize care delivery at your hospital," June 2019, http://www.healthcarebusinesstech.com/drones-care-hospital/

[9] M. Blau, "Condom drops and airborne meds: 6 ways drones could change health care," June 2017, https://www.statnews.com/2017/06/13/drones-health-care/

[10] S. J. Kim et al., "Drone-aided healthcare services for patients with chronic diseases in rural areas," *Journal of Intelligent Robotic System*, (2017) vol. 88, 2017, pp. 163–180.

[11] "Drone delivery models for healthcare," https://adalidda.com/posts/9ckvrmyhrA7Rp7zHK/drone-delivery-models-for-healthcare

[12] R. Sokullu, A. Balcı, and E. Demir, "The role of drones in ambient assisted living systems for the elderly," in I. Ganchev et al. (eds.), *Enhanced Living Environments: Algorithms, Architectures, Platforms, and Systems.* Springer, 2019, pp 295-321.

[13] P. V. de Voorde, "The drone ambulance [A-UAS]: Golden bullet or just a blank?" Resuscitation, vol. 116, July 2017, pp. 46-48.

[14] B. McCall, "Sub-Saharan Africa leads the way in medical drones," *World Report*, vol 393, January 2019, pp. 17-18.

[15] "World Bank president hails Rwanda's use of drones in healthcare delivery," http://www.xinhuanet.com//english/2017-03/22/c_136148796.htm

[16] R. Sengupta, "Drones deliver medicines in Africa," June 2019, https://www.downtoearth.org.in/news/health-in-africa/drones-deliver-medicines-in-africa-64832

[17] "Singapore to use drones to transport medicine," July 2018, http://www.healthcareasia.org/2018/singapore-to-use-drones-to-transport-medicine/

[18] R. Khan, S. Tausif, and A. J. Malik, "Consumer acceptance of delivery drones in urban areas," *International Journal of Consumer Studies*, vol. 43, no. 1 January 2019, pp. 87-101.

[19] Mario, "The pros and cons of drones (UAVs)," https://www.dronetechplanet.com/the-pros-and-cons-of-drones/

[20] A. Alexandrou, "A security risk perception model for the adoption of mobile devices in the healthcare industry," *Doctoral Dissertation*, Pace University, July 2015.

[21] T. Kille, P. R. Bates, and S. Y. Lee, *Unmanned Aerial Vehicles in Civilian Logistics and Supply Chain Management.* IGI Global. 2019.

CHAPTER 14

AMBIENT INTELLIGENCE IN HEALTHCARE

"It is not the strongest of the species that survives, nor the most intelligent, but the one most responsive to change." - Charles Darwin

14.1 INTRODUCTION

Health plays a major role in the our life. A major concern of the healthcare industry today should be how to use AI and other disruptive technologies to create the healthcare of the future. One of such technologies is ambient intelligence. The continuous advances in information technology (IT) have led to ambient intelligence, in which people are empowered through a digital environment that is sensitive, adaptive, and responsive to human needs, habits, and emotions. Ambient Intelligence is an environment that intelligently supports people inhabiting in it. It proposes a new way to interact between humans and technology.

Ambient intelligence is regarded as one of the emerging technologies that support hospitals, patients, and healthcare practitioners with the aid of artificial intelligence techniques and wireless sensor networks. The transformation of healthcare will be built around ambient intelligence, which is sensitive and responsive to the presence of people and their needs, habits, gestures, and emotions. Ambient systems can enhance the efficiency and effectiveness of medical treatment [1].

Ambient intelligence (AmI), also known as intelligent environments (IEs), refers to electronic environments that are sensitive and responsive to the presence of people (patients, doctors, nurses, and informal caregivers). Ambient describes a physical space (hospitals, clinics, and assisted living facilities, etc.) and its internal and external surroundings [2]. The ambient devices offer interfaces that are easy to use and do not require prior learning. Ambient intelligence may be regarded as a data-intensive environment that senses changes in state and responds appropriately to correct, act or alert decision makers. It is any digitized working environment that is designed with embedded technology and AI to assist people. The environment is unobtrusive, interconnected, embedded, and intelligent. The environment is sensitive to the needs of its inhabitants, and capable of anticipating their needs and behavior.

Ambient intelligence (AmI) is the vision of a future in which environments support the people inhabiting them. It refers to an intelligent, embedded, digital environment that is sensitive and responsive to the presence of people. It is intelligence gathered from a wide variety of sources in our personal environment, such as sensors, wearables, and smart devices. AmI infrastructures have emerged in healthcare for providing effective solutions. AmI requires integrating software, hardware, and networks to support humans in the environment.

This chapter provides an introduction on the use of ambient intelligence in healthcare. It begins by explaining the concept of ambient intelligence and the enabling technologies. It presents some applications of AmI. It considers AmI in the global context. It addresses the benefits and challenges of AmI. The last section concludes with comments.

14.2 CONCEPT OF AMBIENT INTELLIGENCE

Ambient Intelligence (AmI) is a new paradigm in information technology. It is simply intelligence embedded in the environment. It may be perceived as an evolution of smart environment systems. It may also be regarded as a computing paradigm wherein conventional input and output media no longer exist. This fundamentally changes the human-machine interaction: the traditional PC input and output media such as mice, keyboards, and screens are disappearing. Instead, sensors, and processors are integrated into conventional objects that harmonize with people in their living environment [3]. Figure 14.1 shows what ambient intelligence is all about [4].

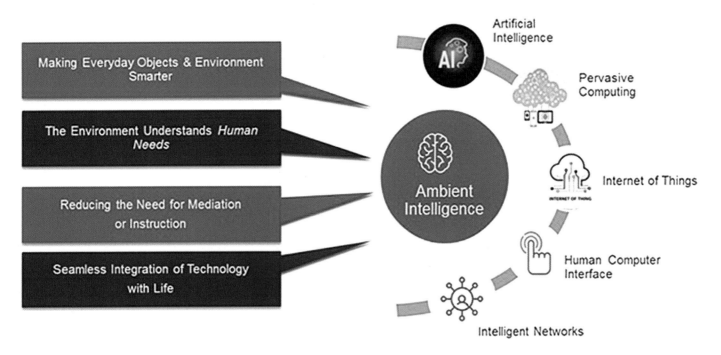

Figure 14.1 What is ambient intelligence [4].

The term "ambient intelligence" was coined by the European Commission in 2001. The concept of ambient intelligence was developed in the late 1990s in a series of internal workshops conducted by Philips (headquartered in Eindhoven, The Netherlands). The workshops were aimed at understanding the need to put the user in the center of product development. It soon became apparent that a single company could not possibly turn the broad concept of ambient intelligence into reality. Although it was originally envisioned for consumer electronics, ambient intelligence has grown into other areas such as healthcare, public, and productivity domains. AmI will be one of the key elements of the fourth industrial revolution.

Ambient intelligence (AmI) is a multi-disciplinary approach which aims to enhance the way environments and humans interact with each other. It is essentially a technology that combines Internet of things (IoT) and artificial intelligence (AI). It is intrinsically connected with AI. Intelligence refers to man's or machine's ability to learn and apply knowledge in new situations. While "artificial" refers to something made by human beings, "ambience" refers to something that surrounds us. AI and AmI are everywhere, making a big impact on our daily lives. Practically, AmI may be roughly regarded as the opposite of virtual reality. While virtual reality puts people inside a computer-generated world, AmI puts the computer inside the world to help people.

An AmI system has following characteristics [5,6]:

- *Context aware*: It can recognize the situational context of subject;
- *Personalized:* It is personalized and tailored to the needs of each individual;
- *Anticipatory:* It can anticipate the needs or desires of an individual without the conscious mediation of the individual;
- *Adaptive*: It adapts to the changing needs of individuals;
- *Ubiquity:* It is embedded and is integrated into our everyday environments;
- *Transparency:* It recedes into the background of our daily life in an unobtrusive way;
- *Intelligent:* It uses intelligence gathered from a wide variety of sources in our personal environment.

14.3 ENABLING TECHNOLOGIES

Ambient intelligence is a technology-enriched environment which involves extensive and invisible integration of technologies in our everyday lives: smart phones, tablets, wireless sensor network (Wi-Fi, Bluetooth, NFC, RFID, etc.), Internet (Facebook, WhatsApp, Twitter, You Tube, Blogs, Cloud Computing, etc.), data acquisition systems, robotic systems, communication technology, wearable devices, decision support, analytics, machine actuators, machine learning, AI, human-computer interaction (HCI), wireless sensor networks (WSNs),and other capabilities [4]. Its five components are: (1) IoT sensors, (2) human computer interactions, (3) pervasive computing, (4) AI frameworks, and (5) invisible intelligent network. Figure 14.2 shows the confluence of different areas into ambient intelligence [7].

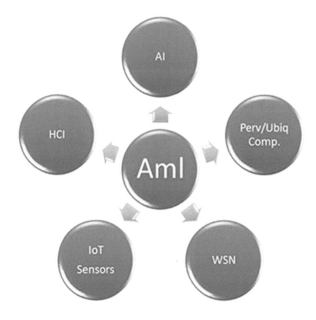

Figure 14.2 Areas related to ambient intelligence [7].

Wireless sensor networks (WSNs) are used for gathering the information needed by AmI environments. Typical examples of wireless technologies are radio frequency identification tags (RFID), Wi-Fi, ZigBee or Bluetooth [8]. Standards such as ZigBee, ZWave, Bluetooth provide wireless communication interfaces between the devices. The principal device in a WSNs is the network node. This device has RFID for the transmission and the reception of information. Sensor data is collected from several sources and later analyzed to produce accurate information.

14.4 APPLICATIONS

Ambient intelligence has several potential applications in diverse areas such as a smart home, an office, transportation, entertainment, tourism, recommender systems, safety systems, ehealth, supported living, medicine, e-learning, education, culture, entertainment, robotics, smart classrooms, and smart cities [9]. Ambient Intelligence healthcare systems are increasingly being deployed in hospitals, clinics, and nursing homes. Common healthcare applications include monitoring the status of patients with chronic diseases, assistive care, persuasive services for encouraging healthier lifestyles, rehabilitation, and emergency services. It is also applicable to patient monitoring and neuroscience research, which require large biomedical data sets. Figure 14.3 illustrates some AmI health services [5].

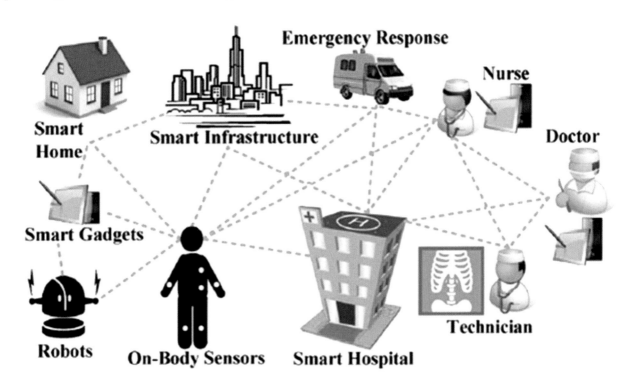

Figure 14.3 Interconnected world of AmI health service [5].

Some of these are explained as follows.
- *Health Monitoring:* Ambient intelligence enhances the quality of healthcare monitoring systems. Traditional healthcare services are inefficient to handle diseases we can prevent in advance. Today one can observe monitoring of persons in many environments. AmI for health monitoring may be an effective solution to treat elderly, disabled, and people with chronic

illness anytime, anywhere, and in an unobtrusive way with low cost. Vision-driven ambient intelligence serves as a constant and fatigue-free observer at the patient bedside. Home based care services that enable the provision of effective care within the home environment, thereby avoiding early hospitalization, which would be more cost intensive [10].

• *ALZ-MA:* This is an AmI-based multi-agent system aimed at enhancing the assistance and healthcare for Alzheimer patients. The health monitoring system embedded in the environment is useful for aged persons to check their health without entering a hospital. Ambient intelligence can assess our cognitive capability by using many sensors [11].

• *Ambient Assisted Living* (AAL): As the world's population ages, there is a driving need for assisted living solutions to help manage the lives of the elderly. Ambient assisted service anywhere and anytime is an AI-based technology that provides safe, high-quality, and independent lives for the frail and elderly to ensure their health and improve their quality of lfie. Assisted living systems must monitor, control, and interact with a number of different components of the living environment, without interfering with the lives of those being monitored [12]. Elderly and disabled people would benefit much from AmI if it is accessible. Individuals with disabilities can live independently using home automation that provides constant monitoring. In AAL environment, different ways of collecting data about its inhabitants include cameras, microphones, and other sensors. Figure 14.4 depicts the levels of abstraction in elderly in-home assistance (EHA) [13].

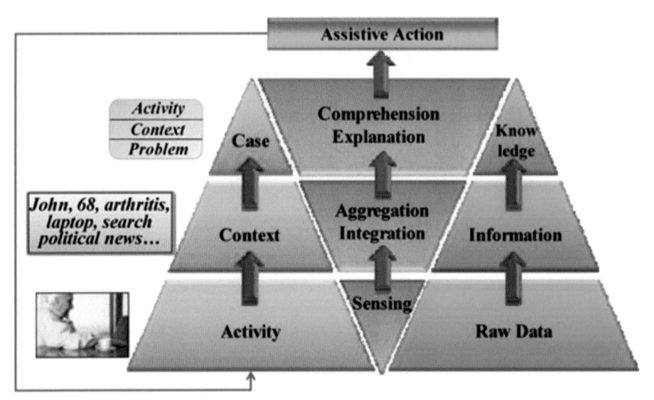

Figure 14.4 Levels of abstraction in elderly in-home assistance [13].

- *Rehabilitation:* The number of people who need rehabilitation services is continuously increasing. AmI can help meet the demand for therapeutic and rehabilitative care. It may be used to support people with special requirements. Its main role in rehabilitation is related to its ability to support the use of other assistive devices. AmI assistive tools are designed to compensate or expand the activity of a disabled person [14]. AmI would be an effective resource for rehabilitation.

- *Smart hospital:* In traditional hospitals, healthcare practitioners must navigate the hospital to gather information about patients and control their status. Ambient intelligence is capable of creating environments that are smart and proactive. These days, things are becoming smart: smart cities, smart hospital, smart environments, smart technologies, smart data, smart phones, smart rooms, smart homes, smart building, smart mobility, smart airports, smart nations, etc. A smart hospital is a smart environment that employs ambient intelligence technologies in order to augment a typical hospital room with smart features that assist both patients and medical staff. This environment allows the patient to control the environment and interact with the hospital facilities [15]. Healthcare in hospitals demands work conditions that differ from those of other sectors. Healthcare practitioners may be served by AmI through improved communications.

Other areas of application of AmI in healthcare include patient monitoring, patient identification, allergy management, collaboration with other medical specities, nursing training, emotional well-being, and cardiology [16].

14.5 GLOBAL AMBIENT INTELLIGENCE IN HEALTHCARE

The concept "ambient intelligence" was introduced by the European Commission's Information Society Technologies Advisory Group (ISTAG) in 2001. Ambient Intelligence is a new paradigm in information technology compliant with the international Integrating Healthcare Enterprise (IHE) board. AI is considered the backbone of the Ambient intelligence technology. AmI seeks to effect a significant change in the way people live their daily life. In this section, we examine how cultural, social, and environmental factors determine the evolution of ambient intelligence in different parts of the world. Although Western and Eastern cultures are different, AmI in both cultures has similar approach on assuring the safety of users. However, there are some differences which allow us to explore the idea of localized ambient and aesthetic intelligence [17].

The segment of population that will benefit most from AmI systems are the elderly and people with disabilities. It will improve important aspects of their life, especially healthcare. There is an ever growing need to provide effective and affordable care and support to the disabled and elderly. Today, the number of Europeans over 60 years represents more than 25% of the population. In the U.S., it is expected that in 2020 people aged 60 and above will represent about 1 of 6 citizens.

Chronic Disease (CD) is becoming the major causes of the death worldwide. In EU countries, cardiovascular disease is the most common cause of death. Ambient Intelligence provides noninvasive monitoring of physiological signs which can benefit patients with chronic diseases. Continuous monitoring may be obtained at various locations within or outside the hospital by RFID technology [18].

The AmI vision has been used by Philips Research laboratories to establish new and promising collaborations with other strong players in the field. Personalization and context-awareness have been some of the objectives of AmI technologies developed at Philips, which has established itself as the intellectual leader in the field of ambient intelligence [19].

14.6 BENEFITS

Ambient intelligence has the potential for vast and varied applications, bringing with it both promise and peril. Since AmI and AI are closely connected, AmI is sharing its fate and fame with AI. AmI technologies are used to support ageing-in-place and they can contribute to an increased safety and security at home. Ambient intelligence can help alleviate loneliness and work in ways that are largely non-intrusive. Other benefits include the following:

- *Technology Integration*: The main objective of ambient intelligence is to integrate technology into every aspect of our lives and to improve the quality of our life. Ambient intelligence serves humans, society, and the planet. It is a fantastic tool for improving and simplifying our everyday.
- *Monitoring:* AmI for healthcare monitoring and personalized healthcare is a promising solution to provide efficient medical services, which could substantially reduce the cost of healthcare.
- *Smart Environment:* Ambient intelligence based systems can be developed to create smart environments for user and environmental monitoring.
- *Productivity:* Ambient intelligent environment enhances the productivity and decision-making process of the healthcare facility managers, who work in complex and dynamic environments where critical decisions are constantly being made. Digital assistance through AmI can help to free healthcare practitioners so that they can have more time to take of care of patients.
- *Elderly Care*: Elderly citizens can benefit from the AmI concept. AmI technology is a tool that can provide cost-effective ways to support the elderly individuals by monitoring them in their homes. The elderly can take advantage of the use of AmI systems because they can focus on their other needs. They are given an opportunity to live more independently and for a longer time in their home rather than in healthcare facilities. Independent living of elderly can be supported with mobile-centric ambient intelligence services.

14.7 CHALLENGES

Ambient intelligence requires new software architectures that support large, distributed, and heterogeneous systems. It is beset by problems such as lack of sustainability and cost inefficiencies. The process of implementing an ambient system is a great challenge. Some other challenges include the following [20]:

- *Trust and Confidence:* AmI needs to gain the confidence and trust of the public before it can be widely adopted. Individuals should be able to trust the intelligent world that surrounds them and through which they move.
- *Security & Privacy:* Ambient Intelligences also gives rise to security and privacy concerns due the collection of large amounts of personal data involved. The success of ambient intelligence will be dictated by on how secure it can be made. Security issues are related to the health

status of the patient, who may be frail and afraid that they are more vulnerable in cases of emergency. Privacy is also a major concern as ambient intelligence becomes more prevalent and able to uniquely track people. Although monitoring of patients is of vital importance for the security of some disabled and elderly, these techniques are intrusive and must be used only with the consent of the user or his/her relatives.

- *Safety:* We are gradually moving into a new era where artificial intelligent agents become intertwined with our daily living. There is no guarantee that these agents can cooperate appropriately and safely.
- *Ethical Concern:* AmI has some serious ethical challenges. It is important for us to consider the ethical implications of using "hidden" intelligence to collect, process, analyze and share personal data. A number of questions relating to home monitoring technologies have been raised. These include questions on how much surveillance is helpful, when does technology start infringing on personal dignity, and whether home automation can improve human condition without frustrating the user.

It is challenging to manage heterogeneity of devices that are present in AmI environments. Some of other concerns are listed as follows [21]:

- *Reliability,* including manageability, predictability, and dependability.
- *Delegation of control,* including content control, system control, and accountability.
- *Social compatibility,* including transparency, knowledge sustainability, fairness, and universal access.
- *Acceptance,* including feasibility and credibility, artefact autonomy, impact on health and environment, and the relationship between man and the world.

These challenges must be addressed in order to develop flexible and evolvable AmI applications.

14.8 CONCLUSION

Ambient intelligence refers to a system and information technology that can adapt to human activities in living environment. It is an emerging field that aims to bring intelligence to our everyday environments and make those environments sensitive to the inhabitants. It is one of the recent technologies that support hospitals, patients, and healthcare professionals for personal healthcare with the aid of AI techniques and wireless sensor networks.

An ambient intelligence (AmI) revolution is already taking place. By transforming our ways of thinking and our interactions with the environment, the ambient intelligence opens up unprecedented new perspectives. The interest in ambient intelligence has increased drastically and worldwide due to the widespread use of portable devices. More information about ambient intelligence can be found in the books in [22-34] and the following closely related journals:

- *International Journal of Ambient Computing and Intelligence*
- *AI Communications*
- *Journal of Ambient Intelligence and Humanized Computing*
- *Journal of Ambient Intelligence and Smart Environment*

REFERENCES

[1] M. Bick1, T. F. Kummer, and S. Ryschka, "Determining anxieties in relation to ambient intelligence—Explorative findings from hospital settings," *Information Systems Management*, vol. 32, 2015, pp. 60–71

[2] M. N. O. Sadiku, S. M. Musa, and A. Ajayi-Majebi, "Ambient Intelligence: A Primer," *International Journal of Trend in Research and Development*, vol. 7, no. 5, August 2020, pp. 71-74.

[3] J. Esch, "A survey on ambient intelligence in healthcare," *Proceedings of the IEEE*, vol. 101, no. 12, December 2013, pp. 2467-2469.

[4] M. López et al., "The awareness of privacy issues in ambient intelligence," *Advances in Distributed Computing and Artificial Intelligence Journal*, vol 3, no 2, 2014.

[5] G. Acampora et al., "A survey on ambient intelligence in healthcare," *Proceedings of the IEEE*, vol. 101, no. 12, December 2013, pp. 2470-2494.

[6] M. N. O. Sadiku, S. M. Musa, and A. Ajayi-Majebi, "Ambient Intelligence in Healthcare," *International Journal of Trend in Research and Development*, vol. 7, no. 5, August 2020, pp. 68-70.

[7] J. C. Augusto, "Ambient intelligence: Opportunities and consequences of its use in smart classrooms," *Innovation in Teaching and Learning in Information and Computer Sciences*, vol. 8, no. 2, 2009, pp. 53-63.

[8] A. A. M. Salih and A. Abraham, "A review of ambient intelligence assisted healthcare monitoring," *International Journal of Computer Information Systems and Industrial Management Applications*, vol. 5, 2013, pp. 741-750.

[9] F. Sadri, "Ambient intelligence: A survey," *ACM Computing Surveys*, vol. 43, no. 4, October 2011.

[10] O. Aouedi, M. A. B. Tobji, and A. Abraham, "Internet of things and ambient intelligence for mobile health monitoring: A review of a decade of research," *International Journal of Computer Information Systems and Industrial Management Applications*, vol. 10, 2018, pp. 261-271.

[11] O. Garcıa e tal., " ALZ-MAS 2.0; A distributed approach for alzheimer health care," in J. M. Corchado, D. I. Tapia, and J. Bravo (eds.), *3rd Symposium of Ubiquitous Computing and Ambient Intelligence 2008*. Berlin: Springer-Verlag, 2009, pp. 76-85.

[12] A. F. Harris, R. Kooper, and R. Kravet, "Meditrina: Addressing the system-level challenges to ambient assisted living," *HealthNet'07: Proceedings of the 1st ACM SIGMOBILE International Workshop on Systems and Networking Support for Healthcare and Assisted Living Environments*, June 2007, pp. 79-82.

[13] F. Zhou et al., "A case-driven ambient intelligence system for elderly in-home assistance applications," *IEEE Transactions on Systems, Man, and Cybernetics—Part C: Applications and Reviews*, vol. 41, no. 2, March 2011, pp. 179-189.

[14] F. Morganti and G. Riva, "Ambient intelligence for rehabilitation," in G. Riva, F. Vatalaro, F. Davide, M. Alcañiz (eds.), *Ambient Intelligence*. IOS Press, chapter 15, 2005, pp. 283-295.

[15] S. Kartakis, "Enhancing health care delivery through ambient intelligence applications," *Sensors*, vol. 12, 2012, pp. 11435-11450.

[16] M. Bick, T. F. Kummer, and S. Ryschka, "Determining anxieties in relation to ambient intelligence—explorative findings from hospital settings," *Information Systems Management*, vol. 32, no. 1, 2015, pp. 60-71.

[17] C. L. Kaiyinga, D. A. Plewea, and C. Röckerb, "The ambience of ambient intelligence: An Asian approach to ambient systems?" *Procedia Manufacturing*, vol. 3, 2015, pp. 2155 – 2161.

[18] L. Pignolo et al., "Ambient intelligence for monitoring and research in clinical neurophysiology and medicine: The Mimerica project and prototype," *Clinical EEG and Neuroscience*, vol. 44, no. 2, 2013, pp. 144-149.

[19] B. de Ruyter and E. Aarts, " Ambient intelligence: visualizing the future," *Proceedings of the Working Conference on Advanced Visual Interfaces*, Gallipoli, Italy, May 2004, pp. 203-208.

[20] J. van Hoof et al., "Ageing-in-place with the use of ambient intelligence technology: Perspectives of older users," *International Journal of Medical Informatics*, vol. 80, no. 5, May 2011, pp. 310-331.

[21] E. Kosta, "Mobile-centric ambient intelligence in health- and homecare—anticipating ethical and legal challenges," *Science and Engineering Ethics*, vol. 16, no. 2, June 2010, pp 303–323.

[22] J. C. Augusto et al. (eds.), *Handbook of Ambient Assisted Living; Technology for Healthcare, Rehabilitation and Well-Being*. IOS Press, 2012.

[23] K. Curran (ed.), *Recent Advances in Ambient Intelligence and Context-Aware Computing*. Information Science Reference, 2015.

[24] E. H. L. Aarts and J. L. Encarnacao, *True Visions: The Emergence of Ambient Intelligence*. Springer, 2005.

[25] A. Salih and A. Abraham, *Ambient Intelligence Assisted Healthcare Monitoring*. LAP LAMBERT Academic Publishing, 2016.

[26] J. M. Corchado, D. I. Tapia, and J. Bravo (eds.), *3rd Symposium of Ubiquitous Computing and Ambient Intelligence 2008*. Berlin: Springer-Verlag, 2009.

[27] J. Arends et al., *Recent Advances in Ambient Assisted Living - Bridging Assistive Technologies, E-Health and Personalized Health Care*. IOS Press, 2015.

[28] A. Aztiria, J.C. Augusto, and A. Orlandini (eds.), *State of the Art in AI Applied to Ambient Intelligence*. IOS Press, 2014.

[29] H. Nakashima, H. Aghaja, and J. C. Augusto, *Handbook of Ambient Intelligence and Smart Environments*. Springer, 2010.

[30] S. Mukherjee et al., *AmIware Hardware Technology Drivers of Ambient Intelligence*. Dordrecht, The Neverlands, Springer, 2006.

[31] Y. Cai and J. Abascal (eds.), *Ambient Intelligence in Everyday Life*. Springer Verlag; 2006.

[32] G. Riva et al. (eds.), *Ambient Intelligence: The Evolution of Technology, Communication and Cognition Towards the Future of Human-Computer Interaction*. Amsterdam, The Netherlands: IOS Press, 2005.

[33] N. M. Garcia and J. J. P. C. Rodrigues, *Ambient Assisted Living*. Boca Raton, FL: CRC Press, 2015.

[34] T. Bosse et al. (eds.), Human Aspects in Ambient Intelligence: Contemporary Challenges and Solutions. Atlantis Press; 2013

CHAPTER 15

HEALTHCARE BLOCKCHAIN

"Everything will be tokenized and connected by a blockchain one day." – Fred Ehrsam

15.1 INTRODUCTION

Health is the foundation of a happy life. Healthcare is an important part of life. The healthcare industry is one of the world's largest industries and is resistant to change and innovative practices. Modern healthcare systems have become highly complex and costly. The cost of healthcare delivery is continuously rising, causing a crisis. The healthcare industry is under extreme pressure to both curb the rising cost of healthcare and provide high quality to patients. Currently, sensitive medical records lack a secure structure, causing data breaches. Blockchain technology has some interesting properties, such as its decentralized nature, immutability, decentralization, transparency, and permissionless, that may provide the solution by addressing pressing issues in healthcare [1,2]. Figure 15.1 shows how blockchain meets healthcare requirements [3]. The blockchain technology is disruptive and considered as the fourth industrial revolution that will change the world.

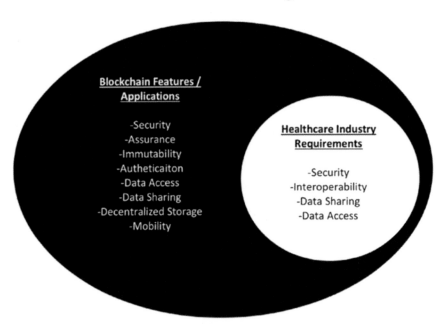

Figure 15.1 How blockchain meets healthcare requirements [3].

Blockchain (BC) consists of a shared or distributed database used to maintain a growing list of transactions, called blocks. Blockchain technology, often called the chain of trust, can support transactional applications and streamline business processes by establishing trust, accountability, and transparency. The so-called digital ledger technology was developed in 2008 by Satoshi Nakamoto, who designed it as the underpinning for the exchange of the digital cryptocurrency known as Bitcoin. BC forms the backbone of cryptocurrencies like bitcoin, Litecoin, and Ethereum. They work by keeping track of transactions in a distributed ledger.

Although blockchain was first largely applied in financial industry as the technology that allowed Bitcoin to operate, it has applications for many industries including healthcare, insurance, pharmacy, manufacturing, healthcare, e-voting, legal contracts, tourism, energy, and travel industry. Healthcare will benefit from the early work in finance and leverage blockchain applications in finance. Appling BC in healthcare serves to improve patient care. BC technology offers patients and care-givers the ability to securely share patient identity and healthcare information across platforms. Imagine a future where patients hold the keys to their healthcare passport. Imagine a better quality of care for both patients and care providers [4].

As a catalyst for change, the blockchain technology is going to change healthcare in major ways. The decentralized ledger can be used to store personal details of the patient. The main motivation for using blockchain in healthcare is to solve the data integrality, data interoperability, and privacy issues in current health systems. Blockchain eliminates the need of a middleman who plays the role of verifying transaction in the healthcare industry [5].

This chapter provides an introduction to the use of blockchain in healthcare. It begins by explaining how blockchain works. It covers the two types of blockchain. It discusses some of its applications in healthcare industry. It covers global blockchain healthcare. It addresses the benefits and challenges of blockchain in healthcare. The last section concludes with comments.

15.2 OVERVIEW OF BLOCKCHAIN

Blockchain technology is a permanent record of online transactions. It is a distributed tamper-proof database, shared, and maintained by multiple parties. It is a new enabling technology that is expected to revolutionize many industries, including healthcare. It has the potential for addressing significant healthcare issues. The BC technology allows participants to move data in real-time, without exposing the channels to theft, forgery, and malice.

The term "blockchain" refers to the way BC stores transaction data – in "blocks" that are linked together to form a "chain." The chain grows as the number of transactions increases. Since every entry is stored as a block on a chain, the care you receive is added to your personal ledger. The first Blockchain was conceived in 2008 by an anonymous person or group known as Satoshi Nakamoto, who published a white paper introducing the concept of a peer-to-peer electronic cash system he called Bitcoin [6].

At its core, blockchain is a distributed system recording and storing transaction records. In a blockchain system, there is no central authority. Instead, transaction records are stored and distributed across all network participants. Rather than having a centrally located database that manages records, the database is distributed to the networks and transactions are kept secure via cryptography. BC eliminates the need for a middleman that traditionally may facilitate such transactions.

Fundamentally, blockchains are distributed digital database that record and maintain a list of transactions taking place in real time. They may also be regarded as decentralized ledgers that sequentially record transactions or interactions among users within a distributed network. They have the following properties [7]:

- Firstly, they are autonomous. They run on their own, without any person or company in charge.
- Secondly, they are permanent. They are like global computers with 100 percent uptime. Because the contents of the database is copied across thousands of computers, if 99 per cent of the computers running it were taken offline, the records would remain accessible and the network could rebuild itself.
- Thirdly, they are secure and tamper-proof. Each record in blockchain is time stamped and stored cryptographically. The encryption used on blockchains like Bitcoin and Ethereum is industry standard, open source, and has never been broken.
- Fourthly, they are open, allowing anyone to develop products and services on them.
- Fifthly, as blockchain is a shared system, costs are also shared between all of its users.

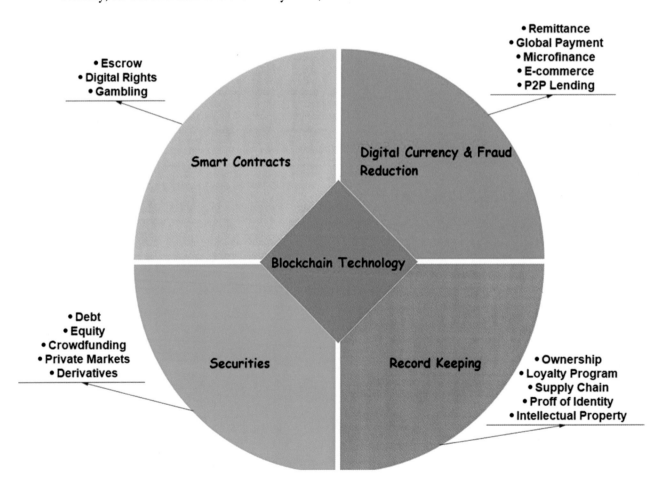

Figure 15.2 General applications of blockchain [8].

The blockchain was designed so transactions are immutable, i.e. they cannot be deleted. Thus, blockchains are secure and meddle-free by design. Data can be distributed, but not copied. When it comes to digital assets and transactions, you can put almost anything on a blockchain. Different scenarios call for different blockchains. Figure 15.2 depicts some general applications of blockchain [8].

The BC technology currently has the following features [9,10]:

1.Peer-to-Peer (P2P) Network: The first requirement of BC is a network, an infrastructure shared by multiple parties. This can be a LAN at a small scale or the Internet at a large scale. All nodes participating in a BC are connected in a decentralized P2P network. Transactions are broadcast to the P2P network. Due to some limitations of P2P networks, some vendors have provided cloud-based BCs.

2. Cascaded Encryption: A BC uses encryption to protect transaction data. Blocks are encrypted in a cascaded manner, i.e. the encryption result of the previous block is used in encrypting the current block. The BC is secured by public key cryptography, with each peer generating its own public-private key pairs.

3. Distributed Database: A BC is digitally distributed across a number of computers. Each party on a BC has access to the entire database and no single party controls the data or the information. Since BC is decentralized, there is no need for central authorizes such as banks.

4. Transparency with Pseudonymity: Each node or participant on a blockchain has a unique 30-plus-character alphanumeric address that identifies it. Users can choose to remain anonymous or provide proof of their identity to others.

5. Irreversibility of Records: Once a transaction is entered in the database and the accounts are updated, the records cannot be altered. Records on the database is permanent, chronologically ordered, and available to all others on the network.

15.3 TYPES OF BLOCKCHAINS

There are two types of blockhains: public and private. Public blockchains are cryptocurrencies such as Bitcoin, enabling peer-to-peer transactions. Private Blockchains use blockchain-based platforms such as Ethereum or blockchain-as-a-service (BaaS) platforms running on private cloud infrastructure. A private BC is an intranet, while a public BC is the Internet. Companies will be disrupted the most by public blockchains.

BCs may be permissioned or permissionless. In a permissioned BC, each participant has a unique identity. Permissionless BCs are appealing because they allow anyone to join, participate or leave the protocol execution without seeking permission from a centralized or distributed authority. However, permissionless BCs, such as Ethereum or Bitcoin, face transaction volume constraints. Both permisisoned and permisionless can be implemented in healthcare [11].

Blockchain technology is emerging and evolving. Its three generations are mentioned here. It was first proposed to support cryptocurrencies like Bitcoin, so cryptocurrency blockchains are known as Blockchain 1.0. All applications of blockchain in the financial area made possible by the union of ethereum smart contracts with digital currencies are labelled Blockchain 2.0. This generation allows customers have a transaction of stock, bill of exchange, intellectual property right or anything related to smart contract. All applications of blockchain technology referable to the wider spectrum of non-cryptocurrency-related uses are usually known as Blockchain 3.0 applications. Blockchain 3.0 applications include electronic voting, healthcare, education, identity management, and decentralized notary [12,13].

MedRec has been proposed as a novel, decentralized record management system to handle electronic health record (EHRs) using blockchain technology. It manages authentication, confidentiality, accountability, and data sharing. It enables patient data sharing and incentives for medical researchers to sustain the system [14] Healthchain is developed on the foundation of blockchain using IBM Blockchain initiative.

15.4 APPLICATIONS

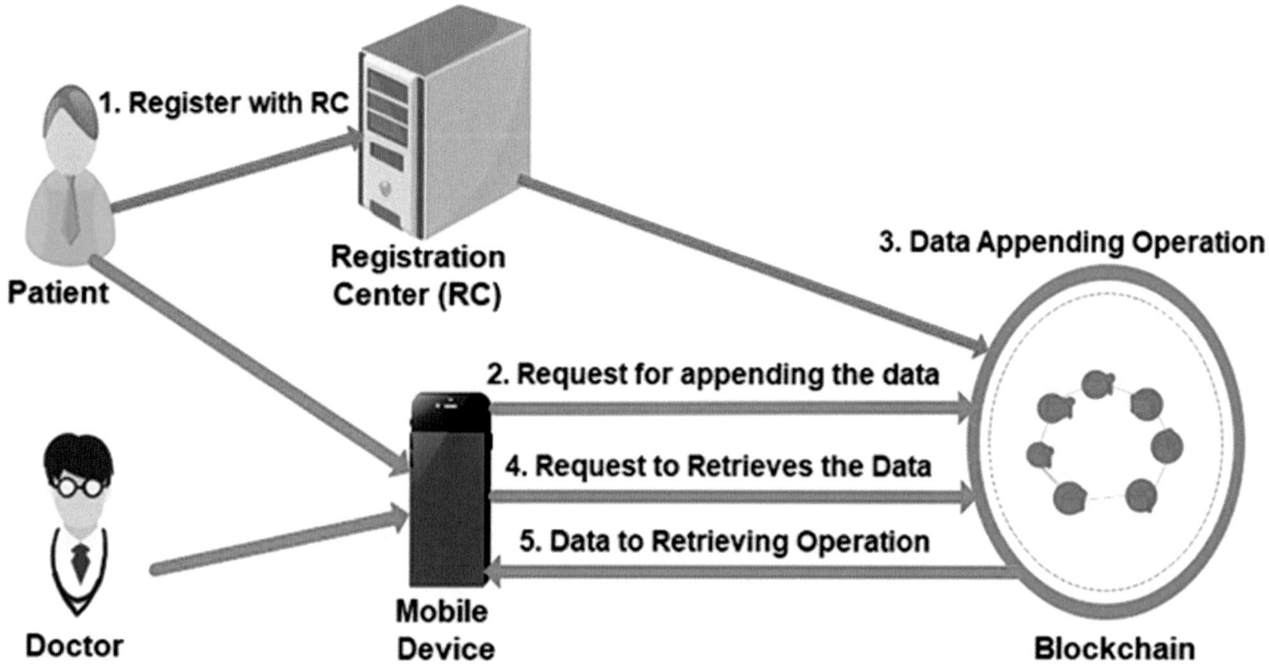

Figure 15.3 A typical blockchain healthcare system [15].

A typical blockchain healthcare system is shown in Figure 15.3 [15]. Blockchain has a wide range of applications in healthcare. It has the potential for addressing significant healthcare issues. Several areas of healthcare can be enhanced using blockchain technologies including medical records or HER systems, device tracking, clinical trials, pharmaceutical tracing, and health insurance. The following are the most likely applications [16]:

- *Medical Data Management:* Healthcare is a data-intensive industry. The healthcare industry is drowning in data— patient medical records, complex billing, clinical trials, medical research, etc. The goal of BC is to give patients and their providers one-stop access to their entire medical history across all providers. Blockchain is able to securely, privately, and comprehensively track patient health records. It makes ERHs more efficient, disintermediated, and secure. Right now, a patient's medical records are dispersed across multiple providers and organizations due to the fact the health systems are fragmented into hospitals, community clinics, general practitioners, specialists, insurance departments, etc. Patient data is one valuable asset of patients, but patients have no control of their personal data. Some of the record pieces are with the primary doctor, some with specialists, and some on devices that track one's health. Every hospital and every doctor's office has a different way of storing the electronic medical records (EMRs), also known as electronic health records (EHRs). For example, in the city of Boston alone, there are 26 different EMRs, each with its own language for representing and sharing data. This situation is costing us money, professional burnout, and sometimes even lives. Blockchain can help us assemble all of these pieces in real-time. This way care providers can have the complete medical history of the patient. For healthcare to reap the benefits of a blockchain-based medical record, it must grant access to everyone that might need patient's information [17,18]. Blockchain can also create a mechanism to access EHRs stored on the cloud.

- *Drug Development:* Blockchains can facilitate new drug development by making patient results more widely accessible. It can help reduce the counterfeit drug implications. The issue of counterfeit medicines has become increasingly pressing in view of the economic cost of the global black market and the risk to human life that comes from taking counterfeit drugs. Blockchain technology is an excellent counter to threats that are rapidly approaching (integrity-based attacks) and it is a good forward-looking tool we might deploy to address them. BC will also enable drug developers to run clinical trials and share medical samples more securely [19].

- *Clinical Trials*: Using blockchain can make clinical trials reliable at each step by keeping track and time-stamping at each phase of the trial. This could reduce waste. Another blockchain use-case would be the adoption of electronic informed consent in clinical trials. BC improves accountability and transparency in the clinical trial reporting process.

- *Data Security:* The perpetrators can steal credit card, banking information, and health records. Sensitive data must be kept safe from hackers and intruders. Blockchain technology has the potential to be the infrastructure that is needed to keep health data private and secure. It makes health information exchanges (HIE) more secure, efficient, and interoperable. BC requires no one central administrator, and it has unprecedented security benefits because records are distributed across a network that are always in sync. For example, Factom employs blockchain technology to securely store digital health records.

- *Pharmaceutical Sector:* Pharmaceutical companies need to have a very secure supply chain because of the kind of product they deal with. Blockchain in healthcare helps pharmaceutical companies create auditable, unalterable, secure, and distributed databases for storing and accessing drug trial data. Blockchain has serious implications for pharmaceutical supply chain management. By scanning the supply chain, the company's app lets patients know if they are taking falsified medicines. Through its app, the company's blockchain-based system can help prevent patients from taking counterfeit medicines. Blockchain can help overcome the increasing risks around counterfeit and unapproved drugs.

- *Medication Adherence:* This is crucial for patient safety. There are blockchain firms like Guardtime, a UK based health tech company, that are already using BC technology to ensure medication adherence.
- *Fraud Detection:* There are risks of using the digital system: fraud and forgery. Fraud detection refers to the process of verifying a document to identify any tampering with the information. Blockchain technology can be in the field of pharmacy with the purpose of detection of counterfeit and poor-quality medicinal products [20].

Other applications of blockchain healthcare include counterfeit drug prevention, validation and payment of claims, clinical trial results, outcome-based payments, reimbursement of healthcare services, exchange of health data, and supply chains [21].

15.5 GLOBAL BLOCKCHAIN HEALTHCARE

Blockchain is one of the most important and disruptive technologies in the world. It can enhance interoperability across the global market overcoming geographical boundaries. The following examples show how blockchain is being deployed around the world.

- *Estonia:* This is the first country to use blockchain on national level. This is a hot spot for digital innovation. Its healthcare system has been revolutionized by e-solutions. Blockchain has been adopted on a large scale by the Estonian government, in partnership with Guardtime, a Netherland-based data security company. The entire country is covered with a broadband connection [22].
- *Tunisia:* Tunisia is in the midst of social, political, and technological transition. As a growing economy, Tunisia encounters related concerns in their healthcare sector. Many of the healthcare issues faced by the country may be solved by the adoption of blockchain technology. The new technology will provide better patient care, improved financial management, and improved patient safety [23],
- *United States:* The healthcare industry in the US consists of complex interconnected entities. Blockchain has the potential to provide answers to many challenges facing the industry.
- *United Kingdom:* Medical records in Britain comprise non-uniform legacy paper records. This restricts doctors in their capacity to provide appropriate care.
- *China:* The blockchain industry has taken off in China, with 456 Chinese blockchain companies. China's government has stated plans to integrate blockchain technology into healthcare.

15.6 BENEFITS

The main benefits of blockchain in healthcare are data interoperability, security, efficiency, and accessibility. Ownership and privacy of data are important issues that blockchain could solve. It holds the promise to unite the disparate healthcare processes, reduce costs, improve regulatory compliance, improve patient experience, provide healthcare at lower costs, and autonomous monitoring and preventive maintenance of medical devices. It ensures the reliability of the stored data, which is determined by the fact that each record is confirmed from several sources. It provides a shared and transparent history of all the transparency, and immutability. Some of these benefits are illustrated in Figure 15.4 and explained as follows [24].

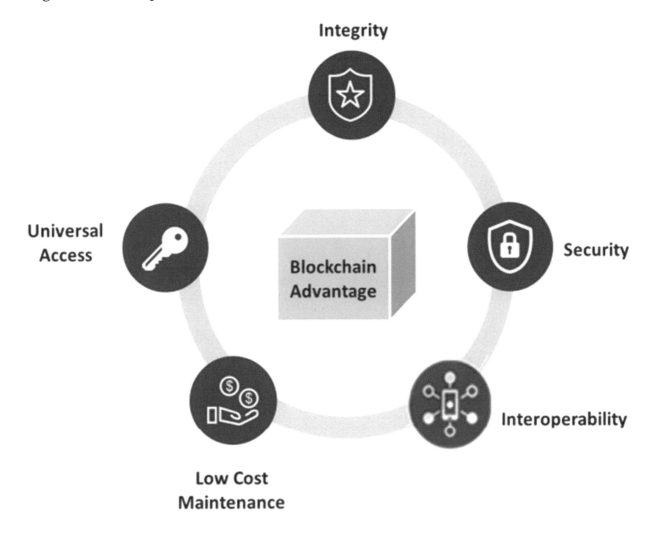

Figure 15.4 Some of the benefits of healthcare blockchain [24].

- *Security:* One of the greatest benefits of blockchain technology is that it is significantly more secure than other data storage platforms. Healthcare generates a massive amount of confidential data that can be detrimental if it falls in the wrong hands. Security should include protecting the confidentiality, integrity, and availability of sensitive data and systems. Blockchain can improve data security since it has no centralized point of failure. This makes it appealing to store and share personal health information (PHI) and stop Cyber-attacks. In January of 2017, IBM Watson partnered with the FDA to develop a secure exchange of health data utilizing blockchain technology. Although the technology provides resilience to certain types of attacks but it is by no means entirely secure. Cybercriminals deliberately target the healthcare industry for the valuable information that they store for individuals. This valuable information includes the names, birth dates, and social security numbers.
- *Interoperability*: This refers to automatic and seamless exchange of health information across health information systems. Seamless exchange of health data across healthcare systems would

be advantageous. In healthcare, interoperability allows two or more systems to exchange and use information. BC can allow improved interoperability as data across multiple systems can be exchanged and accessed simultaneously. It can enhance interoperability across a global market, eliminating system boundaries and geographic limitations. Improved interoperability or cost-effectiveness can result in efficiency [25].

- *Integrity:* BC can help bring some of the data integrity, accessibility, security, privacy, and interoperability needed by pharmaceutical companies, and eliminate falsified medication. Blockchain technology helps ensure data integrity while encryption of data enhances data security across the network. The immutability of a blockchain carries with it inherent integrity, as blocks cannot be rewritten without collaboration of a majority of nodes.
- *Universal Access:* Blockchain provides a possible future solution for data sharing. It has the potential to reduce healthcare costs, streamline business processes, and improve access to information. It ensures that required data is present at every node and is available for use to the authorized entities. Data sharing enables real-time updates. It also enables collaborative clinical decision-making in telemedicine and precision medicine. Healthcare organizations need not compete among themselves because they all have access to the same information. However, the universal availability of patient data poses some challenges [26].
- *Patient-Centered Care:* The healthcare industry is shifting from volume-based care to value-based care that promotes patient-centered care with higher quality. In patient-centered care, patients are given access to their clinical data in real-time, with a comprehensive view of their entire health history. There are ongoing efforts to explore the use of blockchain-based systems to create a more patient-centric environment wherein patients would be in control of their own health data. Interoperability is crucial to support a patient-centric model [27].
- *Cost Saving:* Blockchain technology saves the cost of mediation, as a blockchain involves no mediator. The interfacing of different systems would also save costs.

Blockchain will speed up the R&D cycle and time to market of new drugs. Blockchain technology has the potential to transform healthcare systems because it places the patient at the center of the health care ecosystem. BC is the perfect solution when we need to document a patient's health record or to secure the movement of drugs through the supply chain. BC has the potential of transmitting patent record across geographies without compromising its integrity, privacy, and security. Because of these benefits, blockchain is beginning to declare itself as a potentially game-changing technology in healthcare.

15.7 CHALLENGES

Although blockchain presents many opportunities for healthcare, it is not fully mature yet. Several technical challenges must be addressed before a healthcare blockchain can be adopted nationwide and worldwide[3,28].

- *Integration*: Integrating blockchain into healthcare is an uphill task. The success of in the healthcare industry depends on whether hospitals, clinics, and other organizations are willing to cooperate in building the technical infrastructure required. The system must facilitate the exchange of sensitive health information between patients and providers as well as exchanges between providers, while remaining secure from malicious attacks [29].

- *Data Ownership and Privacy:* Transferring data ownership from the government and organizations to patients make patients to become active agents in their own care, but it would require extensive transformation of legacy systems. Enabling direct patient involvement in controlling the secure use of their records will ensure patient privacy and potentially lead to improved health outcomes. Blockchains are not ideal for storing private information due to the transparency that they provide. Data privacy and the ability to access sensitive patient information are the key challenges in the design of a healthcare blockchain application [30]. As they work today, anyone can look at the bitcoin or Ethereum ledger at any time. If someone can identify your records on the blockchain, they know everything about your medical history. By design, BC technology is distributed and storage space is limited, so small data or metadata is preferable.
- *Regulation:* Some healthcare professionals think that blockchain deployments are held back by regulatory issues.
- *Lack of standardization:* As a relatively new technology, there is a lack of standardization. This hinders its broad acceptance and slows down development.

Critics question the scalability, security, and sustainability of blockchain technology. The security of medical devices cannot be compromised in critical care. These challenges restricting the implementation of blockchain technology need to be addressed.

15.8 CONCLUSION

Although the application of blockchain to healthcare is in its infancy, its adoption has been exponential. The blockchain revolution has made its way to the healthcare industry, and leaders are now wondering what is possible and how blockchain can solve many issues that plague the industry. BC is the technology that will possibly have the greatest impact on the next few decades; not social media or big data or robotics. Although BC is not fully mature, the healthcare system can take advantage of a beneficial disruptive innovation that will stand the test of time like blockchain.

The rapid growth in the deployment of blockchain healthcare warrants keeping a close eye on blockchain in healthcare and the opportunities it will bring. Blockchain has great potential for the future and will cause disruptive changes in the healthcare industry [31]. For more information about blockchain healthcare, one should consult the books in [32-35] and the following related journal: *Blockchain in Healthcare Today* .

REFERENCES

[1] H. S. Chen et al., "Blockchain in healthcare: A patient-centered model," *Biomedical: Journal of Scientific & Technical Research,* vol. 20, no. 3, 2019, pp. 15017-15022.

[2] M. Prokofieva and S. J. Miah, "Blockchain in healthcare," *Australasian Journal of Information Systems*, vol 23, 2019.

[3] T. McGhin et al., "Blockchain in healthcare applications: Research challenges and opportunities," *Journal of Network and Computer Applications,* vol. 135, 2019, pp. 62-75.

[4] S. Manski, "Building the blockchain world: Technological commonwealth or just more of the same?" *Strategic Change*, vol. 26, no. 5, 2017, pp. 511-522.

[5] M. N. O. Sadiku, K. G. Eze, and S.M. Musa, "Block chain technology in healthcare," *International Journal of Advances in Scientific Research and Engineering*, vol. 4, no. 5, 2018, pp. 154-159.

[6] M. N. O. Sadiku, Y. Wang, S. Cui, and S. M. Musa, "A primer on blockchain," *International Journal of Advances in Scientific Research and Engineering*, vol. 4, no. 2, February 2018, pp. 40-44.

[7] S. Depolo, "Why you should care about blockchains: the non-financial uses of blockchain technology," March 2016, https://www.nesta.org.uk/blog/why-you-should-care-about-blockchains-non-financial-uses-blockchain-technology

[8] "Security in blockchain applications," https://cri-lab.net/security-in-blockchain-applications/

[9] M. Iansiti and K. R. Lakhani, "The truth about blockchain," *Harvard Business Review*, Jan./Feb. 2017. https://hbr.org/2017/01/the-truth-about-blockchain

[10] W. T. Tsai et al., "A system view of financial blockchains," *Proceedings of IEEE Symposium on Service-Oriented System Engineering*, 2016, pp. 450-457.

[11] Z. Alhadhrami et al., "Introducing blockchains for healthcare," *Proceedings of International Conference on Electrical and Computing Technologies and Applications*, 2017.

[12] D. D. F. Maesa and P. Mori, "Blockchain 3.0 applications survey," *Journal of Parallel and Distributed Computing*, vol. 138, 2020, pp. 99-115.

[13] T. L. Nguyen, "Blockchain in healthcare: A new technology benefit for both patients and doctors," *Proceedings of PICMET '18: Technology Management for Interconnected World*, 2018.

[14] A. Azaria et al., "MedRec: Using blockchain for medical data access and permission management," *Proceedings of the 2nd International Conference on Open and Big Data*, 2016, pp. 25-30.

[15] V. Ramani et al., "Secure and efficient data accessibility in blockchain based healthcare systems," *Proceedings of IEEE Global Communications Conference*, (GLOBECOM), December 2018.

[16] B. Marr, "This is why blockchains will transform healthcare," https://www.forbes.com/sites/bernardmarr/2017/11/29/this-is-why-blockchains-will-transform-healthcare/#467c7fbe1ebe

[17] "Blockchain in health care: The good, the bad and the ugly," https://www.forbes.com/sites/forbestechcouncil/2018/04/13/blockchain-in-health-care-the-good-the-bad-and-the-ugly/#c00ec6462787

[18] D. V. Dimitrov, "Blockchain applications for healthcare data management," *Healthcare Informatics Research*, vol 25, no. 1, January 2019, pp. 51-56.

[19] "What the hell is blockchain and what does it mean for healthcare and pharma?" http://medicalfuturist.com/what-the-hell-is-blockchain-what-does-it-mean-for-healthcare-and-pharma/

[20] V. Pashkov and O. Soloviov, "Legal implementation of blockchain technology in pharmacy," *SHS Web of Conferences*, vol. 68, 2019.

[21] S. Attili, "Today's healthcare challenges and how blockchain can help solve them – Join IBM for a HIMSS17 breakfast briefing," https://www.ibm.com/blogs/insights-on-business/healthcare/todays-healthcare-challenges-blockchain-can-help-solve-join-ibm-himss17-breakfast-briefing/

[22] "Building blockchain powered trusted digital health services, Estonia," https://blockchainhealthcaretoday.com/index.php/journal/article/view/129/153

[23] A. Rejeb and L. Bell, "Potentials of blockchain for healthcare: Case of Tunisia," July 2019, https://ssrn.com/abstract=3475246

[24] V. Rawal et al., "Blockchain: An opportunity to address many complex challenges in healthcare," May 2018, https://www.healthcare.digital/single-post/2018/05/26/Blockchain-An-opportunity-to-address-many-complex-challenges-in-Healthcare

[25] A. A. Vazirani et al., "Implementing blockchains for efficient health care: Systematic review," *Journal of Medical Internet Research,* vol. 21, no. 2, February 2019.

[26] A. H. Mayer, C. A. da Costa, and R. R. Righi, "Electronic health records in a blockchain: A systematic review," *Health Informatics Journal,* 2019, pp. 1–16.

[27] P. Zhang et al., "Chapter one - Blockchain technology use cases in healthcare," *Advances in Computers,* vol. 111, 2018, pp. 1-41.

[28] M. A. Engelhardt, "Hitching healthcare to the chain: An introduction to blockchain technology in the healthcare sector," *Technology Innovation Management Review,* vol. 7, no. 10, 2017, pp. 22-34.

[29] "Who will build the health-care blockchain?" https://www.technologyreview.com/s/608821/who-will-build-the-health-care-blockchain/

[30] D. Randall, P. Goel, and R. Abujamra, "Blockchain applications and use cases in health information technology," *Journal of Health & Medical Informatics*, vol. 8, no. 3, 2017.

[31] M. Mettler, "Blockchain technology in healthcare: The revolution starts here," *Proceedings of IEEE 18th International Conference on e-Health Networking, Applications and Services*, 2016.

[32] H. Jahankhani et al. (eds.), *Blockchain and Clinical Trial; Securing Patient Data.* Springer, 2019.

[33] D. Metcalf et al., *Blockchain in Healthcare: Innovations that Empower Patients, Connect Professionals and Improve Care.* Merging Traffic Inc., 2019.

[34] P. B. Nichol, *The Power of Blockchain for Healthcare: How Blockchain Will Ignite The Future of Healthcare.* Peter B. Nichol, 2017.

[35] L. Sebastian, *Ultimate Blockchain Technology: Mega Edition – Six Books – Best Deal For Beginners in Blockchain, Blockchain Applications, Cryptocurrency, Bitcoin, Mining and Investing,* 2019.

CHAPTER 16

NANOMEDICINE

"Nanotechnology in medicine is going to have a major impact on the survival of the human race." - Bernard Marcus

16.1 INTRODUCTION

Medicine refers to the science, engineering, and practice of diagnosing, treating, curing, and preventing diseases. One of its ultimate goal is to improve the quality of life. Nanomedicine is a unique branch of medicine that involves the development and application of materials and technologies with nanometer length scales. It is the application of nanoscale materials toward the betterment of human health. It is an interdisciplinary discipline that combines nanoscience, nanoengineering, nanotechnology, nanoelectronics, and life sciences. The interest in nanomedicine spans a wide area in medicine such as drug delivery, vaccine development, antibiotics, diagnosis and imaging tools, wearable devices, implants, and high-throughput screening platforms [1].

Nanomedicine is essentially the medical application of nanotechnology to the diagnosis, management, and treatment of disease. It also can be regarded as the application of nanotechnology to healthcare. It seeks to manufacture drugs and other products that are packaged into nanoscale systems for improved delivery. The most prominent area of nanomedical research and drug approvals is cancer treatment. Although many nanomedicines are already in use or are being studied in clinical trials, many challenges and risks impede bringing these drugs to market [2].

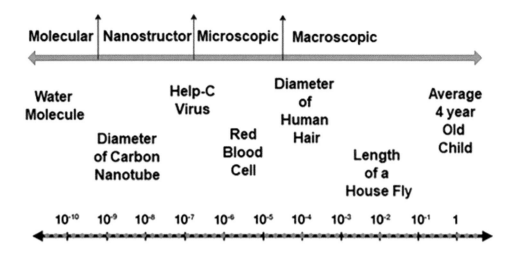

Figure 16.1 Scale of nanoparticles [3].

Nanomedicine is regarded as one of the most promising technologies of the 21st century. It is a rapidly growing area that is focused on developing nanoparticles (NPs) for different applications. Nanoparticles (NPs) are key components of nanotechnology and nanomedicine. Figure 16.1 shows the scale of nanoparticles [3]. They differ in characteristics like shape and size. Types of nanoparticles and their biomedical applications are shown in Figure 16.2 [4]. They are being developed to diagnose and treat various diseases. Some of the nanoscale materials have shape-dependent optical, electronic, and magnetic properties. Nanoparticles such as graphene, carbon nanotubes, and tungsten disulfide are being used in bone tissue engineering applications [5]. Applications for NPs include use in vaccinations, magnetic resonance imaging, pathogen detection, protein identification, DNA structure probing, and tissue engineering. Trials applying nanoparticles on catheters, hand gels, and therapeutic vaccines have been conducted.

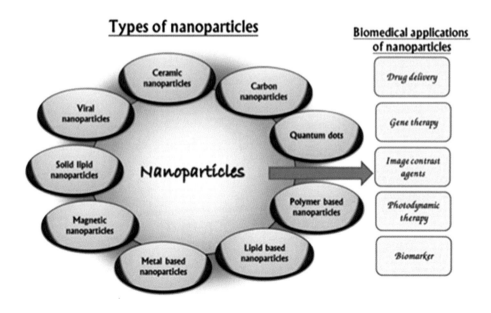

Figure 16.2 Types of nanoparticles and their biomedical applications [4].

This chapter provides an introduction to nanomedicine. It starts with the basics of nanobiotechnology and nanomedicine. It covers some of the applications of nanomedicine. It highlights some of its benefits and challenges. The last section concludes with some comments.

16.2 OVERVIEW OF NANOMEDICINE

Techniques are now available which make it possible to manipulate materials on the atomic or molecular scale to produce objects which are no more than a few nanometres in diameter. The processes used to make and manipulate such materials are known as *nanotechnology*, the materials or objects themselves are called *nanomaterials*, and the study and discovery of these materials is known as *nanoscience*.

Nanotechnology has been introduced in our daily routine. This revolutionary technology has been applied in multiple fields through an integrated approach. Nanotechnology, the engineering of atomically precise structures, has come a long way. Now nanomedicine, a marriage of nanotechnology and medicine, is taking the place of nanotechnology in the fight against unmet diseases. Its aim is preserving and improving human health using engineered nanoparticles and nanodevices. The delivery and targeting of pharmaceutical, therapeutic, and diagnostic agents are at the forefront of research in nanomedicine.

Richard Feymann, the Nobel Prize-winning physicist, introduced the world to nanotechnology in 1959. Nanotechnology involves the manipulation of atoms and molecules at the nanoscale so that materials have new unique properties. Nanotechnology is a multi-disciplinary field that includes biology, chemistry, physics, material science, and engineering. It is the science of small things—at the atomic or nanoscale level [6].

As mentioned earlier, nanomedicine is an offshoot of nanotechnology, the engineering of tiny machines. The control of structures at the nanometer level has allowed nanotechnology to be distinct from other traditional science fields. Nanomedicine is different from traditional medicine in that it potentially touches a wide range of social, ethical, and legal issues. Developing components on the nanoscale allows engineers and scientists to take advantage of physical, chemical, and biological interactions that are not feasible on larger size scales. Nanotechnology has made it possible to deliver drugs to specific cells using nanoparticles. It may be used as part of tissue engineering to help reproduce or repair damaged tissue. It has produced major advances in areas of energy, food, and agriculture.

The characterization of nanomedicine is necessary to understand its behavior in the human body. One way of characterizing nanomedicine is by "tools", "materials", "devices" and "intelligent materials and machines." Compared to conventional medicine, nanomedicine is much better at precise targeting and delivery systems.

16.3 APPLICATIONS

The development of nanomedicine has the potential to revolutionize both diagnostics and therapies. Research in nanomedicine covers a wide range of areas including drug delivery, vaccine development, diagnosis and imaging tools, wearable devices, implants, high-throughput screening, cancer, diabetes, cardiovascular and respiratory diseases, immunological and infectious diseases, and musculoskeletal disorders. Although there are many applications of nanomedicines, there are concerns about their potential side effects when they are used in humans. Success in animal models of disease does not guarantee efficacy in patients [7].

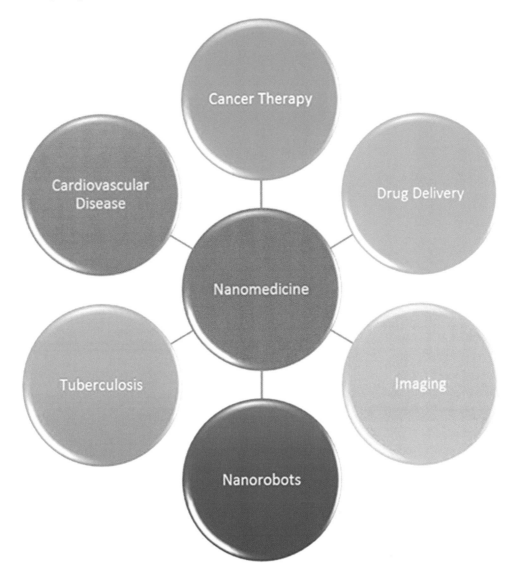

Figure 16.3 Some application areas of nanomedicine.

The most active areas of nanomedical research and development are shown in Figure 16.3 and explained as follows.

- *Cancer Therapy:* Cancer is known as one of the leading causes of death. It is a group of diseases characterized by uncontrolled cell growth. Traditional cancer treatments are limited to surgery, radiation, and chemotherapy. All three methods cause damage to healthy tissues. Nanomedicine is poised as the future of cancer treatment [8]. Application of nanotechnology in cancer is often called nanooncology. Figure 16.4 shows nanoparticles in cancer management [9]. Nanomedical products are prominently used is in the treatment of cancers. The small size of nanoparticles (5 to 100 nanometers) endows them with properties that can be very useful in oncology. Nanoparticles can be designed to deliver anti-cancer drugs directly to tumor cells while leaving healthy cells alone. Nanomedicine is capable of safely treating cancer within the pediatric population. Nanomedicine for cancer therapy is advantageous over traditional medicine because it has the potential to enable the preferential delivery of drugs to tumors, owing to the enhanced permeability and retention effect [10]. Cancer nanomedicines have been envisioned to overcome the pharmacokinetic limitations associated with traditional drugs. Successful nanomedicines for cancer treatments include Abraxane, Depocyt, Oncospar, Doxil, and Neulasta.

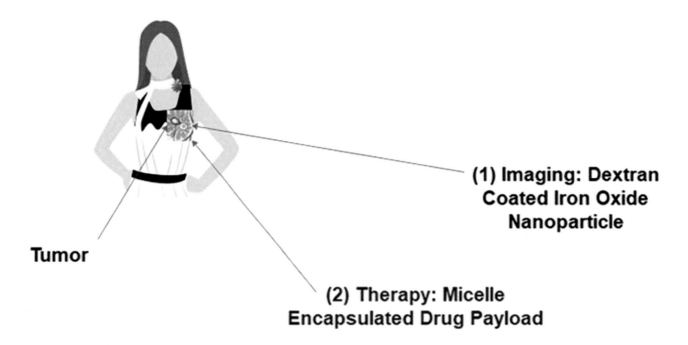

(1) Imaging: Dextran Coated Iron Oxide Nanoparticle

Tumor

(2) Therapy: Micelle Encapsulated Drug Payload

Figure 16.4 Nanoparticles in cancer management [9].

- *Drug Delivery:* The innate properties of nanomaterials have brought many benefits in the pharmaceutical development. It is challenging within the pharmaceutical industry to locate drugs more efficiently to their diseased targets within the human body. Nanoparticles used for drug delivery are usually in the nanometer range. They can be engineered to package and transport drugs directly to where they are needed, enabling more precise targeting with a controlled release. The targeting property of nanoparticles is dictated by certain factors such as particle size, surface charge, and surface modification. Nanomedicines offer many advantageous properties for drug innovation and development: increased solubility/bioavailability, better safety and efficacy profile, targeting specific tissues, crossing biological barriers that conventional products cannot bypass, extended drug exposure with a larger therapeutic window, and other impressive features [11,12].
- *Imaging:* Traditional clinical imaging methods are associated with high costs, low sensitivity, and spatial resolution. Nanoparticles can be used for imaging of diseased cells. Nanotechnologies already offer the possibility of intracellular imaging through attachment of quantum dots. Image-guided nanomedicine can deliver nanoparticles locally using non-invasive imaging. Medical image-guided interventional oncology approaches should be one of the promising solutions for current nanomedicine [13].

- *Nanorobots*: One of early dreams of nanomedicine is the possibility of using tiny nanorobots and related machines to design, manufacture, and perform cellular repairs in the human body at the molecular level. Robots can be programmed to perform routine autonomous surgery inside the human body. Nanomedicine would make use of nanorobots and nanodevices as miniature surgeons. It can also make use of nanorobots (planted in the body) to repair or detect damages and infections. Nanorobots can be introduced into the body to repair or detect damages and infections. Although medical nanorobots are just theory, there is evidence that they are buildable.
- *Tuberculosis:* This is the second leading cause of death from an infectious disease worldwide. Nanomedicines have the potential to improve TB treatment outcomes by providing therapies with reduced drug doses [14].
- *Cardiovascular disease* (CVD): This is another leading cause of death and disability worldwide. It is comprised of a group of disorders affecting the heart and blood vessels of the human body. Nanomedicine has emerged as a potential strategy in addressing challenges encountered in the treatment of CVD. It offers novel tools with high efficacy for biomedical applications, such as radiological imaging, vascular implants, gene therapy, tissue regeneration in myocardial infarction, and targeted delivery systems [15].

Other application of nanomedicine include tissue engineering, respiratory diseases, lab-on-a-chip, regenerative medicine, personalized medicine, rheumatoid arthritis, neuropathic pain, pulmonary diseases, reproductive healthcare, and implanted devices. Nanomedicines have the potential to address challenges encountered in the treatment of cardiovascular disease, tuberculosis, diabetes, and hematological malignancies.

16.4 NANOMEDICINE FOR GLOBAL HEALTHCARE

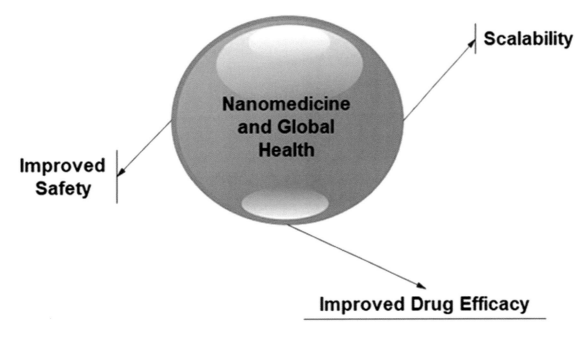

Figure 16.5 Nanomedicine in global health [16].

Nanomedicine refers to the application of nanotechnology for medical purposes. In spite of modern advances, a wide range of diseases continually afflict the global population. The prevalence of communicable and noncommunicable diseases continues to be a major challenge for global health and worldwide commercialization of nanomedicines. In addition to this, the benefits and risks of nanomedicine have led to global indecisiveness regarding a suitable approach for regulating it. Figure 16.5 depicts nanomedicine in global health [16]. We now consider nanomedicine in the following countries:

- *United States:* Applications of nanotechnology for treatment, diagnosis, monitoring, and control of biological systems has recently been referred to as "nanomedicine" by the US National Institutes of Health. Globally, research and development on nanomedicine have been dominated by developed nations of Europe and United States of America. The US is leading nanomedicine research on delivery systems and clinical development of nanodrugs [17]. A significant number of FDA-approved therapeutics, medical devices, imaging agents, and diagnostic devices utilizing nanomaterials have already become available, advancing healthcare.

- *European Union:* Europe has clearly recognized the potential of nanomedicine since an early stage. The use of nanotechnology in the development of new medicines is now part of R&D R&D in the EU. Nanotechnology has been recognized as a key enabling technology, capable of providing innovative solution to address unmet medical needs. The European Commission regards nanomaterial as a natural or manufactured material comprising particles with one or more external dimensions is in the size range of 1–100 nm. The European Committee for Standardization is considering the possibility of introducing nanotechnology standards on quality, safety and efficacy of nanoproducts. The nanomedicine market in EU is composed by nanoparticles, liposomes, nanocrystals, nanoemulsions, and nanocomplexes. It will take some time for nanomedicine to be introduced in the clinical practice in all EU countries [18]. France is a nation where the medical development of nanomedicine is significant, like Germany, the United Kingdom, and Spain.

- *Canada:* In Canada, healthcare is a growing common concern for governments, taxpayers, and the citizens. Canadian legislations are not sufficiently responsive to the challenges of nanomedicine applications. Health Canada is referring to the existing medical system to regulate nanomedicine applications. Under the Canadian regulation, medical devices are categorized into four classes: Class I, Class II, Class III, and Class IV, where Class I represents the lowest risk and Class IV represents the highest risk [19].

- *Africa:* Research efforts on nanomedicine by African researchers has revealed promising approaches for improving treatments of Poverty Related Diseases (PRD), such as tuberculosis (TB), malaria, and HIV. Challenges in drug development towards PRD are considered to be a critical issue in African nations. As such, nanomedicine can play a crucial role towards PRD in Africa, with technologies aimed at targeting issues such as poor solubility and limited bioavailability of medications. In order to accelerate the global contribution of African nations in the field of nanotechnology, the Nanosciences African Network (NANOAFNET) was established in 2005, engaging around 27 African nations. South Africa is one of the nations engaged in nanomedicine research and product development on the continent [20,21].

- *Australia:* In Australia, nanomedicine is regarded as a type of medicine and nanomedical products as a type of therapeutic goods. In Australia, the National Industrial Chemicals Notification and Assessment Schemes (NICNAS) is primarily responsible for regulating the industrial use of nanomaterials. Standards Australia (SA) and Friends of the Earth (FoE) are programs that are related to nanotechnology, which are yet to be implemented. While Australia is eager to encourage nanomedicine production, it requires a regulatory framework that enables companies to produce high-quality nanomedicines and be accountable for mitigating the potential negative impacts of their products [22].

- *Japan:* This nation is breaking ground in areas the rest of the world will soon be addressing: old age, cancer, neuroscience. Japan has invested heavily into pursuing the dream of invisible devices, working from within to detect, diagnose, and treat. Multidisciplinary teams are designing micelles targeted to the right areas of the body to deliver drugs where and when they are needed [23].

- *India:* In India, nanomedicine is still at a technology level with major research and developed concentrated in the academia. The Indian government has been funding R&D in nanomedicine with the intention to address specific societal needs and to be a forerunner in this area. The Department of Science and Technology (DST) established a Nanomission program in 2007 to foster basic research, strike international collaborations, and strengthen the capacity for creating nanoenabled technologies in India. Other government organizations followed suit in funding nanomedicine projects. It is anticipated that more nanomedicine products would be released in the Indian market in the next few years [24].

16.5 BENEFITS

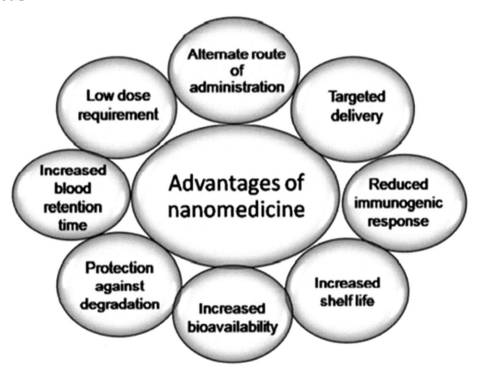

Figure 16.6 Some advantages of nanomedicine [25].

Nanomedicine is disease centered, attempting to do better what physiology, pathology, and the various medical sciences have been doing so far. It has the goal of providing cost effective novel therapies and diagnostics. A major benefit of using nanoscale for medical technologies is that smaller devices are less invasive and can possibly be implanted inside human body. The nanoscale physical properties afford the potential for biomedical applications. Some benefits of nanomedicine are illustrated in Figure 16.6 [25].

- *Various Treatments:* The application of nanomedicine, particularly in cancer treatment, promises to have a profound impact on healthcare. Nanomedicines are also used for treatment of cardiovascular, respiratory, hematological, auto-immune, and infectious diseases.
- *Improve Solubility:* Nanoparticles can help with the solubility of drugs. Due to their tiny size, nanomedicines can readily target difficult-to-reach sites with improved solubility and reduced adverse effects.
- *Targeted Drug Delivery:* Targeting drugs to particular organs or tissues is becoming popular in medicine. Nanomedicine enables for cell-targeted drug delivery, whereby medications can be more efficiently delivered to the site of action using nanotechnology. Drugs could be specifically delivered to organs, tumors, and cells by direct targeting, which can be active or passive. For example, a tumor antigen found on malignant cells can be targeted. Tumor targeting drugs are being developed. A recent first-in-human pilot studies have successfully used both passive and active targeting agents for image-guided surgery of human tumors.
- *Drug Development*: Nanomedicine has been successful through the development of new drug products such as Doxil and Abraxane. It has many impressive applications in drug product development and research since it offers flexible and fast drug design and production.

16.6 CHALLENGES

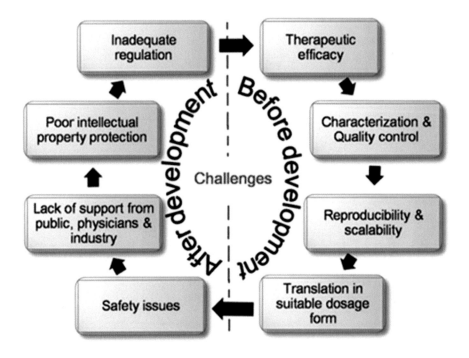

Figure 16.7 Some challenges facing nanomedicine [25].

The nanomedicine research is at a very early stage of development and many challenges need to be overcome. The main drawback of nanomaterials is the difficulty to reproduce all the complex interactions in the human body between sub-cellular levels, cells, organs, tissues and membranes. Nanomedicines present a wide range of technological, scientific, and legal challenges. There are also current challenges in manufacturing, characterization, and regulation. Some nanotechnological-based drug can be toxic and not biodegradable. Nanomedicines need to pass through stringent clinical trials to ensure safety and minimize risks. Patient backgrounds constitute the greatest of challenges for new technologies in term of improving bioavailability and dosage. Some challenges facing nanomedicine are illustrated in Figure 16.7 [25].

- *Privacy and Ethics:* In using nanomedicine, ensuring privacy and confidentiality is of utmost importance. The protection and maintenance of health information of the patient is an ethical issue. For example, applications of nanotechnology to RFID tags raise privacy concerns, particularly given the expected proliferation of tags (what does this actually mean?). There is a need for a forum to discuss the potential effects of nanomedical products including toxicity [26].

- *Uncertainties:* There are a lot uncertainties concerning safety and ethics as it pertains to nanomedicine. This may cause innovators to stay close to what is approved and already on the market. Investors are very cautious about making large investments in nanomedicine partly because they are concerned about whether the FDA will be stringent in regulating nanomedicines. Some critics have urged government agencies and private companies to proactively address the ethical, social, and regulatory aspects of nanomedicine.

- *Lack of Regulations:* There is currently a lack of a globally accepted approach for regulating nanomedical products and this has some serious consequences. FDA is being asked to develop regulatory guidelines that are specific to nanomedical products since current FDA regulations were written before the advent of nanotechnology. The potential risks of nanomedicine should be openly researched, debated, and regulated.

Because of these challenges, nanomedical products currently occupy only a tiny niche of the biotech market.

16.7 CONCLUSION

Nanomedicine is an interdisciplinary research field that results from the application of nanotechnology to medicine. It is focused on medical intervention at the molecular scale. It has the potential to address many of the challenges facing global healthcare in the future. Despite the variety of challenges that impede the development of nanomedicines, research and investments are expected to increase, causing them to become part of mainstream medicine in the future. Nanomedicine will lead to many more exciting medical breakthroughs. The full promise of nanomedicine will perhaps not arrive until after the development of programmable medical nanomachines and nanorobots.

It is crucial for our future medical physicians to have a solid understanding of the potential for nanomedicine to revolutionize therapeutics and diagnostics. There is a need for more formal interdisciplinary training to support the rapidly developing field of nanomedicine. Although many impressive achievements have been made on nanomedicine, there is much more to learn. Nanomedicine will change medicine greatly in the coming decades. More information about nanomedicines can be found in the books in [7, 27-45] and the following journals on the topic:

- *Nanomedicine*
- *Nanomedicine Journal*
- *Nanomedicine: Nanotechnology, Biology and Medicine*
- *International Nano Letters*
- *Global Journal of Nanomedicine*
- *Nanomedicine Research Journal*
- *Journal of Nanomedicine & Nanotechnology*
- *International Journal of Nanomedicine*
- *Journal of Interdisciplinary Nanomedicine*
- *American Journal of Nanotechnology & Nanomedicine*
- *The Open Nanomedicine and Nanotechnology Journal*
- *Advances in Nanomedicine and Nanotechnology Research*
- *Annals of Nanomedicine and Nanotechnology*
- *Archives of Nanomedicine: Open Access Journal*
- *Journal of Nanoscience, Nanomedicine & Nanobiology*
- *Journal of Nanotechnology: Nanomedicine & Nanobiotechnology*

REFERENCES

[1] B. Pelaz et al., "Diverse applications of nanomedicine," *ACS Nano*, vol. 11, no. 3, 2017, pp. 2313–2381.

[2] M. N. O. Sadiku, T. J. Ashaolu, and S. M. Musa, "Nanomedicine: A primer," *International Journal of Trend in Research and Development*, vol. 6, no. 1, Jan.-Feb. 2019, pp. 267-269.

[3] "Explainer: What is nanomedicine and how can it improve childhood cancer treatment?" May 2017, https://theconversation.com/explainer-what-is-nanomedicine-and-how-can-it-improve-childhood-cancer-treatment-69897

[4] R. Gaurab et al., "Nanomedicine: Therapeutic applications and limitations," in S. Soni, A. Salhotra, and M. Suar (eds.), *Handbook of Research on Diverse Applications of Nanotechnology in Biomedicine, Chemistry, and Engineering*. Hershey, PA: IGI Global, 2015, chapter 5, pp. 64-86.

[5] "Nanomedicine," *Wikipedia*, the free encyclopedia https://en.wikipedia.org/wiki/Nanomedicine

[6] M. N.O. Sadiku, M. Tembely, and S.M. Musa, "Nanotechnology: An introduction," *International Journal of Software and Hardware Research in Engineering*, vol. 4, no. 5, May. 2016, pp. 40-44.

[7] S. Soni, A. Salhotra, and M. Suar, *Handbook of Research on Diverse Applications of Nanotechnology in Biomedicine, Chemistry, and Engineering*. Hershey PA: Engineering Science Reference, 2015.

[8] R. Sebastian, "Nanomedicine - the future of cancer treatment: A review," *Journal of Cancer Prevention & Current Research*, vol. 8, no. 1, 2017.

[9] O. Lloyd-Parry et al., "Nanomedicine applications in women's health: State of the art," *International Journal of Nanomedicine*, vol. 13, 2018, pp. 1963–1983.

[10] R. K. Jain and T. Stylianopoulo, "Delivering nanomedicine to solid tumors," *Nature Reviews*, vol. 7, Nov. 2010, pp. 653-664.

[11] B. Flühman et al., "Nanomedicines: The magic bullets reaching their target?" *European Journal of Pharmaceutical Sciences,* vol. 128, Feb. 2019, pp. 73-80.

[12] S. B. Somwanshi et al., "Nanomedicine drug delivery system," *Asian Journal of Biomedical and Pharmaceutical Sciences*, vol. 3, 2013, pp. 9-16.

[13] D. H. Kim, "Image-guided cancer nanomedicine," *Journal of Imaging,* vol. 4, no. 18, 2018.

[14] A. Dube et al., "State of the art and future directions in nanomedicine for tuberculosis," *Expert Opinion on Drug Delivery*, vol. 10, no. 12, October 2013, pp. 1725-1734.

[15] A. Trisolino, "Nanomedicine: Governing uncertainties," *Master's Thesis,* University of Toronto, 2010.

[16] Z. M. Binsalamah et al., "Nanomedicine in cardiovascular therapy: Recent advancements," *Expert Review of Cardiovascular Therapy*, vol. 10, no. 6, 2012, pp. 805-816.

[17] N. Tsai et al., "Nanomedicine for global health," *Journal of Laboratory Automation,* vol. 19, no. 6, 2014, pp. 511–516.

[18] S. M. Moghimi, "Nanomedicine: Current status and future prospects," *The FASEB Journal,* vol. 19, March 2005, pp. 311-330.

[19] S. Soares et al., "Nanomedicine: Principles, properties, and regulatory issues," *Frontiers in Chemistry*, vol. 20, August 2018.

[20] T. Saidi, J. Fortuin, and T. S. Douglas, "Nanomedicine for drug delivery in South Africa: A protocol for systematic review," *Systematic Reviews*, vol. 7, 2018.

[21] M. Saravanan et al., "Barriers for the development, translation, and implementation of nanomedicine: An African perspective," *Journal of Interdisciplinary Nanomedicine*, vol. 3, no. 3, September 2018, pp. 106-110.

[22] M. M. Rahim, "Nanomedicine regulation in Australia," *Alternative Law Journal*, vol. 44, no. 2, 2019, pp. 133–137.

[23] "Nanomedicine in Japan," November 2018, https://www.nature.com/collections/zmpvwjpfpd

[24] P. Bhatia,, S. Vasaikar, and A. Wali, "A landscape of nanomedicine innovations in India," *Nanotechnology Reviews,* vol. 7, no. 2, 2018, pp. 131–148

[25] P. Bidve et al., "Emerging role of nanomedicine in the treatment of neuropathic pain," *Journal of Drug Targeting,* vol. 28, no. 1, 2020, pp. 11-22.

[26] F. Allhoff, "The coming era of nanomedicine," *The American Journal of Bioethics,* vol. 9, no. 10, 2009, pp. 3-11.

[27] A. K. Mishra, *Nanomedicine for Drug Delivery and Therapeutics.* Scrivener/Wiley Publishing, 2013.

[28] T. Webster (ed.), *Nanomedicine: Technologies and Applications.* Woodhead Publishing, 2012.

[29] S. Brenner, *The Clinical Nanomedicine Handbook.* Boca Raton, FL: CRC Press, 2014.

[30] D. Pan (ed.), *Nanomedicine: A Soft Matter Perspective.* Boca Raton, FL: CRC Press, 2015.

[31] M. Hehenberger, *Nanomedicine: Science, Business, and Impact.* Pan Stanford Publishing, 2015.

[32] R. Burgess, *Understanding Nanomedicine: An Introductory Textbook.* Singapore, Pan Standard Publishing, 2012.

[33] K. K. Jain, *The Handbook of Nanomedicine.* Humana Press, 3rd edition, 2017.

[34] M. Sebastian et al. (eds.), *Nanomedicine and Cancer Therapies.* Apple Academic Press, 2013.

]35] A. M. Nyström et al., *Update on Polymer Based Nanomedicine.* Smithers Rapra, 2012.

[40] S. Bhattacharjee, *Principles of Nanomedicine.* Jenny Stanford Publishing, 2019.

[41] A. Kumar et al. (eds.), *Nanomedicine in Drug Delivery*. Boca Raton, FL : CRC Press, 2013.

[42] V. Torchilin and M. M. Amiji (eds.), *Handbook of Materials for Nanomedicine*. Pan Stanford Publishing, 2011.

[43] L. A. Le, R. J. Hunter, and V. R. Preedy (eds.), *Nanotechnology and Nanomedicine in Diabetes*. Boca Raton, FL: CRC Press, 2012.

[44] C. R. Martin et al. (eds.), *Nanomedicine and the Nervous System*. Science Publishers, 2012.

[45] N. A. Monteiro-Riviere and C. L. Tran, *Nanotoxicology: Progress Toward Nanomedicine*. Boca Raton, FL: CRC Press, 2nd edition, 2014.

CHAPTER 17

VIRTUAL AND AUGMENTED
REALITY IN HEALTHCARE

*"VR at its best shouldn't replace real life, just modify it, giving us
access to so much just out of reach physically, economically. If you
can dream it, VR can make it."* — Matthew Schnipper

17.1 INTRODUCTION

The effectiveness of the healthcare system is highly dependent on its use of cutting-edge technologies. Virtual reality (VR) and augmented reality (AR) technologies offer feasible solutions to the many challenges of the healthcare system. They are two contemporary simulation models that are used in different areas in healthcare and medicine. They can drastically affect the overall effectiveness and efficiency of the healthcare services. Implementing VR and AR in healthcare system can be game-changing.

Human beings are visual creatures. Both hearing and seeing are central to our sense of space. As we've been spending an increasing amount of time in front of computers, the need for exploring more of the role of virtual environments needs to be increased as well. Virtual reality is the key technology for experiencing sensations of sight, hearing and touch of the past, present, and future.

Virtual reality (VR), also known as virtual environment, is a computer simulation system that can create and simulate virtual worlds. It promises to extend human experience to new possibilities. Virtual reality has existed in various forms since the late 1960s. Since then, VR has played a role in the automobile and military sectors.

Mankind has senses for interacting with the environment. Advances in technology has made the acquisition, recording, and manipulation of virtual 3D data technically affordable. Augmented Reality (AR) is any case in which a real environment is "augmented" or "enhanced" by means of virtual (computer graphic) objects. It is a visualization technique that superimposes computer generated data (such as text, video, graphics, and GPS data) on top of the real-world view.

Augmented reality (AR) refers to technology that overlays information and virtual objects on real-world scenes in real-time. With the help of advanced AR technologies, the information about the real-world surrounding the user becomes interactive. AR is rapidly becoming popular because it brings elements of the virtual world into our real world, thereby enhancing one's perception of reality and the things we see, hear, and feel. AR apps are being developed at a rapid pace for many industrial applications. Many developers, such as Apple and Google, are creating powerful tools for augmented reality apps.

This chapter provides an introduction on the use of virtual reality and augmented reality in healthcare. It starts with explaining the basic concepts of VR and AR technologies. It considers the relationship between VR and AR. This is followed by covering some specific applications areas of VR and AR in healthcare. It addresses global augmented reality and virtual reality in healthcare. It highlights the benefits and challenges of VR and AR in healthcare. The last section concludes with comments.

17.2 CONCEPT OF VIRTUAL REALITY

The term "virtual reality" essentially means "near-reality." Virtual reality has been known by different names such as synthetic environment, cyberspace, artificial reality, virtual environments, and simulator technology. The two terms, "virtual reality" and "cyberspace," are often used interchangeably. A cyberspace may be regarded as a networked virtual reality. Virtual reality is a simulated experience that can be similar to or different from the real world. It is a computer generated, 3D environment that completely immerse the senses of sight, sound, and touch. The complete immersion of the senses literally overwhelms users, totally engrossing them in the action [1].

Virtual reality (VR) describes a three-dimensional (3D), computer generated environment which can be explored and interacted with by a person. Once entered, it becomes reality to the person. Instead of viewing a screen in front of them as when using traditional interfaces, users are immersed and able to interact with 3D worlds.

Virtual reality is the simulation of a real environment using visual, auditory, and other stimuli. It involves using computer technology to create a simulated environment. VR technology creates an enjoyable, interactive world for the user. It has a variety of applications from education to entertainment. Although there are limitations to most VR systems, VR remains a powerful tool for studying the interaction between perception and action.

Based on data entered by programmers, computers create virtual environments by generating 3D images (3rd time repeating this sentence). Users can view these images by using a head-mounted device, which can be a helmet or goggles. Mobile VR glasses enable users to be present in any environment they want at any time and at any place. Users may use a joy stick or track ball to move through the virtual environment. A person using virtual reality equipment can dive into a complete, fully immersive 3D environment, look around the artificial world, move around in it, and interact with virtual objects. The virtual environment can be viewed using a cell phone screen, monitor, projector, or head-mounted display (HMD). As the person is immersed in the computer-generated environment, the brain is deluded into thinking the virtual world is reality.

VR has three main characteristics [2]: interaction, immersion, and imagination. Interaction refers to the natural interaction between the user and the virtual scene. Immersion means that the user feel that they are part of the virtual world as if they are immersed. Imagination refers to the use of multi-dimensional perception information provided by the VR scenes.

Virtual reality technology includes multiple components which can be divided into two main groups: the hardware components and the software components [3].

- *Hardware Components:* The hardware components consist of computer workstation, sensory displays, tracking system, wearable devices, and input devices. Sensory displays are used to display the simulated virtual worlds to the user. The most common type is the head-mounted displays (HMDs), which is used in combination with tracking systems. A typical head-mounted display is shown in Figure 17.1 [4]. Users interact with the simulated environment through some wearable devices. VR depends on special responses such as raising hands, turning the head, or swinging the body. A wearable device is important in making these effects realistic. Special input devices are required to interact with the virtual world. These include the 3D mouse, the wired glove, motion controllers, and optical tracking sensors. These devices are used to stimulate our senses together in order to create the illusion of reality.

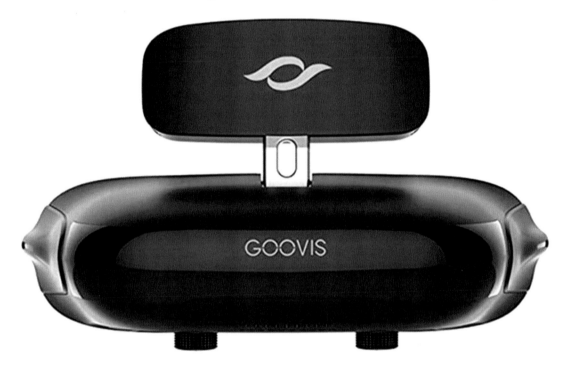

Figure 17.1 Head-mounted display [4].

- *Software Components:* Besides the hardware, the underlying software plays a very important role. It is responsible for the managing of I/O devices and the time-critical applications. The software components are 3D modeling software, 2D graphics software, digital sound editing software, and VR simulation software. VR technology has been designed to ensure visual comfort and ergonomic usage.

17.3 CONCEPT OF AUGMENTED REALITY

The term "augmented reality" was coined in 1990 by Tom Caudell, a former Boeing researcher. Since then the technology has vastly improved. The rise in AR usage stems from four main developments [5]: (1) the pervasiveness of low-cost visual sensors, such as phone cameras, (2) progress in environmental perception algorithms, such as visual simultaneous localization and mapping, (3) advances in optics, and (4) the maturity of multimedia techniques.

Augmented reality (AR) is a technology which combines real-world environments with computer-generated information such as images, text, videos, animations, and sound. It has the ability to record and analyze the environment in real time. The technology is accessible for the ordinary user. It is becoming more attractive as a mainstream technology mainly due to the proliferation of modern mobile computing devices like smartphones and tablet computers with location-based services. For example, AR allows consumers to visualize a product in more detail before they purchase it. This enhances consumer's interaction and prevents them from buying the wrong product.

The key objective of AR is to bring computer generated objects into the real world and allow the user only to see it. In other words, we use AR to track the position and orientation of the users head in order to augment his or her perception of the world. Projected images are overlaid on top of a pair of goggles or glasses, which allow the images and interactive virtual objects to lay on top of the user's view of the real world. Thus, augmented reality involves extending the real-time environment with a digital overlay, in which real life is enhanced by computer-generated images and sound. The digital overlay scene appears on the actual scene the user is experiencing.

Augmented reality falls into two categories: 2D information overlays and 3D presentations, like those used with games. It combines multiple technologies allowing users to interact with virtual entities in real time. Various technologies used for augmented reality include a processor, monitors, handheld devices, display systems, sensors, and input devices. Modern mobile computing devices like smartphones and tablet computers contain these elements also, making them suitable AR platforms.

To obtain a sufficiently accurate representation of reality, AR needs the following components [6]:

- *Sensors:* AR needs suitable sensors in the environment and possibly on a user including (what does this mean?) fine-grained geolocation and image recognition. These are activating elements that trigger the display of virtual information.
- *Image augmentation:* This requires techniques such as image processing and face recognition.
- *Head-mounted Display:* HMDs are used to view the augmented world where the virtual computer-generated information is properly aligned with the real world. Display technologies are of two types: video display and optical see-through display.
- *User Interface:* This includes technologies for input modalities that include gaze tracking, touch, and gesture. AR is a user interface technology in which a camera-recorded view of the real world is augmented with computer-generated content such as graphics, animations, and 2D or 3D models.
- *Information Infrastructure:* AR requires significant computing and communications infrastructure undergirding all these technologies. The infrastructure determines what real-world components to augment, with what, and when.

The AR systems, based on these technologies, should be more accurate, smaller, lighter, faster, simpler, cheaper, and convenient for the users. Google Glass was the first AR platform to get wide public exposure.

17.4 RELATIONSHIP BETWEEN VIRTUAL AND AUGMENTED REALITY

Augmented reality (AR) should not be confused with virtual reality (VR). AR and VR rely on similar technologies, but they provide a different kind of visual feedback. AR is a more recent technology than VR. VR attempts to replace a world, while AR seeks to add to it instead. Unlike VR, AR uses visual inputs to enhance a user's natural vision rather than completely replace it. AR alters a person's perception of a real-world environment, whereas virtual reality completely replaces the person's real-world environment with a simulated one.

The use of AR and VR in healthcare was discovered in the late 1990s. Virtual reality creates immersion in an artificial environment, but augmented reality heightens an experience in the real world by layering additional information atop it. Haptic perception of virtual objects is different in augmented reality compared to virtual reality [7]. Many computer assistance systems rely on either virtual reality (VR) or augmented reality (AR) approach.

The terms virtual reality, augmented reality, and mixed reality are related. They are explained as follows [8]:

- *Virtual Reality:* VR immerses a user in a virtual environment, excluding them from their current physical environment. It essentially places the user in another world. The purpose of VR is to allow a person to experience the environment as if it were the real world. It consists of a computer-generated simulation that produces sight, sound, and touch stimuli so that individuals experience a completely separate environment.

- *Augmented Reality:* AR is essentially a modified form of VR which includes a combination of both real and virtual elements. AR blends the virtual and physical, providing an overlay. AR renders 3D virtual components in the context of a user's physical environment. In AR, the users can see their own body in the environment. The most popular example of this is Pokémon Go.

- *Mixed Reality:* This is a combination of real content, and digital content that sometimes consists of, for instance, two types of video essentially layered over each other. With mixed reality (MR), users can quickly and easily interact with digital objects to enhance their experience of reality. MR can be a safer way for patients to relearn tasks.

All three have their own distinct advantages. They are illustrated in Figure 17.2 [9]. In VR, people are immersed in virtual environments and are allowed to interact with it. AR is an extension of the real world, mixing real and artificial reality where people keeping the opportunity to see their own body, which is not possible with VR. Technologies such as VR/AR/MR alter our perception of the world around us and are becoming a reality of everyday life. Healthcare is one of the main application areas for VR/AR/MR technologies.

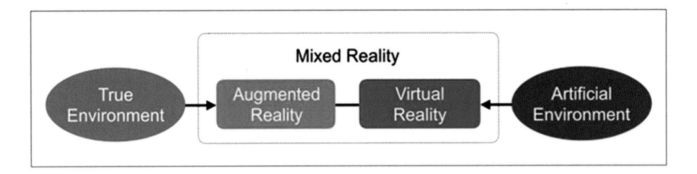

Figure 17.2 Reality-virtuality continuum [9].

17.5 APPLICATIONS OF VIRTUAL REALITY IN HEALTHCARE

Virtual reality is an interactive, simulated visual and audio environment generated by computer. The most common way of applying VR is using a VR headset to display a realistic visual environment. Virtual reality is often used in entertainment applications such as video gaming and 3D cinema. It is also used in social sciences, medicine, education and training, simulation, marketing, commerce, architecture, arts, sport, fashion, engineering, construction, environmental navigation, factory, tourism, archaeology, military, media, music, cinema, scientific visualization, telecommunication, and programming languages. The possibilities are endless [10]. VR has been widely applied in numerous applications in healthcare and medicine. Some of the applications in healthcare are presented as follows.

- *Pharmacy*: VR technology can potentially be applied as a replacement for pharmacotherapy; in drug design and discovery. It has been used in pharmacy education to engage in learning. There is also the potential for using VR in pharmacy for clinical, research, and educational applications [11]. VR will not replace drug therapy, but it can help patients rely less on drugs by patient counseling and behavior modification.

- *Mental Health:* The World Health Organization has reported that one in four people in the world will be affected by mental health disorder at some point in their lives. Unfortunately, nearly two-thirds of people with mental problem fail to seek help. VR and AR technologies have been used for treating several mental disorders such as anxiety disorders, alcohol abuse disorder (AADs), posttraumatic stress disorder (PTSD), depression, eating disorders, phobias (e.g., specific phobias, social phobia, agoraphobia), addiction disorders. The virtual environment generated by VR can help patients relax their body and mind.

- *Clinical psychology:* The artificial environment generated from virtual and augmented reality is closer to daily life people experience. AR enables us to study behavioral, cognitive, and emotional aspects that were hard to realize before. VR technology has been used by mental health providers as a therapeutic modality for those who are diagnosed with a phobia disorder. A patient would be virtually exposed to their fear slowly (i.e., being in enclosed spaces seen agrophobia) in a safe environment over several sessions until they become desensitized.

- *Dentistry:* Dental healthcare issues are becoming increasingly important due to the crisis of aging populations. VR can be used as an effective treatment of patients with dental phobia, a common problem in our society . The VR-based procedure is accurate, noninvasive, and time saving. Both AR and VR systems have a wide range of applications in the manually dominated medical disciplines such as dental medicine. Their applications are of increasing importance in dental education [9].

• *Pain Reduction:* VR environment can be used as a pain reduction technology and improvement of sleep habits. Immersive VR helps with pain reduction by distracting the mind. It can reduce the quantity of pain medications and prevent overuse of opioids.

• *Education and Training:* Concerning healthcare education, several requests have been made to eliminate outdated, inefficient, and passive learning approaches and embrace newer methodologies of learning such as VR and AR. The use of VR and AR devices allows learning to occur through hands-on immersive experiences. They are ideal for training in hands-on procedures without harming actual patients. VR is becoming useful for training physicians through visual simulation technology. It can be used to train medical students and resident physicians for surgeries in a risk-free environment without physically being in an operating room. VR trainers are available for various medical procedures. VR and AR technologies will play an increasing role in teaching, surgery, learning anatomy, anesthesia, and dentistry.

• *Improved Patient Experience:* Patient experience is the one of the areas that get the most out of the implementation of VR and AR in healthcare. Immersion and engagement matter a lot for successful treatment. AR can also help the patient to stay tuned with their therapy progress in an engaging manner.

• *Surgery:* Physicians can produce a three dimensional model of a particular patient's anatomy and map out the surgery ahead of time. Figure 17.3 shows virtual reality in surgery [12].

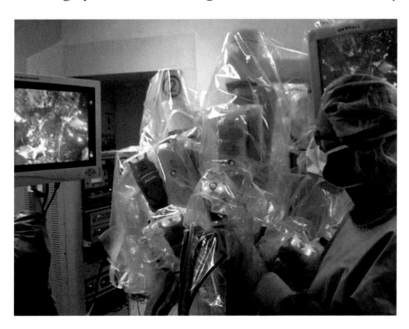

Figure 17.3 Virtual reality in surgery [12].

• *Robotics:* Virtual reality has been used in robotics development. It can control robots in telepresence and telerobotic systems. VR environment can be wired to a remote-controlled robot which will handle the actual operation, while the surgeon performs the routine elsewhere.

VR has been used to support children and adults with disabilities to improve their health or physical condition. VR is also gaining traction as promising tool in forensic psychiatry, which is the interface of law and mental health. VR can be applied to other areas of healthcare such as neuroscience, neuropsychology, radiology, telemedicine, preventive medicine, and urology.

While virtual reality is becoming more popular, their applications are rocketing through the market. Amazon, Apple, Facebook, Google, Microsoft, HP, Levono, Sony, Ebay, Samsung, and several other companies have developed VR-related products with the hope of grabbing a piece of the still-burgeoning market.

17.6 APPLICATIONS OF AUGMENTED REALITY IN HEALTHCARE

Augmented reality applies displays, cameras, and sensors to overlay digital information onto the real world. The concept of augmented reality can be applied to any technology that combines virtual and real information. Commercial augmented reality experiences were first introduced in entertainment and gaming businesses. Since then, AR has been explored for many applications including medicine, education, librarian services, military, business, archaeology, architecture, pattern recognition, translation, commerce, visual arts, fashion, social interaction, journalism and media, tourism, navigation systems, robots, driver-assistance systems, advertising, manufacturing, smart cities, social networking, and communications. There are several exciting applications for augmented reality in healthcare. Tools that will improve visualization of anatomy and orientation are invaluable, especially when pathologies obscure natural anatomy. Some of the applications in the healthcare sector are explained as follows [13]:

- *Education and Training:* Education is a common application of augmented reality in the healthcare field. AR is useful in healthcare education because it helps the healthcare learner to understand spatial relationships and concepts, to acquire skills and knowledge, to capture learner's attention, to shorten their learning curve, and to prolong learning retention, [15] which is helpful in learning anatomy and physiology. Figure17.4 shows augmented reality in medical education [14]. Compared to paper-based training, AR allows medical professionals to continuously observe and give feedback to students during their practice. It can also be used to provide feedback from students.

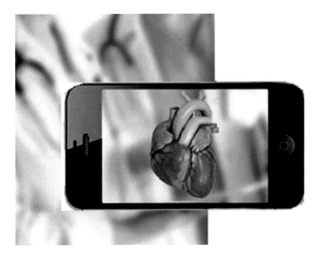

Figure 17.4 Augmented reality in medical education [14].

- *Surgery:* When it comes to surgery, precision is paramount. Surgeons use several techniques to visualize the area they operate on. Surgery is an exciting area where AR is predominantly implemented. AR devices increase the success rate and decrease certain complications from surgery. AR can assist surgical professionals by providing things such as interfaces to operating room (what is this?) and instant access to patient records. AR can project three dimensional representations of the patient's anatomy for the surgeon to view, thereby improving accuracy of the procedure [16]. Surgeons have started using Microsoft's HoloLens AR glasses during reconstructive surgery.
- *Diagnosis:* Diagnostics is a critical aspect of healthcare which often relies on close evaluation of various signs and symptoms. Sometimes patients cannot accurately describe their symptoms to doctors. AR makes it possible for doctors to better assess their patients' symptoms and accurately diagnose them. AR also plays a significant role in more efficient detection, prevention, and treatment of many diseases.
- *Data Visualization:* Visualization techniques help to visualize the innumerate amount of the analytical results as diagrams, tables, and images. VR and AR are fast developing technologies that allow the 3D visualization of digital information or data, especially big data. AR technology enables healthcare practitioners to view precise images of body structures without using intrusive methods. Visualization, which in an interactive way, can improve understanding and literacy among those who use medications [17].

Other specific areas of application of AR in healthcare include psychiatry, telemedicine, radiology, joint injection, tumor resection, administering local anesthetics, forensic medicine, diathermy, tissue engineering, disease outbreak, clinical breast examination, cardiologic data, and life support training.

17.7 GLOBAL AUGMENTED REALITY AND VIRTUAL REALITY

AR and VR can play a significant role in global healthcare as it seeks to reduce risk. Increasing cost of healthcare, rapid digitization of the healthcare sector, and the need for cutting-edge technologies for diagnostics and treatment have propelled the need for integrating AR and VR technology in the healthcare industry. Researchers, engineers, and healthcare professionals worldwide confirm that VR and AR handsets are effective, efficient, and widely accessible tools in mental healthcare interventions.

The global virtual reality and augmented reality market in healthcare is witnessing several changes and is expected to grow significantly. The market is segmented into software, hardware, and services. In terms of the regional segmentation, the VR and AR market has been segregated into North America, Europe, APAC, and the Rest-of-the-World (ROW). In 2018, North America dominated the AR and VR market in healthcare [18]. Owing to the immersive nature of VR and AR, the UK National Institute of Health Research awarded £4 million to fund the development of VR treatments.

17.7 BENEFITS

Changes are always made in healthcare to improve patient care. VR and AR technologies are new tools that can help in maximizing the quality of learning and proficiency of patient care. With VR and AR, patients can feel "as if they are" in a reality that does not exist in the external world. Immersion in virtual reality can change the way a patient behaves in the real world. It gives the patient with the strong illusion of being somewhere else. VR and AR are poised to disrupt healthcare, because they will change the way doctors view data and their patients.

Virtual reality is the creation of a virtual environment which is presented to our senses in a way that we experience it as if we were really there. What distinguishes VR from other media is the sense of presence. It has an advantage to create a safe virtual world where the patient can experience "new realities." The virtual environment is both realistic and enjoyable. VR offers the human factors professional an important new tool of investigation. VR provides realistic, safe, and cost-effective training for professional such soldiers, police officers, and firefighters. This gives VR a great advantage over conventional training methods. VR technology has become affordable, flexible, and portable, enabling its use for therapeutic purposes.

Augmented reality (AR), the overlaying of computer graphics onto the real worldview, has the potential to provide a competitive advantage in globalizing markets in industrial applications. AR can provide immense benefits and efficiencies to both patients and healthcare providers. It can greatly enhance the viewer's perception of reality. It is very effective at increasing employee learning and accuracy by delivering guides for learning and performing on the job. It helps to present information succinctly. It allows nurses to find veins easier, for insertion of intravenous catheters. It allows the patients to see how the drug works in 3D in their body.

It may shape the competitive advantage of companies by providing various benefits for the consumers. AR devices have the potential to mediate interpersonal communication. It is an interactive technology which is attractive to consumers due to the variety of possible applications, ranging from education to healthcare [19].

17.8 CHALLENGES

The widespread adoption of AR and VR technologies has been hindered by some factors such as health risks, possibility of information security leak, privacy issues, lack of proficiency among medical practitioners to adopt new technologies, and social issues such as public acceptance. The feasibility, affordability, and accessibility challenges of VR and AR applications often hinder broad global adoption. With VR and AR, it is becoming increasingly difficult for the human brain to separate digital encounters from real-world occurrences. Critics are concerned that virtualized experience featuring violence or pornography can lead to inappropriate behaviors in the real world.

VR technology is yet to develop to a point where many of these applications are readily available or affordable. Costs can be prohibitive. Virtual reality interfaces are difficult and expensive to make. Prolonged use of virtual reality has caused adverse effects such as headache, seizures, eye fatigue, discomfort, and stress injury [20]. The virtual reality world may lead to false hope or misconception. It has been said that VR has finally reached the "plateau of productivity." Regardless of the VR application, there are challenges to address, including cost, lack of standardization, and resistance from critics. Another major challenge is cybersickness (CS), the bodily discomfort associated with exposure to VR content. It is a form of visually induced motion sickness. These challenges have slowed proliferation of VR technology.

Technological limitations remain the major obstacle for AR systems. Developing successful AR applications is a challenging task because applications are both hardware and software intensive. Right now, developing or prototyping AR-applications remains a challenge because there are no standards for AR user interfaces, which provide the right information at the right moment and the right place. Since there are no fixed surfaces, devices like mice and keyboards are not practical. The ergonomics of holding a smartphone to "look through it" while using an AR application are problematic and socially awkward. Social issues such as technology transfer may need to be addressed.

17.9 CONCLUSION

VR and AR are emerging technologies that alter the way humans interact with computers. They involve using computer, software, display device, and tracking sensors. They are increasingly becoming available, accessible and affordable. Virtual reality is a digitally simulated environment that can be used to manipulate our perception of the physical surrounding. It should expand beyond sight and sound "touch." VR is posed to influence your workplace, hobbies, and social life in the future. VR challenges the concept of reality, but it will never replace reality. VR is the art of the twenty-first century just as cinema was for the twentieth [21].

Augmented reality is a real environment being augmented by virtual objects. It presents a view of the real, physical world that incorporates additional information to enhance or augment this view. In the future, AR technology may allow multiple users to share the experience, thereby enabling collaborative work.

Some academic institutions are already offering introductory courses that will equip the students with the basics of VR and AR technologies. This includes students in engineering, business, educations, and social sciences. In view of the students' proficiency for the use of smartphones, Internet, and of continuously refreshing applications, AR is very suited for teaching or training students [22].

Virtual reality is rapidly becoming one of the most exciting computer technologies of our modern society. It is no longer a promise of the future, but has become a reality in many different fields. Although AR is still its early stages, it is really blurring the lines of reality. It is becoming pervasively used due to the application of mobile devices. VR and AR will become mainstream technologies for healthcare. They will play a significant role in training the next generation of healthcare professionals. The future of VR and AR appears to have limitless possibilities. More information about VR and AR can be found in the books in [22-37] and a related journal: *Journal of Healthcare Engineering*

REFERENCES

[1] M. N. O. Sadiku, K. G. Eze, and S. M. Musa, "Virtual reality: A primer," *International Journal of Trend in Research and Development*, vol. 7, no. 2, March-April 2020, pp. 160-162.

[2] Y. Li et al., "Gesture interaction in virtual reality," *Virtual Reality & Intelligent Hardware*, vol.1, no.1, February 2019, pp. 84-112.

[3] M. O. Onyesolu and F. U. Eze, "Understanding virtual reality technology: Advances and applications," *Advances in Computer Science and Engineering*, March 2011, pp. 53-70.

[4] "Five ways virtual reality is improving healthcare," June 2017, https://theconversation.com/five-ways-virtual-reality-is-improving-healthcare-79523

[5] H. Ling, "Augmented reality in reality," *IEEE MultiMedia*, July–September 2017, pp. 10-15.

[6] M. Singh and M. P. Singh, "Augmented reality interfaces," *IEEE Internet Computing*, November/December 2013, pp. 66-70.

[7] Y. Gaffary, B. L. Gouis, and M. Marchal, "AR feels 'softer' than VR: Haptic perception of stiffness in augmented versus virtual reality," *IEEE Transactions on Visualization and Computer Graphics*, Vol. 23, No. 11, November 2017, pp. 2372-2377.

[8] P. Milgram et al., "Augmented reality: A class of displays on the reality-virtuality continuum," *Telemanipulator and Telepresence Technologies*, vol. 2351, 1994, pp. 282-292.

[9] T. Joda et al., "Augmented and virtual reality in dental medicine: A systematic review," *Computers in Biology and Medicine*, vol. 108, May 2019, pp. 93-100.

[10] "Applications of virtual reality," *Wikipedia*, the free encyclopedia https://en.wikipedia.org/wiki/Applications_of_virtual_reality

[11] C. L. Ventola, "Virtual reality in pharmacy: Opportunities for clinical, research, and educational applications," *PT*, vol. 44, no. 5, May 2019, pp. 267-276.

[12] "In a first, British hospital livestreams surgery in virtual reality," April 2016, https://www.indiatoday.in/world/story/in-a-first-british-hospital-livestreams-surgery-in-virtual-reality-318214-2016-04-15

[13] "Augmented reality," Wikipedia, the free encyclopedia https://en.wikipedia.org/wiki/Augmented_reality

[14] "Virtual, augmented reality revolutionizing med education, anatomy imaging," https://medicalvirtualreality.org/virtual-augmented-reality-revolutionizing-med-education-anatomy-imaging/

[15] E. Zhu et al., "Augmented reality in healthcare education: An integrative review," *PeerJ*, July 8, 2014.

[16] K. Wong et al., "Applications of augmented reality in otolaryngology: A systematic review," *Otolaryngology– Head and Neck Surgery*, vol. 159, no. 6, 2018, pp. 956–967.

[17] BIS Research, "Virtual reality and augmented reality in healthcare: A market overview," May 2019, https://blog.marketresearch.com/virtual-reality-and-augmented-reality-in-healthcare-a-market-overview

[19] E. Olshannikova et al., "Visualizing big data with augmented and virtual reality: Challenges and research agenda," *Journal of Big Data*, 2015.

[20] T. Grzegorczyk, R. Sliwinski, and J. Kaczmarek, "Attractiveness of augmented reality to consumers," *Technology Analysis & Strategic Management*, 2019.

[21] "Virtual Reality," *Wikipedia*, the free encyclopedia https://en.wikipedia.org/wiki/Virtual_reality

[22] M. L. Ryan, *Narrative as Virtual Reality: Immersion and Interactivity in Literature and Electronic Media*. Baltimore, MD: The Johns Hopkins University Press, 2001.

[23] A. Klimova, A. Bilyatdinova, and A. Karsakov, "Existing teaching practices in augmented reality," *Procedia Computer Science*, vol. 136, 2018, pp. 5-15.

[24] F. Hu, J. Lu, and T. Zhang (eds.), *Virtual Reality Enhanced Robotic Systems for Disability Rehabilitation*. Medical Information Science Reference, 2017.

[25] P. Fuchs et al. (eds.), *Virtual Reality: Concepts and Technologies*. Boca Raton, FL: CRC Press, 2011.

[26] G. C. Burdea and P. Coiffet, *Virtual Reality Technology*. Hoboken, NJ: John Wiley & Sons, 2003.

[27] J. Vince, *Introduction to Virtual Reality*. London, UK: Springer, 2004.

[28] A. B. Craig, *Understanding Augmented Reality: Concepts and Applications.* Morgan Kaufmann Pub., 2013.

[29] G. Kipper and J. Rampolla, *Augmented Reality: An Emerging Technologies Guide to AR.* Syngress Media, 2013.

[30] H. Altinpulluk and G. Kurubacak (eds.), *Mobile Technologies and Augmented Reality in Open Education.* IGI Global, 2017.

[31] W. Barfield (ed.), *Fundamentals of Wearable Computers and Augmented Reality.* Boca Raton, FL: CRC Press, 2nd edition, 2017.

[32] B. Furht (ed.), *Handbook of Augmented Reality.* Springer, 2011.

[33] S. K. Ong and A. Y. C. Nee (eds.), *Virtual and Augmented Reality Applications in Manufacturing.* London, UK: Springer-Verlag, 2004.

[34] G. Guazzaroni, *Virtual and Augmented Reality in Mental Health Treatment.* Hershey, PA : IGI Global, 2019.

[35] M. Ma, L. C. Jain, and P. Anderson (eds.), *Virtual, Augmented Reality and Serious Games for Healthcare.* Springer, 2014.

[36] T. Jung and M. C. tom Dieck (eds.), *Augmented Reality and Virtual Reality: Empowering Human, Place and Business.* Springer, 2018.

[37] D. N. Le et al., *Emerging Technologies for Health and Medicine: Virtual Reality, Augmented Reality, Artificial Intelligence, Internet of Things, Robotics, Industry 4.0.* Hoboken, NJ: John Wiley & Sons, 2018.

CHAPTER 18

HEALTHCARE BUSINESS INTELLIGENCE

"A customer is the most important visitor on our premises, he is not dependent on us. We are dependent on him. He is not an interruption in our work. He is the purpose of it. He is not an outsider in our business. He is part of it. We are not doing him a favor by serving him. He is doing us a favor by giving us an opportunity to do so." — Mahatma Gandhi

18.1 INTRODUCTION

In the United States, healthcare is undergoing dramatic change. The industry is shifting from historical fee-for-service to fee-for-value and is in the middle of a digital revolution with massive amounts of data generated daily. Today's healthcare providers are facing the demand for information to comply with legal and customer requirements. Hospitals have their data spread out and residing in several databases in the form of clinical data, administrative data, and external data [1]. Business intelligence (BI) is considered a possible solution to these challenges. It is a term used to represent tools, techniques, and systems that are useful in making informed, better decisions. BI system is developed to support decision-making domains such as hospital management, clinical decision support, and clinical research.

To turn any business into a profit-making enterprise requires that the work force make wise decisions, which depends on the available information. This is where business intelligence comes in. It is a broad term to describe a set of methods, processes, and technologies that transform raw data into meaningful and useful information to support business operations. It may also be regarded as a collection of decision support technologies for the enterprise aimed at enabling professionals make better and faster decisions. The purpose of BI is to support better business decision-making. Business Intelligence (BI) refers to technologies, applications and practices for the collection, integration, analysis, and presentation of business information and also sometimes to the information itself [2]. Business intelligence (BI) also refers to a broad category of analytics, data warehousing, and visualization tools. The purpose of BI is to support better business decision-making. BI is a concept that can be applied in almost any area of work. Although BI is designed for the business environment, it can be used by government, universities, healthcare, and security.

This chapter begins by explaining business intelligence. It provides an examination of the deployment and constraints of business intelligence in healthcare. It also explains the current state of BI in global healthcare. It covers some applications of BI, the increased need for it, and highlights the benefits and challenges of business intelligence in healthcare. The last section concludes with comments.

18.2 BUSINESS INTELLIGENCE CONCEPT

To succeed in a modern digital world, healthcare industry must be data-driven. Hospitals and healthcare institutions desire to make their workflows more efficient in order to meet demand. One way they can achieve this is with the help of business intelligence (BI) software. BI refers to the acquisition, correlation, and transformation of data into insightful and actionable information through analytics. Utilizing a BI software is an indispensable part of the growth process toward becoming data-driven. In the modern healthcare environment, almost all BI initiatives will be driven by data analytics.

The concept of business intelligence (BI) refers to the tools and systems that play a major role in the planning process of an organization. The tools represent BI in customer support, customer profiling, market research, product profitability, and business analysis.

The main objective of business intelligence is to enable business managers to have easy access to data, conduct analysis, allow them to convert data into useful knowledge, and then make faster, better decisions [3]. BI software supports reporting, interactive analyses, visualization, and statistical data mining. People use business intelligence for many reasons such as the need to seek improvements in decision-making, competition, and the need to seek efficiency.

Different types of data analytics can help hospitals and other healthcare organizations better serve patients in several ways [4]:

- *Descriptive analytics:* Shows what is happening or has been happening.
- *Diagnostic analytics:* Evaluates correlation and causation. Ie, tracing hyperlipidemia or diabetes mellitus type 2 back to poor diets.
- *Predictive analytics:* Indicates what will likely happen
- *Prescriptive analytics:* Recommends specific actions in response to individual patient symptoms.

BI system is an integrated set of tools, technologies, and programmed products, which are used to collect, integrate, analyze, and share data. BI system has following components [5]:

- *Extraction-Transformation-Load* (ETL): ETL tools that are responsible for data transfer from operational or transaction systems to data warehouses.
- *Data Warehouse*: Data Warehouse (DW) is the core of any solid BI solution. It provides storing of aggregated and analyzed data. It allows reports to be produced at a reasonable cost for community. A good data warehouse should ensure data protection and security.
- *Data Management and Integration:* This component prepares data to be ready for analysis and reports. It involves analyzing, reporting, and presenting tools such as on-line analytical processing (OLAP), which allow users access to analyze and model business problems and share information.
- *Presentation:* This component is a focused layer which helps bring discernment to make better decisions to users. Presentation layers include customized graphical and multimedia interfaces or dashboards to provide users with information in a comfortable and accessible form.

Business specific applications require all components above to work together to produce a complete solution.

18.3 BUSINESS INTELLIGENCE IN HEALTHCARE

Business intelligence (BI) is a fast growing field with significant benefits and opportunities for healthcare workers. The healthcare industry must be innovative in the way they operate. This will avoid being data rich but information poor. To maintain competitive advantage, healthcare providers must excel in four key areas: optimum care delivery, developing a reliable financial baseline, employing rigorous business planning, and increasing market share. It is equally important to empower healthcare workers for strategic decision making through data warehousing based on critical thinking. They need fast, responsive, and user-friendliness in using BI software to maximize the value of their data and support critical areas of decision making. BI tools are must-haves for any long-term and sustainable analytics foundation. The healthcare organizations may need to acquire expertise and technology for business intelligence. Figure 18.1 shows a typical healthcare business intelligence [6].

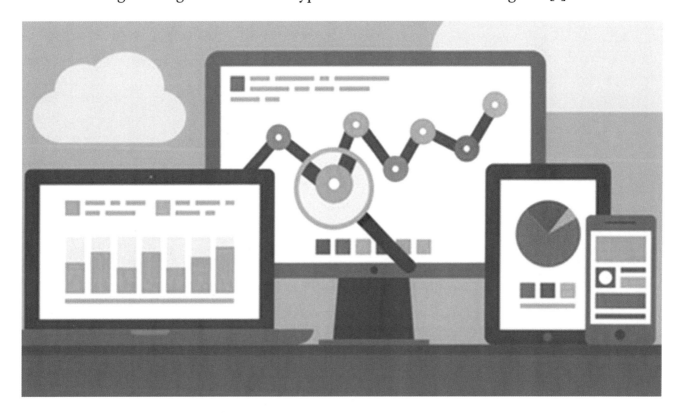

Figure 18.1 Healthcare business intelligence [6].

BI is important to healthcare because healthcare organizations generate a lot of data. The healthcare industry is heading toward the data-driven world. It is shifting from fee-for-service to fee-for-value. Business intelligence can disrupt the processes through which healthcare services are provided.

Healthcare business intelligence solutions rely on big data, which is the ever-growing volume of digital information that healthcare providers and related industries generate. The increase in volume of data is a significant trend in healthcare. Just imagine keeping patient records (geographics, vital signs, diagnosis, imaging, labs, treatment details, administrative details, etc.) for several millions of patients lying in different hospitals, clinics, skilled nursing facilties all across the world.

18.4 APPLICATIONS

Interest in implementation of business intelligence (BI) technologies in different sectors has been increasing from year to year. BI is applied in various areas such as finance, retail, insurance, healthcare, etc. All these areas are entering a new era that is data-driven.

Healthcare organizations are adopting BI tools to get data-driven insights and improve patient care. This approach has been called healthcare BI or clinical business intelligence. Healthcare has the most complex data of any industry, both structured and unstructured data. For example, the hospital collects data from different sources such as from sensors on patient vital signs, labs, pharmacy, claims, billing, CRM, EMR, HMS, etc. These data can be grouped into three categories: financial, operational, and clinical. Business Intelligence is needed in healthcare to manage the sheer amount of data being generated by hospitals and healthcare organizations daily. Incorporating the BI technology into deploy electronic health record (EHR) and electronic medical record (EMR) will improve the quality and safety of healthcare delivery [7,8].

As illustrated in Figure 18.2, applications of business intelligence in healthcare can be categorized into two major sets of solutions: Technology solutions and business solutions [9,10].

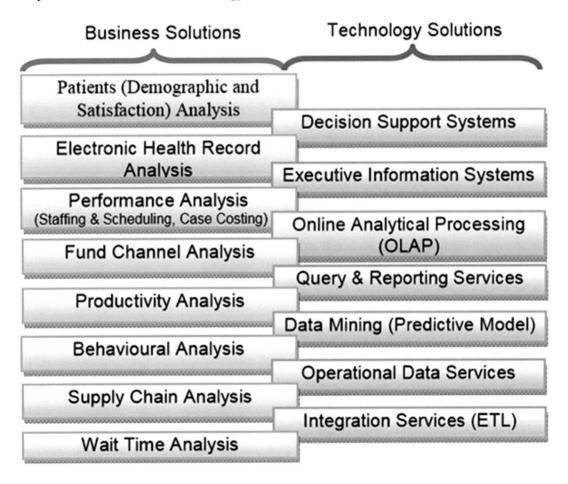

Figure 18.2 BI applications in healthcare [9].

A. Technology Solutions: It is data and information tools and services, as follows:

(1) Decision Support Systems (DSS): Support managerial decision making, usually day-to-day tactics. BI enables the right people to access the right information at the right time for better decision-making.

(2) Executive Information Systems: Support decision making at the senior management level which provide metrics-based performance information.

(3) Online Analytical Processing (OLAP): Support analysts with the capability of perform multi-dimensional analysis of data.

(4) Query and Reporting Services: Provide quick and easy access to the data with predefined report design capabilities.

(5) Data Mining: Examines data to discover hidden facts in databases using different techniques.

(6) Operational Data Services: Collect data from end users, organizing data, establishing solid data structures and store them in multiple databases.

(7) Integration Services: Design and implement process flow of data extracting, transforming, and loading to the data warehouse.

B. Business Solutions: Business focused analytical applications as follows:

(1) Patient Analysis: Focuses on analysis of patients' demographic and satisfaction processes.

(2) Electronic Health Record Analysis: Focuses on analysis of the quality of clinical data. Only 35% of healthcare systems in the US have transitioned to electronic health records (EHRs). "Ninety-nine percent of hospitals across the country now use electronic health record systems (EHRs), compared to about 31 percent in 2003" -

(3) Performance Analysis: Streamline and optimize the way that a business uses its resources. BI enables healthcare providers to use dashboards to indicate which products and services are profitable.

(4) Fund Channel Analysis: Devise, implement, and evaluate fund strategies, then use the corporate metrics to continuously monitor and enhance the fund process

(5) Productivity Analysis: Focuses on building business metrics for activities such as quality improvement, risk mitigation, asset management, capacity planning, etc.

(6) Behavioral Analysis: Understanding and predicting trends and patterns that provides business advantage.

(7) Supply Chain Analysis: Monitor, benchmark, and improve supply chain activities from materials ordering through service delivery.

(8) Wait Time Analysis: Focuses on the factors that are associated with longer waiting times and the effects of delays in scheduling and operation.

In addition to these applications, the following applications also employ BI:

- *Hospital:* Business intelligence helps hospitals to establish best practices in both care and management. A patient receives acute care in hospitals and sees many specialists in a hospital. The number of patients in the hospitals are increasing due to various illnesses, diseases, accidents, aging, and other factors. Hospital administrators are caught in complex web of resource optimization since resources are limited and budgets are tight. They need to use all the tools available to operate more efficiently and effectively. There is a constant demand for accurate information from health insurance. Healthcare business intelligence may be the answer that hospitals are looking for. BI improves patient care while limiting expenses by giving the right treatment at the right time. BI technology helps to monitor cases for insurance companies. Hospitals desire to make their workflows more efficient in order to meet demands. This can be achieved with the help of BI software [11].

- *Patient Care and Satisfaction:* BI has been one of the figurative lifesavers in the healthcare arena. Emergency clinics and other medical services need a situation that supports the day-to-day practices of surgeons, physicians, and all other healthcare personnel. BI consolidates and presents all the cases to a doctor which can be obtained via electronic health record. The BI software keeps track of all the patient data. The doctor can access every single test and treatment reports of the patient. Patient data is becoming more accessible and accessing the information is easier than ever before using BI. Treatment regimens are now able to move out of a one-size-fits-all category to remedy based on each patient's medical history and health concerns. BI enables the prediction of some diseases [12].

- *Cost Reduction:* BI is useful in analyzing the most useful profit strategies and marketing campaigns. It is also useful in locating sources with the best ROI rates and also reducing the cost of an organization. Business intelligence can be aimed at improving the quality of patient care, so the resources are directed in the right direction. With big data, it is increasingly easy to monitor the most useful aspects of medical care that can be implemented in cutting costs, improving waste management, and managing overhead spending [13].

- *Claims Management:* BI technology helps to screen and monitor cases for health insurance companies. It can help improve reaction times against claims. It can also help insurance agencies to safeguard themselves against fraudulent claims.

18.5 GLOBAL HEALTHCARE BUSINESS INTELLIGENCE

The healthcare industry is the most lucrative sector in the world because it meets the essential needs of human beings. Healthcare providers use BI software to gain insights into patient satisfaction and to make smart financial decisions. The BI industry is expanding in various industries around the world. The healthcare business intelligence (BI) market is divided based on component, function, application, and deployment model. Based on component, the global healthcare business intelligence market can be divided into the platform, software, and services. Based on the function, the market can classified into query and reporting, OLAP and visualization, and performance management. Based on the application, the market is divided into financial analysis, operational analysis, patient care, and clinical analysis. Based on the deployment model, the market has been divided into the on-premise model, cloud-based model, and hybrid model [14]. Understanding the segments helps in identifying the importance of different factors that foster the market growth and also in understanding the industry's future trends.

The global (North America, South America, Europe, Africa, Middle East, Asia, China, Japan) market for BI tools in healthcare is booming. The Asia Pacific is expected to witness the fastest growth in the global healthcare business intelligence market. The region is anticipated to witness significant growth due to increasing penetration, spreading IoT connectivity, and growing investment in healthcare infrastructure. SPEC INDIA studies BI techniques adopted by hospitals across the world to assist the adoption of healthcare business intelligence solutions. We now consider the BI market in the following nations:

- *United States:* The United States healthcare system is known to be a high-cost, low-yield investment. The US is ranked as the top nation in the world in healthcare expenditures. It accounts for the largest share of the healthcare business intelligence market due to increased implementation of healthcare BI solutions. This may be attributed to the local presence of major software and service providers for healthcare industry such as Microsoft Corporation, Oracle Corporation, and SAS Institute. In spite of this, a third of healthcare organizations in US are not using BI tools. The US healthcare industry follows certain national standards to process electronic healthcare transactions. Healthcare providers across America use BI to monitor patient diagnoses and improve patient care. They work tirelessly to remain effective and improve their efficiency. The top players of the global healthcare business intelligence (BI) market include BOARD International, IBM, Information Builders, Microsoft, MicroStrategy Incorporated, Oracle, Information Builders, Acmeware, Datawatch, Epic Systems, Getwellnetwork, Inovalon, SAS, SAP AG, Medhost, Siemens Medical Solutions USA, Sisense Inc., Tableau Software, Yellowfin BI, and Strata Decision Technology [15].
- *Netherlands:* An electronic health record (EHR) can be regarded as a systematic collection of electronic health information about individual patients or populations. An EHR of a local general practitioner can be linked with the EHR of the local pharmacy. In 2008 about 98% of the healthcare professionals in the Netherlands already made use of some sort of HER. A recent study indicates that the Netherlands is a key player in adopting EHRs in ambulatory healthcare and hospital settings. The Dutch Ministry of Health aimed to establish a national infrastructure for data exchange between electronic patient records (EPRs). This will provide up-to-date information about a patient. EHRs are a very hot topic in the Netherlands because of those relatively recent changes in the development of the national EHR [16]. The management of healthcare institutions in the Netherlands is changing focus.
- *Egypt:* Healthcare providers in Egypt are proactively approaching IT-based business strategies. Applications of business intelligence in different areas of the economy have been increasingly. BI provides an effective methods and robust environment in the growing healthcare industry in Egypt [17].

18.6 BENEFITS

The benefits of applying BI in healthcare are tremendous. BI provides full transparency, analysis, and delivery of financial and operational data. It allows organizations to build a reputation around patient and clinical care. BI adoption helps healthcare organizations manage the untapped potential of their massive amounts of data. Other benefits of using Business intelligence in a healthcare include [1,18,19]:

- *Making Better Decisions:* The main purpose of BI is to support better business decision-making. BI applies data to make better and quicker decisions. It accelerates and improves healthcare decision making. Gathering high quality data faster and receiving a meaningful analytical report production helps in decision support. BI systems also enable healthcare organizations to gather their data in a single repository. They can allow decision makers to use and alter data and models in real time to support decision making.

- *Protection of Data:* Since there would be a single point of access to data, access is only provided to those with appropriate access authorization. All healthcare organizations need a data governance system to protect the privacy of patients' health records.
- *Increased Profits and Reduced Costs*: The need to reduce costs across all areas of operations is becoming necessary. BI allows healthcare providers to reduce waste and minimize the costs of healthcare specialists, lab equipment, medical materials, lab consumables, and treatment per diagnosis.
- *Enhanced Patient Care:* With BI, healthcare professionals have easy access to patient's data and can make decisions based on demographic data, sex, age, etc. All reports can be collated and presented in a visual format, providing detailed insight on every aspect of the patient's health and also a 360-degree view of data at all times. Health care providers can use this information to prescribe medications, access labs or imaging to properly diagnosed a patient. Timely and effective clinical decisions are better facilitated by using BI.
- *Reduction of Medical Errors:* Providing safe, quality care is a top priority for the healthcare industry. BI enables organizations to track large amounts of information and identify the most efficient practices. It also helps providers identify trends and anomalies, and analyze risk in clinical care. For an example, Prescription Drug Monitoring Programs, is a statewide electronic database that tracks all controlled substance prescriptions. Authorized users can access prescription data such as medications dispensed and doses to help identify patients who are obtaining opioids from multiple providers. (source: https://www.cdc.gov/drugoverdose/pdf/pdmp_factsheet-a.pdf)
- *Prediction:* Application of BI in healthcare will give healthcare providers the power to address the future, not just simply relying on historical data to make decisions. BI software (such as data visualization tools, discovery tools) also gives them the tools necessary to make accurate predictions regarding patients. Making such prediction may require time, relevant data, sufficient information, and experience.
- *Integration:* There is a need for better integration and sharing of data within and across health care entities. In the past, it was common for healthcare organizations to store patient data, financial data, and operations data in different locations. BI software for healthcare settings combines these data sources in one location and integrates all tools in one, easy-to-use platform. This consolidation impacts patient care and increases the efficiency of medical staff. It promotes consistency of data and trust in the data. It is also useful in supporting disease management, patient satisfaction, cost reduction, waste minimization, and predictive analysis.

18.7 CHALLENGES

Applying business intelligence to the healthcare sector faces several challenges including the following [20]:

- *Lack of funds:* Adopting and shifting to such a complex technology requires a lot of initial capital. Such a complex system requires availability of equipment like server, fast computing machines, and expensive software. Some healthcare organizations are challenged by limited budgets and ineffective management.

- *Complexity of IT Equipment:* Technically, healthcare based business intelligence systems are complex to build and maintain. Healthcare organizations have many complex machines e.g. ventilators, MRI, CT scans etc. so combining and studying data from such complex systems can be difficult. Healthcare organizations find it difficult to keep up with fast changing technologies. It may also be difficult to segregate between relevant and irrelevant data. The implementation of a BI project for healthcare organizations is a challenge due to the nature of the data involved.

- *Lack of knowledge:* Advanced technology requires the availability of the knowledgeable personnel who can help others to learn and use the technology appropriately and effectively.

- *Data Standards:* Organizations need to have a standard according to which such complex data can be structured. Interoperability is needed to allow sharing electronic health records with physicians, pharmacists, and hospitals.

- *Interoperability.* This refers to the ability of healthcare information systems to connect across health organizations for care delivery for individuals. Interoperability is needed to make it easier to share electronic health records with physicians, pharmacists, and hospitals. Lack of interoperability can lead to information silos and process inefficiency. Implementing a BI software can help health organizations with their interoperability initiatives and, and achieve their goals.

18.7 CONCLUSION

The delivery of healthcare has always been information intensive. The volume of information created, shared, and stored is growing at a rapid rate. Healthcare is changing very fast and so is the industry's need for business intelligence. One may regard BI as a new methodology to maximize the benefits for healthcare organizations. BI provides a means to see the hidden meaning of the data. It helps to transform raw data into smart, actionable information. It empowers an organization to get the right data and information, to the right people, at the right time, in the right format, through the right channel.

Today, healthcare industry is under pressure to improve operational efficiency, patient care, and economic sustainability. It is growing to include not only the traditional information systems, but also a business intelligence platform. Forward-thinking healthcare companies realize that data and business intelligence play a crucial role in precise decision-making that will improve patient care. The level of involvement of business intelligence healthcare will dictate the difference between surviving and thriving in the new data-driven era. BI will continue to play a crucial role in the future of the healthcare industry as the industry is moving into the data-driven world.

Some universities are now offering courses on business intelligence. More information about healthcare business intelligence can be found in the books in [21-24] and one related journal: *Business Intelligence Journal.*

REFERENCES

[1] Nikhilesh, "Importance of business intelligence in healthcare," November 2012, https://www.helicaltech.com/blogs/importance-of-business-intelligence-in-healthcare/

[2] T. Mettler and V. Vimarlund, "Understanding business intelligence in the context of healthcare," *Health Informatics Journal*, vol. 15, no. 3, 2009, pp. 254-264.

[3] M. N. O. Sadiku, M. Tembely, and S. M Musa,"Toward better understanding of business intelligence," *Journal of Scientific and Engineering Research*, vol. 3, no. 5, 2016, pp. 89-91.

[4] I. Hertz, "Healthcare and BI: How can analytics improve patient care?" March 2018, https://technologyadvice.com/blog/healthcare/healthcare-bi/

[5] C. M. Olszak and K. Batko, "The use of business intelligence systems in healthcare organizations in Poland," *Proceedings of the Federated Conference on Computer Science and Information Systems*, 2012, pp. 969–976.

[6] S. Y. Lee, "Architecture for business intelligence in the healthcare sector," *IOP Conference Series: Materials Science and Engineering*, 2018.

[7] "Healthcare business intelligence market 2019 precise outlook – IBM Corporation, Information Builders, Microsoft Corporation,," February 28, 2019, https://erpinnews.com/healthcare-business-intelligence-market-2019-precise-outlook-ibm-corporation-information-builders-microsoft-corporation

[8] W. Bonney, " Applicability of business intelligence in electronic health record," *Procedia - Social and Behavioral Sciences*, vol. 73, no. 27, February 2013, pp. 257-262.

[9] M. N. O. Sadiku, A. A. Omotoso, and S. M. Musa, "Healthcare business intelligence: A primer," *International Journal of Trend in Scientific Research and Development*, vol. 4, no. 2, February 2020.

[10] O. T. Ali, A. B. Nassif, and L. F. Capretz, " Business intelligence solutions in healthcare a case study: Transforming OLTP system to BI solution," *Computational Intelligence Applications in Software Engineering*, Beirut, 2013.

[11] S. Y. Lee, " Architecture for business intelligence in the healthcare sector," *Proceedings of the 4ᵗʰ International Conference on Advanced Engineering and Technology*, 2018.

[12] "Role of business intelligence in healthcare industry," https://www.knowledgenile.com/blogs/business-intelligence-healthcare-industry/

[13] R. Sharma,"4 Ways business intelligence is revolutionizing healthcare management," April 2020, https://www.upgrad.com/blog/business-intelligence-in-healthcare-management/

[14] "Healthcare business intelligence market value hit US$ 12.7 Bn by 2026," April 2020, https://www.prnewswire.com/news-releases/healthcare-business-intelligence-market-value-hit-us-12-7-bn-by-2026--300990436.html

[15] K. Monica, "Top healthcare business intelligence companies by hospital users," May 2017, https://healthitanalytics.com/news/top-healthcare-business-intelligence-companies-by-hospital-users

[16] M. Spruit and M. Lammertink, "Effective and efficient business intelligence dashboard design: Gestalt theory in Dutch long-term and chronic healthcare," in *Applying Big Data Analytics in Bioinformatics and Medicine*. IGI Global, Chapter 10, 2018, pp. 243-271.

[17] D. A. Magdi, "Enhancing Egyptian healthcare industry based on customized business intelligence solution," in X. S. Yang et al. (eds.), *Third International Congress on Information and Communication Technology*. Springer, 2018. pp 95-105.

[18] "The relevance of BI in healthcare industry," https://www.appsvolt.com/the-relevance-of-business-intelligence-in-healthcare-industry/

[19] N. Ashrafi, L. Kelleher, and J. P. Kuilboer, "The impact of business intelligence on healthcare delivery in the USA," *Interdisciplinary Journal of Information, Knowledge, and Management*, vol. 9,2014, pp. 117-130.

[20] A. Khanna and D. Bhasin, "Business intelligence in healthcare industry," *International Journal of Science and Research*, vol. 4, no. 12, December 2015, pp. 2136-2139.

[21] L. B. Madsen, *Healthcare Business Intelligence: A Guide to Empowering Successful Data Reporting and Analytics* Hoboken, NJ: John Wiley & Sons, 2012.

[22] J. Khuntia, X. Ning, and M. Tanniru *Theory and Practice of Business Intelligence in Healthcare.* IGI Global, 2019.

[23] J. Machado and A. Abelha (eds.), *Applying Business Intelligence to Clinical and Healthcare Organizations (Advances in Bioinformatics and Biomedical Engineering).* IGI Global, 2016.

[24] S. J. Miah and W. Yeoh, *Applying Business Intelligence Initiatives in Healthcare and Organizational Settings.* IGI Global, 2018.

CHAPTER 19

HEALTHCARE 4.0

"There's nothing more important than our good health - that's our principal capital asset." - Arlen Specter

19.1 INTRODUCTION

Healthcare plays a major role in the growth and well being of any nation. It is an important component of the infrastructure that supports a smart society or a smart city. The healthcare industry sector can be divided into four segments [1]: (1) Health care services and facilities; (2) Medical devices, equipment, and hospital supplies manufacturers; (3) Medical insurance, medical services and managed care; (4) Pharmaceuticals. The digitalization of healthcare is progressing steadily and the digital revolution is arriving at a hospital near you. The Internet of things (IoT), big data analytics, artificial intelligence, robotics, and blockchain are being used to create digitalized healthcare products and services.

The rapid increase in population, rising burden of noncommunicable chronic diseases (such as diabetes and hypertension), care costs skyrocketing, and the global shortage of doctors, nurses, and technicians are leading to an increased demand for resources to support healthcare. These global challenges will seriously affect the healthcare delivery in the US and around the world. The current technological advancements are leading to the emergence of the so-called Health 4.0 revolution. Healthcare 4.0 has the potential to enable new healthcare-related processes (such as home care and personalized treatments) and transform them into services [2].

Healthcare is under tremendous pressure to deliver superior health outcomes, comply with regulations, achieve customer satisfaction, reduce cost of care, ensure patient safety, and handle financial constraints and budget reductions. Some of the challenges are illustrated in Figure 19.1 [3]. The healthcare industry is in dire need of the improvements that digitalization will bring in terms of saving costs, improved diagnostics, and more effective care. Healthcare 4.0 has the potential to offer realistic solutions to handle these challenges.

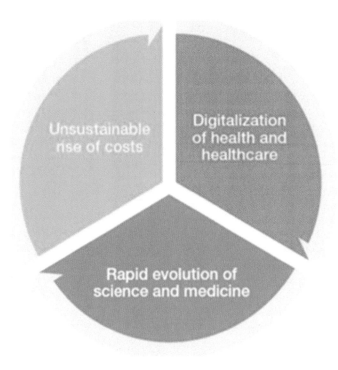

Figure 19.1 Some healthcare challenges [3].

This chapter provides an introduction to the emerging area of Healthcare 4.0, derived from Industry 4.0. It begins by providing the fundamentals of Fourth Industrial Revolution (or Industry 4.0), which inspired Healthcare 4.0. It discusses the concept of Healthcare 4.0. It covers some of the applications of Healthcare 4.0 in the healthcare industry. It addresses some benefits and challenges of Healthcare 4.0 in the industry. It covers Healthcare 5.0, the relatively new concept. The last section concludes with comments.

19.2 FUNDAMENTALS OF INDUSTRY 4.0

The Fourth Industrial Revolution is commonly referred to as Industry 4.0 (or I4.0). The term "Industry 4.0" came from the German term "Industrie 4.0," which was first used in 2011 in a project sponsored by the German government that was meant to promote the computerization of manufacturing.

Industry 4.0 is powered by the technologies originated from manufacturing industries. These technologies include the Internet of things (IoT) or Internet of medical things (IoMT), Internet of services (IoS), industrial Internet of things (IIoT), big data analytics, artificial intelligence (AI), cloud computing, cyber and physical systems (CPS), robotics, advanced materials, additive manufacturing, machine learning, cybersecurity, and mobile devices. Some of these technologies are shown in Figure 19.2 [4]. They help reate digitized healthcare products and technologies, as well as digitized healthcare services and enterprises.

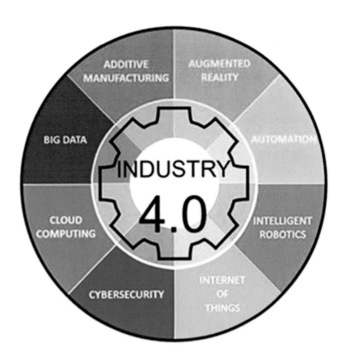

Figure 19.2 Key technologies for Industry 4.0 [4].

Industry 4.0 refers to the current trend of automation and employment of Internet technologies in manufacturing. This includes using machine-to-machine and Internet of things (IoT) deployments to help manufacturers provide increased automation, and improved communication and monitoring. This trend of the Industry 4.0 affects most people and processes throughout the society. Industry 4.0 is an emerging network approach where components, processes, and machines are becoming smart. It enables companies to achieve faster innovation, increase efficiencies, produce customized products of higher quality, and expand the boundaries of new innovative new manufacturing opportunities. Factories will gradually become automated and self-monitoring as the machines are given the ability to communicate with each other and their human co-workers. The major applications of Industry 4.0 are smart factory, manufacturing, smart product, and smart city [5].

19.3 CONCEPT OF HEALTHCARE 4.0

The healthcare extension of Industry 4.0 is known as Healthcare 4.0 or Health 4.0 in short. Healthcare 4.0 extends the concept of Industry 4.0 in a scenario where healthcare organization is an integrated center capable of providing the patient with a personal care. The scope of Healthcare 4.0 is broad and is characterized by a fusion of technologies across physical, digital, and biological domains. The major technologies that can significantly contribute in realizing the objectives of Healthcare 4.0 include [6]:

- *The Internet of Medical Things* (IoMT): This is a healthcare application of IoT technologies and envisions a network of connected devices that sense vital data in real time. It drives the next generation of connected healthcare, with the capability to store and process scalable sensor data (big data) for health care applications. The Internet of services (IoS) paradigm can connect gadgets intelligently. IoMT is driving the next generation of connected healthcare. IoMT facilitates the assessment and monitoring of illnesses. It will allow patients to consolidate their data and help healthcare providers to understand a more accurate picture of a patient's health.

- *Artificial Intelligence* (AI): In AI, machines are programmed to develop cognitive functions for learning and problem solving. AI uses the power of predictive analytics to accelerate healthcare. It has the ability to sift through large amounts of information. AI-based technology has the potential to assist physicians in diagnosing diseases. Without doubt, AI will drive the healthcare of tomorrow.

- *Cybersecurity:* Healthcare is one the most targeted industries when it comes to cyberattacks. This could put patients in danger. Patient records, such as EHRs, are sought after by hackers. It is up to suppliers and the hospitals to work together to deliver security to the patient's identity. For example, a rural hospital had to replace its entire computer network after a ransomware cyber-attack froze the hospital's electronic health record (EHR) system. In ransomware schemes, attackers may hold a hospital's data hostage until some prescribed amount of money is paid, interrupting services and putting patients' lives at risk [7].

Other technologies include genetic engineering, synthetic biology, nanotechnology, data science, bioinformatics, the healthcare informatics, the cyber-physical systems, the Internet of things (IoT), robotics, drones, blockchain, cloud computing, 3D printing (additive manufacturing), and the information security. These technologies are shaping the way we treat patients. One may describe Healthcare 4.0 as [8]:

Healthcare 4.0 = (IoT + AI + Omics) x (Platform) x (Patient Experience)

Putting the patient at the center with a focus delivering a superior experience is probably the most critical factor of the Healthcare 4.0 equation.

19.4 APPLICATIONS

Healthcare 4.0 is a disruptive process of transformation of the entire healthcare value chain ranging from medicine, medical equipment production, hospital care, remote care, healthcare logistics to healthy living environment. However, the implementation of Industry 4.0 in healthcare will be a transitional process for the healthcare industry because of the importance in retaining compliance and the need to prove quality systems. The following are common applications of H4.0 [9]:

- *Personalized Medicine:* This is tailoring of disease treatment to a specific person, taking into account their genetics, the environment in which they live. It also identifies what the best sequence of care is for a given patient. Collaboration, coherence, and convergence will make healthcare more predictive, precise, and personalized. Healthcare 4.0 promises to transform health by providing more accurate and personalized service. This can be achieved through the integration of medical devices, with cyber-physical systems, big data tools, IoT, 5G, blockchain, etc. [10]. Personalized healthcare could fundamentally change both the patient and care giver's experience.

- *Medical Device Manufacturing:* More and more technologies incubated in manufacturing industries driven by Industry 4.0 are being adopted in healthcare industries and services.

Industry 4.0 manufactures high-quality medical devices which are highly customized as per patient requirements. For example, Industry 4.0 shows the extensive capability of manufacturing newly customized implants. Medical device manufacturers are facing challenges in terms of price, speed to market, increased product complexity, and more stringent regulatory compliance. The pharmaceutical manufacturing has paid much attention on producing safe and quality products. The manufacturing control of pharmaceutical production should be self-organized and flexible enough to meet external market's demands. Providers of service and goods need to work together with consumers to ensure their adaptability to smart product characteristics.

- *Smart Hospitals:* Hospitals are complex entities and are difficult to manage. The application of Healthcare 4.0 technologies can make a great impact on hospitals. Many hospitals are still working towards becoming "connected" or smart. The digital revolution is arriving at a hospital near you. Hospital 4.0 or Smart Hospitals can be regarded as healthcare facilities that seek to optimize resources for better organization of information, patients, healthcare practitioners, and staff. Smart hospitals are dictating the way in which they purchase equipment. There is a demand on hospitals to make them an integrated center that provides patient with personalized care service. Besides improving patient outcomes, leveraging on Healthcare 4.0 will help hospitals address global operational challenges. Intelligent care beds are becoming more and more popular in hospitals and nursing homes. Figure 19.3 shows nursing beds in Hospital 4.0 [11].

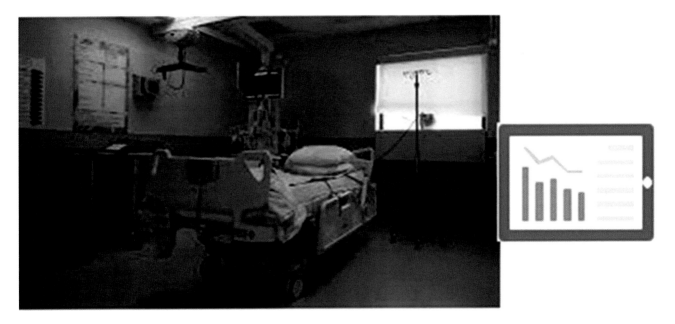

Figure 19.3 Nursing beds in Hospital 4.0 [11].

Some of these applications of Healthcare 4.0 are shown in Figure 19.4. Other applications include Intensive Care Unit (ICU), telemedicine, and digitalized surgery (or surgery 4.0).

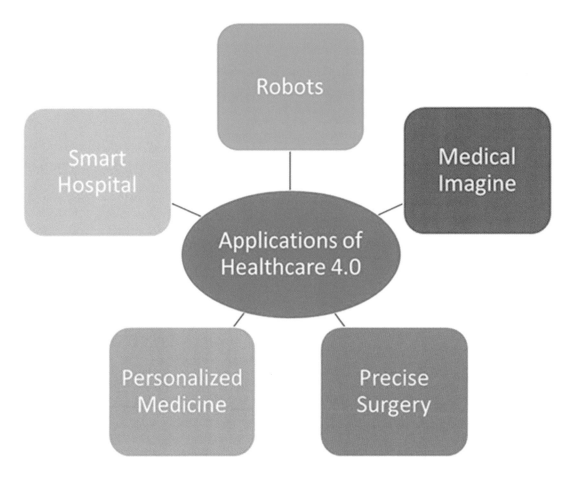

Figure 19.4 Applications of Healthcare 4.0.

1.5 GLOBAL HEALTHCARE 4.0

As new technologies (AI, IoT, robotics, blockchain, etc.) revolutionize industrial production, the German government launched to promote the computerization of manufacturing, which was named the fourth industrial revolution (Industry 4.0). China developed its own initiative, Made-in-China 2025, as a strategic plan announced in 2015 to increase competitiveness in cutting-edge industries including the manufacturing sector [12,13].

There has been an exponential increase in the usage of Healthcare 4.0-based systems around the world. Unfortunately, a large part of the world population still does not have access to the Internet. While developed nations have an Internet penetration rate of 81%, only 17.5% of the population in less developed nations have internet access. Health 4.0 needs to focus on inclusion of less developed nations in the digital age. A major challenge is language barriers, since medical terminologies are often hard to translate. We now consider how Healthcare 4.0 is deployed in the following nations:

- *United States:* Healthcare in the United States is a big business. Healthcare facilities are largely owned and operated by private businesses. The healthcare industry is moving forward into a new era of smart hospitals and healthcare 4.0. Employment in the health sector has increased in recent years. The high cost of healthcare is the primary reason Americans have problems accessing healthcare sector. The United States spends more money per capita on healthcare than any other developed country. Another problem in the US healthcare system is apparent racial and gender bias in the system. People-centric healthcare is gaining traction with people once value is perceived and trust is nurtured by giving enough attention to ethics [14].

- *European Union:* The European Commission outlined three priorities for the European Union (EU) in this field: (1) Cooperation at EU level, (2) Accelerating personalized medicine and creating infrastructure that allows data sharing, (3) Citizen empowerment. The Commission intends to publish policy recommendations on the sharing of patient data across borders. Citizens can get secure access to electronic health records and they will be empowered to take responsibility for the management of their own health. There is the need to develop standards. The European Commission promotes the OpenNCP as an environment connecting National Health Systems (NHS) cross European nations in order to create a network for sharing patient's health records. The OpenNCP platform constitutes the backbone for exchanging patient's health records across EU nations since it connects different national healthcare systems. IoT systems are being integrated with NHS. The NHS addresses the transfer of treatments from the hospital to the home, without disruption in outpatient services [15,16].

- *Thailand:* Millions of people already visit Thailand every year not just for medical tourism, but for medical treatment. Thailand is emerging as a global medical hub hoping to attract patients from around the globe. As part of its ambitious Thailand 4.0 initiative, the Thai government aims at making Thailand a leading destination for pharmaceuticals and medical devices and a world-class provider of medical care. Thailand is proactively dealing with two major issues confronting its medical system: (1) its aging population, (2) rising rates of non-communicable diseases. The country's compliance with the manufacturing standards will make it an attractive partner for multinational pharmaceutical manufacturers looking for Asian distribution partners [17].

- *India:* Medical tourism is a growing sector in India. India is a preferred medical tourist destination for cardiology, orthopedics, transplants, and ophthalmology, with offerings in wellness, preventive, and alternative medicine. The main advantages of receiving medical treatment in India include reduced costs, high quality care, the availability of latest medical technologies, and a growing compliance on international quality standards [18]. Key states and cities that are becoming well known for medical tourists include Chennai, Mumbai, Goa, New Delhi, and Ahmedabad. India faces some challenges including slow infrastructural development, government support, accreditations and promotions, insurance and allied services. These challenges tend to hinder the full-fledged growth of the medical tourism in India [19].

- *Japan:* Japan is eyeing a transformation that is more radical than any the industrialized world has ever seen. Japan's initiative is to create a new socio-economic model by fully incorporating the technological innovations of the fourth industrial revolution. Japan has advantages that make Society 5.0 or Healthcare 5.0 possible. Society 5.0 addresses a number of key pillars: infrastructure, finance tech, healthcare, logistics, and AI. Japan's advanced technology and several years of basic research will work toward creating products using information technologies like Big data and AI. Japan will overcome social challenges (such as aging society and security expenses) and experience a vibrant economy by improving productivity and creating new markets. By doing this Japan will play a key role in expanding the new Society 5.0 model to the world [20,21].

19.6 CHALLENGES

Healthcare 4.0 faces some significant challenges including the reliability and latency issues of high speed data networks. Other challenges include the following [22]:

- *Security and Safety:* When it comes to exchanging and sharing of information, security is the biggest concern. In spite of delays caused by the time it takes technologies to leave the lab and reach the population, it is prudent that such technologies are properly regulated, with a balance between safety and development. Healthcare 4.0 should guarantee the safety of data, and safety of patients.

- *Self-diagnosis Systems for Patients*: Patients through wearable devices can monitor their health conditions without having to go to the clinic or hospital.

- *Patient Monitoring*: In today's hospitals, the ability to have continuous life parameter assessments is crucial and the need to guarantee remote access by doctors is important.

- *Digital Data Archive:* The goal is to integrate the devices with the digital medical records in order to guarantee a constant and automatic update of the patient's vital conditions.

- *Acceptance of Artificial Intelligence* (AI): AI is beginning to play an increasingly important and crucial role in diagnoses and therapies. Sharing information is fundamental. Some challenges include the acceptance of robotics in clinical practice, the human safety issue during human-robot interaction, and the corresponding legal issues.

- *Regulatory Compliance*: The field of healthcare is burdened with regulatory compliance and strict regulation. Healthcare organizations, governmental agencies, and healthcare professionals need to discuss the challenges involved in implementing Healthcare 4.0.

19.7 HEALTHCARE 5.0

The future of healthcare industry is known as Health 5.0 or Healthcare 5.0, the fifth stage of the healthcare sector. By incorporating the innovations of the fourth industrial revolution, the society of the future will be one in which people 's lives are more conformable and sustainable. This will lead to Society 5.0, a super-smart society. Japan will take the lead to realize this ahead of the rest of the world.

The five stages of evolution of the healthcare sector are presented as follows [23].

- *Healthcare 1.0- Production:* In the first stage, an industry emerges. Evidence-based treatment was the focus. This first stage may also be regarded as the hunter-gatherer stage of human development. Vaccines become gradually available and the epidemics of dangerous infectious agents were prevented and controlled (i.e., small pox).

- *Healthcare 2.0 - Industrializing:* The focus shifts toward creating an ecosystem of partners, bringing them together, to provide better services. An example of such approach in healthcare was the emergence of in-patient clinics and hospitals. The second stage of the health industry introduced the integration of patient-care services.

- *Healthcare 3.0 – Automation:* The third stage focuses on automation of its activities — seeking productivity gains, improving efficiency and throughout, reducing cost and waste. In the healthcare industry, the cost to serve efficientlyy became the strategic focus. This way, the services became available for more citizens, increasing access to health services.

- *Healthcare 4.0 - Digitalization:* The fourth stage of industrial evolution is digitalization. It focusses on new and better *business models*, providing unique services. Digitization is the way forward in healthcare and promises care to be more precise and personalized. Digital technologies can offer unlimited possibilities to improve health. The focus is on collaboration, coherence, and convergence. [24].
- *Healthcare 5.0 - Personalization*: The fifth stage recognizes the main role of patients. In the healthcare, the fifth stage gravitates toward patient-centric wellbeing services. Healthcare providers are seeking ways to fit in their customers' lives. The traditional one-size-fits-all approach could lead to fewer ineffective interventions. Personalized care is tailored to the unique needs, genetic makeup, and lifestyle of each patient.

Figure 19.5 illustrated four stages of evolution of the healthcare [25].

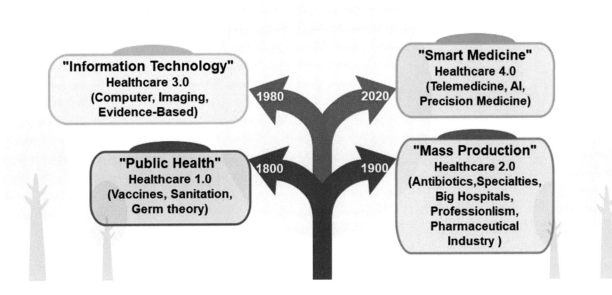

Figure 19.5 The four stages of evolution of the healthcare [25].

Health 5.0 will give rise to digital wellness, which refers to increasing, maintaining or restoring physical, mental, or emotional well-being. Healthcare 5.0 is gradually entering a digital healthcare system and it will supersede its predecessor of the Industry 4.0. It will ultimately digitally transform society, reduce the overload on acute care, and allow communities to strengthen health with a faster response time [25].

19.8 CONCLUSION

The digital age has arrived. Digitalization of healthcare may be denominated as "healthcare 4.0." The digital revolution is arriving at a hospital or clinic near you. Healthcare 4.0 is a strategic concept derived from the Industry 4.0 concept. It is currently being hailed as the industrial revolution in the healthcare sector. The digitization of healthcare will fundamentally change medicine in general and laboratory medicine in particular.

Those who ignore the opportunities I4.0 offers will be in serious danger of not being able to compete in the near future as others drive down manufacturing costs. More information on Healthcare 4.0 can be found in the books in in [26-28].

REFERENCES

[1] M. Bause et al., "Design for Health 4.0: Exploration of a new area," *Proceedings of the International Conference On Engineering Design*, Delft, The Netherlands, August 2019, pp. 887-896.

[2] M. N. O. Sadiku, A. A. Omotoso, and S. M. Musa, "Healthcare 4.0: An introduction," *International Journal of Trend in Scientific Research and Development*, vol. 4, no. 2, February 2020.

[3] M. Wehd, "Healthcare 4.0," *IEEE Engineering Management Review*, vol. 47, no. 3, Third Quarter, September 2019, pp. 24-28.

[4] A. Luque et al., "State of the industry 4.0 in the Andalusian food sector," *Procedia Manufacturing*, vol. 13, 2017, pp. 1199–1205.

[5] M. N. O. Sadiku, S. M. Musa, and O. M. Musa, "The essence of Industry 4.0," *Invention Journal of Research Technology in Engineering and Management*, vol. 2, no. 9, September 2018, pp. 64-67.

[6] "Health and healthcare in the fourth industrial revolution global future council on the future of health and healthcare 2016-2018," April 2019, https://www.weforum.org/reports/health-and-healthcare-in-the-fourth-industrial-revolution-global-future-council-on-the-future-of-health-and-healthcare-2016-2018

[7] "Health industry cybersecurity practices: Managing threats and protecting patients," https://www.phe.gov/Preparedness/planning/405d/Documents/HICP-Main-508.pdf

[8] F. Kumli, "Healthcare 4.0: The patient experience imperative," August 2016, https://www.linkedin.com/pulse/healthcare-40-patient-experience-imperative-frank-kumli

[9] Z. Pang et al., "Introduction to the special section: Convergence of automation technology, biomedical engineering, and health informatics toward the Healthcare 4.0," *IEEE Reviews In Biomedical Engineering*, vol. 11, 2018, pp. 249-259.

[10] E. M. Dias, "Health 4.0: Challenges for an orderly and inclusive innovation," September 2019, https://technologyandsociety.org/health-4-0-challenges-for-an-orderly-and-inclusive-innovation/

[11] "Healthcare 4.0 - Nursing beds in digital age," https://www.wi-bo.com/en-DE/news-room/news-and-press-releases/2018/Caritas_Wallenfels

[12] M. Javaid and A. Haleem, "Industry 4.0 applications in medical field: A brief review," *Current Medicine Research and Practice*, vol. 9, no. 3, May–June 2019, pp.102-109.

[13] T. Ruppert et al., "Enabling technologies for Operator 4.0: A survey," Applied Sciences vol. 8, 2018.

[14] T. Rice et al., "United States of America: Health system review," *Health Systems in Transition*, vol. 15, no. 3, 2013.

[15] X. Larrucea et al., "Towards a GDPR compliant way to secure European cross border Healthcare Industry 4.0," *Computer Standards & Interfaces*, vol. 69, March 2020.

[16] A/C. B. Monteiro et al, "Health 4.0: Applications, management, technologies and review," *Medical Technologies Journal,* vol. 2, no. 4, January-March 2018, pp. 262-276.

[17] The Thailand Board of Investment, "Here's Thailand's plan to transform into Asia's next big medical hub," October 2018, https://qz.com/1397519/heres-thailands-plan-to-transform-itself-into-asias-next-big-medical-hub/

[18] "Medical tourism in India," Wikipedia, the free encyclopedia, https://en.wikipedia.org/wiki/Medical_tourism_in_India

[20] "5 Emerging healthcare hubs in India," June 2019, https://www.imtj.com/news/5-emerging-healthcare-hubs-india/

[20] "Realizing Society 5.0," https://www.japan.go.jp/abenomics/_userdata/abenomics/pdf/society_5.0.pdf

[21 M. Minevich, "Japan's 'Society 5.0' initiative is a road map for today's entrepreneurs," February 2019, https://techcrunch.com/2019/02/02/japans-society-5-0-initiative-is-a-roadmap-for-todays-entrepreneurs/

[22] L. Cassettari, C. Patrone, and S. Saccaro, "Industry 4.0 and its applications in the healthcare sector: A sistematic review," https://www.summerschool-aidi.it/cms/extra/papers/441.pdf

[23] M. Kowalkiewicz, "Health 5.0: The emergence of digital wellness," November 2017, https://medium.com/qut-cde/health-5-0-the-emergence-of-digital-wellness-b21fdff635b9

[24] M. Bause et al., "Design for Health 4.0: Exploration of a new area," *Proceedings of International Conference on Engineering De*sign, Delft, The Netherlands, August 2019,

[25] N. Amunugama, "Healthcare 5.0 and the age of analytics," https://www.hhmglobal.com/knowledge-bank/articles/healthcare-5-0-and-the-age-of-analytics

[26] C. Thuemmler and C. Bai (eds.), *Health 4.0: How Virtualization and Big Data are Revolutionizing Healthcare.* Springer, 2017.

[27] J. Chanchaichujit et al., *Healthcare 4.0: Next Generation Processes with the Latest Technologies.* Singapore: Springer, 2019.

[28] D. G. Pascual, P. Dapante, and U. Kumar, *Handbook of Industry 4.0 and SMART System*s. Boca Raton, FL: CRC Press,2020.

CHAPTER 20

3D PRINTING IN HEALTHCARE

20.1 INTRODUCTION

Due to the individualized nature of healthcare, it is often necessary that customized medical devices or human parts are tailored to each individual patient. Before, conventional manufacturing may have struggled to create the custom part. Also donor shortages for organ transplantations are a major clinical challenge worldwide and replacement can be time consuming and expensive post-operative, due to frequent doctor visits and medications to prevent organ rejection. Three-dimensional (3D) printing technology holds the potential to solve these limitations. It is a new manufacturing technique in which material is laid down, layer by layer, to form a three-dimensional object. It is becoming one of the main tools of the medical industry.

3D printing is the means of producing three dimensional solid objects from a digital model. It has been regarded as one of the pillars of the third industrial revolution. No industry has embraced the 3DP technology more enthusiastically than healthcare, especially surgery. With healthcare industry under political and economic pressure to perform, 3D printing allows manufacturers to cost effectively produce customized medical devices. 3DP has the potential to change healthcare by making care it more affordable, accessible, and personalized [1].

This paper provides a brief introduction on how 3DP is used in healthcare industry. It begins by explaining in detail what 3-D printing is. It presents some applications of 3DP in healthcare. It addresses the benefits and challenges of 3DP. It highlights the global 3DP. It covers the relatively new concept of 4D printing, which adds the fourth dimension of time. The last section concludes with comments.

20.2 CONCEPT OF 3D PRINTING

Three-dimensional printing (3DP) is a manufacturing procedure in which an object is fabricated by depositing materials—such as plastic, metal, ceramics, powders, liquids, or even living cells—using additive processes in which successive layers of material are assembled on top of one another to produce the desired 3D object. In other words, 3D printing instructs a computer to apply layer upon layer of a specific material (such as plastic or metal) until the final product is built. This is distinct from conventional manufacturing methods, which often rely on removal (by cutting, drilling, chopping, grinding, forging, etc.) instead of addition. Figure 20.1 shows the 3D printing procedure [2].

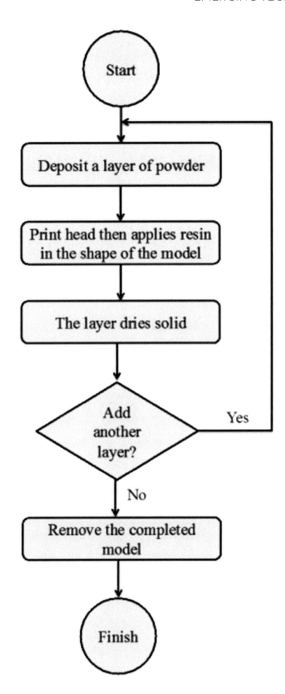

Figure 20.1 3D printing procedure [2].

Models can be multi-colored to highlight important features, such as tumors, cavities, and vascular tracks. 3DP technology can build a 3D object in almost any shape imaginable as defined in a computer-aided design (CAD) file. It is *additive* technology as distinct from traditional manufacturing techniques, which are s*ubtractive* processes in which material is removed by cutting or drilling [3].

3D printing translates computer-aided design 3D models into physical objects in a layer-by-layer fashion. It enables designers to have fully functional prototype a few hours after the design is completed. A new industrial revolution is around the corner as commercial 3D printers become smaller, portable, and cheaper. The healthcare industry must implement 3D printing as part of their overall digital transformation process.

3D printing (also known as additive manufacturing (AM) or rapid prototyping (RP)) was invented in the early 1980s by Charles Hull, who is regarded as the father of 3D printing. Since then it has been used in manufacturing, automotive, electronics, aviation, aerospace, aeronautics, engineering, architecture, pharmaceutics, consumer products, education, entertainment, medicine, space missions, the military, chemical industry, maritime industry, and jewelry industry. It is a technology perfectly tailored for the healthcare industry. It offers a range of precision healthcare solutions, including tissue and organ fabrication; creation of customized prosthetics, implants, and anatomical models, drug delivery, and testing, as well as in clinical practice.

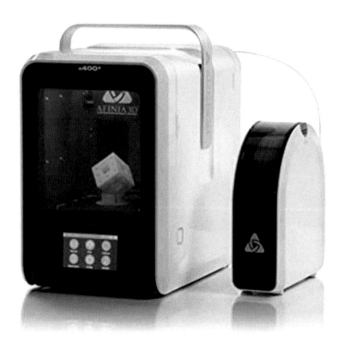

Figure 20.2 A typical 3D printer [4].

There are several types of 3D printers that are commercially available, each with its own advantages and disadvantages. Figure 20.2 shows a typical 3D printer [4]. The 3D printing technologies can be classified into three groups: extrusion printing, photopolymerization, and powder-based printing. Based on this, the main types of 3D printing include [5]:

a. *Stereolithography* (SLA): An SLA apparatus creates 3D objects by polymerizing a bath, or "vat" of photosensitive polymer resin. SLA is the most common method and has become widely accepted as the easiest method for printing surgical models quickly and accurately.

b. *Selective Laser Sintering* (SLS): SLS is a method of 3D printing that does not use photosensitive layers of liquid resin, but instead used powder which solidifies into layers.

c. *Inkjet:* This technique uses methods similar to 2D desktop inkjet printers.

d. *Fused Deposition Modeling* (FDM): Like an inkjet printer, FDM uses printer heads to deposit melted lines of plastic onto a platform in layer

e. *Sheet Lamination* (SL): This bonds sheets of material together to form objects from synthetic polymers or paper.

20.3 APPLICATIONS

3D printing has found numerous applications in healthcare, manufacturing, automotive, electronics, aviation, aerospace, defense, consumer products, education, entertainment, jewelry industries, military, engineering, libraries, food industry, dental, human medicine, and veterinary medicine. The biggest driver of adoption of 3D printing is the manufacturing world. Perhaps the most exciting 3DP applications can be found in the world of healthcare. The applications of 3DP in healthcare are already in the mainstream. These include medical device manufacturing, tissue engineering, pharmacology, surgery, anatomy, dentistry, orthopedics, prosthodontics, periodontics, personalized care, research and development, education and training, and medical imaging. Figure 20.3 depicts the 3D printing of human body [6]. Here we present some 3DP applications in healthcare that are revolutionizing the industry [7,8]:

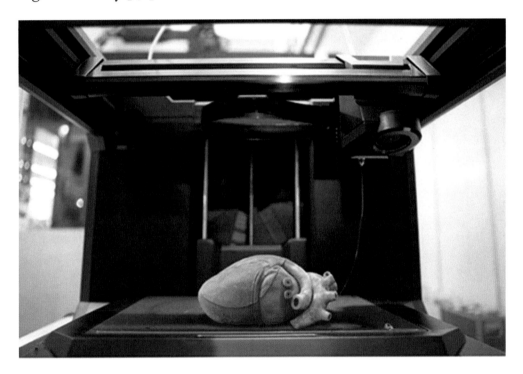

Figure 20.3 3D printing of human body [6].

- *Manufacturing of Medicines:* 3DP has become a leading manufacturing method in healthcare for a wide range of applications in medicine. It allows on-demand fabrication with high productivity in a cost-effective manner. It also allows for more accurate personalized manufacturing of medical devices across all medical fields created to the patient's own specifications. Several medical products manufactured by 3D printing are currently available in the market.
- *Tissue Engineering:* 3DP has emerged as a powerful tool for tissue engineering (or bioprinting) whether it is about blood, bones, heart or skin. Manufacturing a human tissue by 3D printing cells is an exciting, booming area. This allows the hospitals to print human tissue structures that could eliminate the need for some transplants. Flat tissues such as skin, tubular structures, and complex organs such as the liver have been 3D bioprinted. The main objective of 3D bioprinting is to reduce the shortage of supply in the organ donor market. The recent focus

of tissue engineering has been to create functional tissues and organs for implantation and to develop tissue models. Bone tissue engineering is a promising approach to bone repair and reconstruction [9].

- *Pharmacology:* 3D printing is the epitome of precision. It enables the precise deposition of drug. It is helping pharmaceutical companies to create more specific drugs. It opens up a field of personalized pharmacology. It has enabled the fabrication of prototypes of patient-specific drug delivery devices (DDD) with varying complexity and shows that customization of drug products is possible. 3D printing of drugs could enable companies to create multi-drug capsules that release different compounds at different times.

- *Anatomical models*: These are structures of anatomy used in training, surgical planning, and medical imaging research. Imaging studies such as CT and MRI can be converted to blueprints of a patient's internal anatomy. 3DP anatomical models can help surgeons better prepared to perform surgery, which will result in improved surgical outcome. Anatomical models are needed in bone construction and tumor treatments. Vessels, tumors, and skulls are just a few of the anatomical models created in a variety of materials. Figure 20.4 illustrates a 3D-printed brain model [10]. The use of 3DP in spine surgery is rapidly evolving. The advantages of using 3D-printed spine model in anatomic research include the following [11]: (1) accurate morphometry of osseous spine; (2) acceptable price; (3) readily available data using the CT or MRI data from hospital's picture archiving and communications system; (4) consistent morphometric models from the same patient's data of CT or MRI; (5) avoiding ethical problem of using cadaveric specimen; (6) overcoming limited availability of cadaveric specimens in countries with lower rate of body donation.

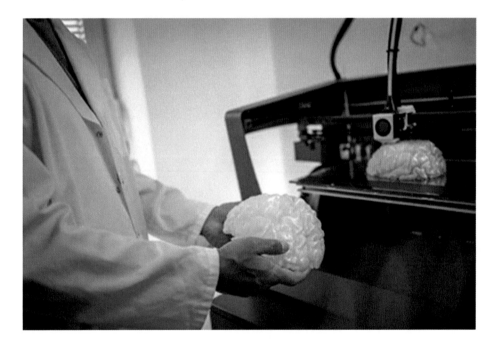

Figure 20.4 *A 3D-printed brain model [10].*

- *Prosthetics:* Prosthetics provide improved quality of life to patients suffering from a loss of limb. Millions of people worldwide need mobility devices such as prosthetics. 3DP allows the creation of custom-fit prosthetics for a patient's specific anatomical needs. 3D printed prostheses are fully customized to the wearer and are affordable. Figure 20.5 displays examples of personalized prosthetics [6].

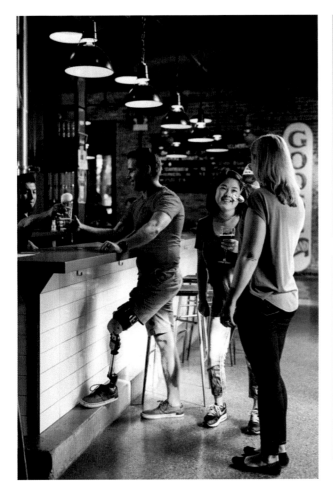
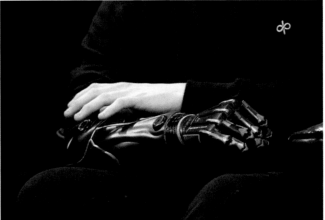
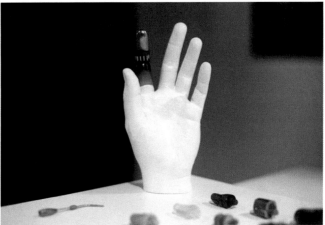

Figure 20.5 Examples of personalized prosthetics [6].

- *Dentistry*: 3D printing is making an impact in the dental sector. It can create sophisticated components in mass production, which makes it an attractive technique for dentistry. By combining oral scanning, CAD/CAM design and 3DP, dental labs can accurately produce crowns, bridges, plaster/stone models, and a range of orthodontic appliances such as surgical guides and aligners [12]. Several dentists are enthusiastic about incorporating 3-D printing into their practice. 3D printing has the potential to revolutionize dentistry.
- *Implants*: The human body is complex and traditional implants often require fit-up and care during implantation. 3DP allows the complex shapes to be designed, optimized and fabricated to the exact dimensional requirements [13]. There are several manufacturers using 3D printing to produce commercial implant products as spinal, hip, knee, skull implants, hearing aids, and vaginal rings. 3D printers can induce several desirable properties in such medical implants. 3D printed implants have been used across a variety of surgical specialties. 3D printers can induce several desirable properties in implants.

- *Personalized Care:* Personalized, precision care is on the rise. 3D printing is being leveraged to create personalized patient care. It allows medical professionals to create patient-specific devices at an affordable cost. 3D printing and advanced visualization techniques can assist clinicians in developing tailored surgical approaches for patients. Implementing a 3D printing technology in a medical center is called Point-of-Care 3D Printing, which is used for personalizing patient care. This increases patient safety, reduce length of stay, and reduces readmissions.

- *Research & Development:* 3DP technology is poised to revolutionize research and teaching medical laboratories. Printing prototypes on site speeds the R&D development cycle and shortens time to market. Prototypes can be made, tested, and finalized in a matter of days instead of weeks. Researching and developing the right formulas to create these new materials offers an opportunity for constant innovation within the healthcare industry.

- *Medical Education and Training.* With 3D technology, one can rapidly create prototype devices and anatomy-based models for testing and training. For example, viewing a model from different angles helps students understand the steps involved in surgery more clearly. 3DP models allow students to view a patient's anatomy. They enhance the students' ability to provide out-of-the-box solutions for unusual challenges that require patient personalization. 3D printing is the ultimate tool for education and training in surgery.

Other areas of applications include radiology images, breast phantom construction, medical imaging, medications, spinal anatomy, assistive technology, and clinical care.

20.4 BENEFITS

3D printing has emerged as a disruptive technology in healthcare. It is being leveraged to create personalized medical devices and provide training to future medical professionals. 3D printers are beginning to infiltrate homes and enter the mainstream. It has created a new generation of at-home and do-it-yourself manufacturers and children are starting to adopt it.

Benefits of 3DP includes rapid prototyping, rapid manufacturing, mass production, mass customization, economies of scale, use of unique materials, customization and personalization of medical products, drugs, and equipment, cost-effectiveness, increased productivity, the democratization of technology, and enhanced collaboration. 3DP will help healthcare organizations increase profitability by lowering costs, improving operational efficiency, improving patient satisfaction, reducing recovery time, and creating new opportunities [14]. The technology allows for cheaper production costs, patient-specific devices, and a just-in-time manufacturing approach. Hospitals could potentially create items on demand and this would significantly alter the healthcare supply chain. 3DP benefits patients, providers, and payers. It provides healthcare practitioner with new tools that can ultimately result in a higher standard of care.

Other benefits of 3DP include [15,16]:

1. *Customized products:* Perhaps the greatest advantage that 3D printers in healthcare application is the freedom to produce custom-made medical products and equipment. Almost every 3DP application needs to be tailored to a specific patient and requires a high level of customization because no one's body is identical (with the exception of identical twins). A customized 3DP model of each patient's

heart enables a surgeon to adjust to the unique features of each patient's heart. For example, making prosthetics the traditional way is very expensive and time consuming because they have to be custom made for the patient. 3D printers allow prosthetics to be more widely available at a lower price.

2. *Rapid prototyping:* This is the largest commercial application for 3D printing today. Conventional manufacturing processes, such as casting or forging, waste time in preparing expensive tooling and are expensive. Rapid prototyping shortens the development life cycle, enables easy experimentation, and increases confidence in the final product. The 3DP technology can be used to quickly fabricate components with any shape. Products designed can easily be made into an actual prototype. It reduces time between design iterations.

3. *Reduced Costs:* Even though the initial setup costs are higher, 3D printing has become cheaper than human labor in third world countries. Additionally, the costs of 3D printing are still decreasing, with the potential of 3D printers in homes in the near future. Furthermore, the costs of customized products are the same for mass production products.

4. *Less inventory:* With traditional manufacturing technologies, it is much faster and cheaper to manufacture additional products that you probably know that you will eventually need. However, with 3D printing, only products that are sold need to be manufactured, thus warehousing of excess inventory is significantly less needed.

5. *Jobs opportunities:* 3DP technology creates jobs for highly-skilled designers who are adept at using 3D printers. More engineers are needed to design and build 3D printers, and more technicians are needed to maintain, use, and fix 3D printers.

6. *Medical Devices:* While 3DP usages are still experimental, the potential advantages are huge. Imagine doctors quickly building and replacing critical organs, such as the heart, lungs, or liver that will have almost no chance of donor rejection, since the organs will be built using the patients' unique characters and DNA. 3DP is saving lives and is now a way to create organs, joints and limbs, helping amputees live a normal life. Production and marketing of medical devices are often regulated.

7. *Donor shortage:* Using 3DP technology for medical applications will efficiently solve the donor-shortage issue, which is a major clinical challenge worldwide. The implantation of artificial organs will improve the quality of life of patients.

20.5 CHALLENGES

Although 3D printing has been around for more than 30 years, its widespread adoption has to wait for other areas to catch up, including materials science, engineering techniques, digital transformation of healthcare. The technology is energy-intensive and limited in functionality compared to some traditional methods, As with most new technologies, 3DP technology prompts some challenges for engineers, scientists, and designers. These challenges must be overcome for the 3D printing technology to be widely adopted in the healthcare industry

The challenges facing 3DP should be understood and mitigated against. They include [15,17]:

1. *Fewer Manufacturing Jobs:* As with all new technologies, manufacturing jobs will decrease. This disadvantage will have a large impact on the economies of third world countries, especially China, that depend on a large number of low skill jobs.

2. *Limited Materials:* Currently, 3D printers only manufacture products out of plastic, resin, certain metals, and ceramics. 3D printing of products in mixed materials and technology, such as circuit boards, are still under development.

3. *Copyright and IP:* Most products and devices are not copyrightable. With 3D printing becoming more common, the printing of copyrighted products to create counterfeit items will become more common and nearly impossible to determine. This may require some regulations. Also, intellectual property (IP) battles are brewing in the world of 3DP technology. IP owners as well as trademark owners are worried about 3D printing, which allows anyone to recreate any existing product design. Business leaders, policymakers, legislators, lawyers, and engineers will need to address these issues.

4. *Dangerous Items:* 3D printers can create dangerous items, such as guns and knives, with very little or no oversight. 3D printers have already been employed for criminal purposes, such as printing illegal items like guns and master keys. FDA ensures that hospital-made 3D printed products intended for human body are safe and effective.

5. *Size Limitations:* At present, 3D printers have limitations on the size of the objects created. They are usually small-scale manufacturing facilities in a box. With minimal resources, they enable rapid on-demand production. It has become accessible and affordable. A typical 3D printers can cost anywhere from $5,000 to $50,000. The cost of buying and using the printer has dropped to the point where 3D printers can be purchased on Amazon by hobbyists for as low as $1,500. One can purchase 3D-printer shoes, 3D-jewelry or even 3D-printer cars.

6. *Speed:* The amount of time required to make 3D anatomical models limits the use of these models in time sensitive, emergent situations.

7. *Regulation:* Regulatory issues are slowing the adoption of 3D printer applications. Users can print molds from exact replicas that are protected under copyright, trademark, and patent laws. Patient-specific devices are difficult to regulate. There are legal and regulatory issues that must be addressed. This will require close cooperation between the manufacturers, the printer makers, and healthcare organizations.

8. *Ethics:* 3DP also raises a number of ethical questions that will need to be addressed. The ethical issues include equal access to health care since utilization of 3DP would increase racial and socioeconomic disparities in healthcare, testing for safety and efficacy, and whether or not we should use 3DP for human enhancement.

9. *Materials:* Limitations also exist in terms of materials, which typically can be plastics, metals, polyethylene, ceramics, liquid molecule or powder grains. There is a limited type of materials that can be used in 3D printing. International standards for choosing medical materials for 3D printing are yet to be developed. It is a challenge to print organs with 3D printing technology.

These challenges are slowing down the full implementation of 3DP in the healthcare industry.

20.6 GLOBAL 3D PRINTING

The medical world is poised to be revolutionized by the vast promises of 3D printing. It is regarded as a transformative technology that could disrupt the healthcare industry. Healthcare providers, hospitals, and research organizations across the globe are using 3D printed models.

Almost every week, 3D printing offers more applications in the healthcare helping to save and improve lives and making 3DP applications increasingly more common. Medical device companies around the world use 3D printing to create accurate prototypes of medical devices. They are able to create tissues, blood vessels, and organs on demand. As the costs of 3D printers continue to decrease and material properties improve, 3D printing will play a crucial role in the healthcare industry. Product fabrication using 3DP technology has the potential to allow individuals from variety of socio-economic backgrounds to develop products to suit their personal needs; a process termed the "democratization of technology." Based on region, the global 3D printing medical device market is segmented into North America, Europe, Asia Pacific, Latin America and Middle East & Africa. Here, we will discuss the differences between the use of 3D printing between the developed and developing nations.

In the developed world, 3D printing is making huge leaps forward. 3DP facilities are available for students in medicine and engineering to develop sophisticated prototypes for their design projects. German medical device company, endocon GmbH, has used metal 3D printing to develop a surgical tool for hip cup removal. As healthcare costs continue to skyrocket in the US, 3DP technology can offer relief. The first medicine manufactured by 3DP technology was recently approved by the Food and Drug Administration (FDA). The FDA states that 3D-printed medical devices must meet the same regulations as their non–3D-printed counterparts. A close collaboration between academics, industry, and the FDA ensures safety for the patients who live within the U.S. a quality of life that will be improved by 3D printing [18]. Nike, the footwear company, creates multicolored footwear prototypes using 3DP. Companies making 3D printing medical devices include Stratasys, Envisiontec, 3D Systems Corporation, EOS GmbH Electro Optical Systems, Renishaw, Arcam, 3T RPD, Concept Laser, and Prodways Group [19].

In developing world, there are entrepreneurs that can design and manufacture items but without a large upfront investment; it makes the utilization of 3DP challenging, especially in healthcare. In Uganda, 3DP technology is used to create 3D-printed prosthetic limbs. In South Africa, a company called Robohand used 3DP technology to manufacture prosthetic hand, arms, and fingers. 3DP technology has been applied in Haiti to print shoes for school aged children in need. 3DP technology can be used to print household items like soap holders at low cost using recycled plastics. There is a lack of standard regulation, but the future of 3DP in developing countries is very promising [1].

20.7 4D PRINTING

The rapid advances in shape memory materials (or smart materials) and additive manufacturing have fueled the development of four-dimensional (4D) printing. 4D printing is a relatively a new development. It is an additive manufacturing that integrates smart materials into the printing material for 3D printing. 3DP technology is able to alter the shape or properties of smart materials over time (the 4th dimension) as a response to the applied external stimuli. This gives rise to a new term "4D printing" [20].

4D printing (4DP) may be defined by the equation:

3D Printing + time = 4D Printing. The rapid advances in materials (or smart materials) and additive manufacturing have fueled the development of 4D printing. The 3D printing (also known as additive manufacturing) of smart materials is known as 4D printing. printing" [21].

4D printing has drawn a lot of attention since it was introduced in 2013. It has captured the imagination of everyone, from industry experts to hobbyists. It allows the printed part to change its shape and function with time in response to change in external conditions. While 3D printing produces parts that are static, 4D printing produces parts that can reshape and evolve over time. Unlike 3DP, 4DP is time-dependent and printer-dependent and targets shape evolution. The differences between 3D printing and 4D printing are illustrated in Figure 20.6 [22].

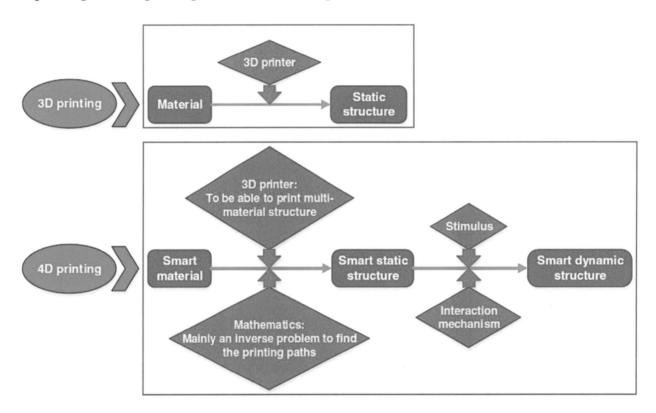

Figure 20.6 The differences between 3DP and 4DP [22].

Two main technologies are responsible for 4D printing: 3D printing and smart materials (SMs); i.e. 4D printing = 3D printing + SMs

- *3D Printing*: In 3D printing, it is common to use modeling software such as 123D Design and AutoCAD. These modeling software can be used for 4D printing too. 3D printing technology involves printing a product in a layer-by-layer manner. In 4D printing, generated 3D objects can change shape automatically and gradually over time [23]. 3D printers are capable of producing complex models from printable materials. 3D printing technology is used in industries and homes across the globe.

- *Smart materials*: Special materials are necessary to enable 4D printing. 4DP involves the creation of smart materials-based 3D objects with novel outstanding features, such as self-transformation over time. The fourth dimension in 4D printing refers to the ability for material objects to change form after they are produced. Smart or intelligent materials are the key technology of 4D printing [24]. Smart materials are materials which sense some stimulus from the external environment and create a useful response. They exhibit certain characteristics which can be exploited in products that in turn exhibit "intelligent" behavior. Smart materials have the ability to change their shape or properties (rigidity, color, texture, transparency, volume) under the influence of external stimuli. Examples of this behavior include responses to external stimuli such as self-sensing, self-healing, self-actuating, self-diagnostic, and shape-changing. Smart materials have the ability to change their shape or property (rigidity, color, texture, transparency, volume) under the influence of external stimuli such as humidity, temperature, light, electricity, and water. Smart materials are chosen based on their physical properties, cost and ease of use [25,26]. Such materials include metamaterials, hydrogels, active origami, shape memory polymers (SMPs), shape memory alloys (SMAs), electroactive polymer (EAP), dielectric elastomers, and nanocomposites [27].

Potential applications of 4DP include bio-printing, shoes, pipes, food, toys, prototypes, solar energy, biomedical devices, soft robotics, wearable sensors, and artificial muscles. 4DP has the economic and environmental implications of additive manufacturing. As an emerging area, 4D printing has a lot of challenges. These challenges can be classified as technological limitation, material limitation, and design limitation.

20.8 CONCLUSION

3DP is an emerging, multidisciplinary field which includes engineering, biology, medicine, material science, and computer science. It is providing healthcare professionals with a powerful tool for rapid prototyping, surgical planning, enhancing students' education, promoting research, and improving patient communication. Although 3DP cannot beat the cost and scale advantage of traditional manufacturing, it is making impact in small scale manufacturing and prototyping. 3DP applications in healthcare industry are booming and may even disrupt many areas of traditional healthcare. It may become a part of mainstream healthcare practice to treat a wide range of people.

Several factors influence global adoption of 3D printing in the healthcare market. These include advances in technology, improvement in the healthcare infrastructure, and reduction in cost of 3DP technology. Healthcare technologies are often expensive when they first enter the market, becoming cheaper over time. As technology develops further, the 3D printing process will become faster and more cost-efficient. With improved technology and an increased range of engineering materials available, this technique is becoming more popular in R&D departments worldwide.

Universities play a major role in the diffusion of 3D printing. Some colleges have started to incorporate 3D printing in their curriculum whereby students are challenged to create a variety of models. 3DP medical models are deployed in the training of surgical residents. This motivates and engages students in learning, while at the same time acquiring the skills of innovation, collaboration, and technological literacy necessary for 21st century professionals [28]. 3DP technology is here to stay. Its use in healthcare is growing every year. 4D printing is basically a renovation of 3D printing and promotes the use of 3D printers for creating final products instead of prototypes. More information about 3DP can be found in the books in [29-33] and the following related journals:

- *3D Printing in Medicine*
- *3D Printing and Additive Manufacturing*
- *Journal of 3D Printing in Medicine*

REFERENCES

[1] M. N. O. Sadiku, J. Foreman, and S. M. Musa, "3D Printing in healthcare," *International Journal of Scientific Engineering and Technology*, vol. 7, no. 7, July 2018, pp. 65-67.

[2] F. R. Ishengoma and T. A. B. Mtaho, "3D printing: Developing countries perspectives computer engineering and applications," *International Journal of Computer Applications*, vol. 104, no. 11, October 2014, pp. 30-34.

[3] M. N. O. Sadiku, S. M. Musa, and O. S. Musa, "3D Printing in the chemical industry," *Invention Journal of Research Technology in Engineering and Management*, vol. 2, no. 2, February 2018, pp. 24-26.

[4] "3D printing," https://skokielibrary.info/services/computers-technology/3d-printing/

[5] P. Hangge et al., "Three-dimensional (3D) printing and its applications for aortic diseases," *Cardiovascular Diagnosis and Therapy*, vol. 8, Suppl 1, 2018, pp. S19-S25.

[6] A. Reichental, "How 3D printing is revolutionizing healthcare as we know it," April 2018, https://techcrunch.com/2018/04/05/bioprinted-organs-skin-and-drugs-how-3d-printing-is-revolutionizing-healthcare-as-we-know-it/

[7] "5 Ways 3D printing will change healthcare," http://www.rapidreadytech.com/2017/09/11806/

[8] E. J. Hurst, "3D printing in healthcare: Emerging applications," *Journal of Hospital Librarianship*, vol. 16, no. 3, 2016, pp. 255-267.

[9] G. Brunello et al., "Power-based 3D printing for bone tissue engineering," *Biotechnology Advances*, vol. 34, 2016, pp. 740-753.

[10] "3D printing in healthcare: Where are we in 2019?" August 2019, https://amfg.ai/2019/08/30/3d-printing-in-healthcare-where-are-we-in-2019/#:~:text=The%20future%20of%203D%20printing%20in%20healthcare&text=Today%2C%20the%20technology%20is%20facilitating,anatomical%20models)%20the%20operating%20room.&text=In%202019%2C%20leading%20hospitals%20and,medical%20practices%20and%20research%20efforts.

[11] A. M. Wu et al., "3D-printing techniques in spine surgery: The future prospects and current challenges," *Expert Review of Medical Devices*, vol. 15, no. 6, 2018, pp. 399-401.

[12] C. Y. Liaw and M. Guvendiren, "Current and emerging applications of 3D printing in medicine," *Biofabrication*, vol. 9, 2017.

[13] "The pros and cons of 3D printing," http://www.philforhumanity.com/3D_Printing.html

[14] C. L. Ventola, "Medical applications for 3D printing: Current and projected uses," *P&T*, vol. 39, no. 10, October 2014, pp. 704-711.

[15] J. U. Pucci et al., "Three-dimensional printing: Technologies, applications, and limitations in neurosurgery," *Biotechnology Advances*, vol. 35, 2017, pp. 521-529.

[16] Q. Yan et al., "A review of 3D printing technology for medical applications," *Engineering*, vol. 4, no. 5, October 2018, pp. 729-742.

[17] D. Thomas and D. Singh, "3D printing in surgery – The evolving paradigm-shift in surgical implants on demand," *International Journal of Surgery*, vol. 42, 2017, pp. 58-59.

[18] A. Christensen and F. J. Rybicki, "Maintaining safety and efficacy for 3D printing in medicine," *3D Printing in Medicine*, vol. 3, no. 1, 2017.

[19] S. Rismani, V. der Loos, and H. F. Machiel, "The competitive advantage of using 3D-printing in low-resource healthcare settings," *International Conference on Engineering Design*, Milano, Italy, July 2015,.

[20] S. K. Leist and J. Zhou, "Current status of 4D printing technology and the potential of light-reactive smart materials as 4D printable materials," *Virtual and Physical Prototyping*, vol. 11, no. 4, 2016, pp. 249-262.

[21] Z. X.Khoo et al., "3D printing of smart materials: A review on recent progresses in 4D printing," *Virtual and Physical Prototyping*, vol. 10, no. 3, 2015, pp. 103-122.

[22] F. Momeni et al., "A review of 4D printing," *Materials and Design*, vol. 122, 2017, pp. 42-79.

[23] S. Chung, S. E. Song, and Y. T. Cho, "Effective software solutions for 4D printing: a review and proposal," *International Journal of Precision Engineering and Manufacturing-Green Technology*, vol. 4, no. 3, July 2017, pp. 359-371.

[24] M. N. O. Sadiku, O. D. Olaleye, A. Ajayi-Majebi, and O. S. Musa, "4D printing: A primer," *International Journal of Trend in Research and Development*, vol. 7, no. 3, May-June 2020, pp. 112-113.

[25] X. Li, J. Shang, and Z. Wang, "Intelligent materials: A review of applications in 4D printing," https://www.emeraldinsight.com/doi/full/10.1108/AA-11-2015-093

[26] G. Sossou et al., "Design for 4D printing: Rapidly exploring the design space around smart materials," *Procedia CIRP*, vol. 70, 2018, pp. 120–125.

[27] Z. X. Khoo et al., "3D printing of smart materials: A review on recent progresses in 4D printing," *Virtual and Physical Prototyping*, vol. 10, no. 3, 2015, pp. 103-122.

[28] O. A. H. Jones and M. J. S. Spencer, "A simplified method for the 3D printing of molecular models for chemical education," *Journal of Chemical Education*, October 2017.

[29] D. M. Lalaskar, *3D Printing in Medicine*. Cambridge, MA: Woodhead Publishing, 2017

[30] A. W. Basit and S. Gaisford (eds.), *3D Printing of Pharmaceuticals*. Springer, 2018.

[31] T. Birtchnell and W. Hoyle, *3D Printing for Development in the Global South: The 3D4D Challenge*. New York: Palgrave Macmillan, 2014.

[32] J. K. Min, B. Mosadegh and S. Dunha (eds.), *3D Printing Applications in Cardiovascular Medicine*. Academic Press, 2018.

[33] D., A.. Kumar, *Four Dimension Printing in Healthcare*. Woodhead Publishing, 2017.

CHAPTER 21

HEALTHCARE SOCIAL MEDIA

"The next generation of healthcare will be decentralized, mobilized, and personalized. Instead of the blunt instruments of the past, we will be giving patients more precise medications and therapies." — Anita Goel

21.1 INTRODUCTION

Societies around the world face an increasing number of health challenges, heightening the importance of social change efforts. Due to human nature, humans tend to group together in order to interact, cooperate, exchange ideas and solve challenges. Social media are web-based and mobile technologies that support interactions within social networks and turn communication into an interactive dialogue. Internet users, worldwide, spend more time on social media sites than on email. Social media are empowering, engaging, and educate patients, as well as healthcare providers. They enable users to create content online.

The Internet now provides health information ranging from factsheet (on health-related information) to videos on how to perform a heart transplant [1]. It has empowered individuals to share health information and interact using social media. The use of social media (SM) has tremendously increased in popularity. Its use by hospitals and health care professionals has grown significantly [2]. It has become vital networks for patients and physicians to communicate with each other. It is becoming increasing important that all healthcare professionals (HCPs) understand the basic function of social media processes.

Social media can be regarded as the collection of Internet-based tools that help a user to connect, collaborate, and communicate with others in real time. In other words, SMs are basically web-based tools used for computer-mediated communication. They comprise of a wide range of services, including forums, blogs and micro blogs, wikis, podcasts, photos, videos, item rating, and bookmarking. Social media is a relatively inexpensive way of delivering health promotion messages. It is a powerful tool that healthcare professionals can use to communicate and interact with patients or people seeking knowledge about their health. It has become an undeniable force that healthcare industry must reckon with. In the near future, healthcare may be more commonly delivered through social media.

This chapter provides an introduction on how, where, and why social media are being used in the healthcare sector. It begins by explaining what social media is all about. It covers popular social media. It presents various applications of social media in healthcare. It addresses some of the benefits and challenges of healthcare social media. It covers how social media are being used in healthcare worldwide. The last section concludes with comments.

21.2 SOCIAL MEDIA BASICS

Traditional social media include written press, TV, and radio. Modern social media, also known as social networking, include Facebook (Facebook, Inc, Menlo Park, California, USA), Twitter (Twitter Inc, San Francisco, California, USA), YouTube (San Mateo, California, USA), LinkedIn (Sunnyvale, California, USA), Instagram (Facebook, Inc, Menlo Park, California, USA), and Pinterest (San Francisco, California, USA). Both the traditional and modern social media are illustrated in Figure 21.1 [3]. Modern social media began in 1978 by Ward Christensen and Randy Suess who created bulletin board to inform friends of meetings, announcements, and share information. Since then, social media has become an integral part of our life [3]. Social media gives companies another means of reaching people in ways that traditional media cannot. They allow your company to boost their brand. Companies that fail to invest in having a strong presence on social media will soon realize they missed out on a serious competitive advantage.

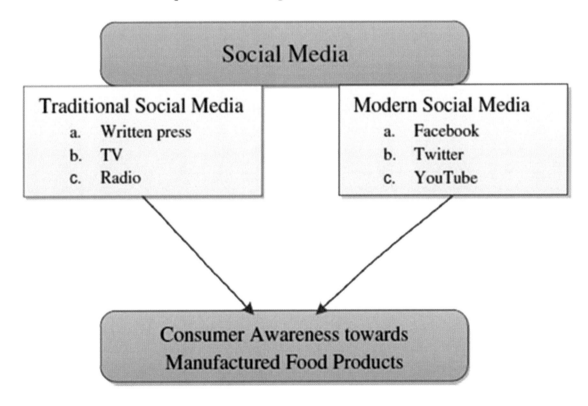

Figure 21.1   Traditional and modern social media [3].

Social media (also called Web 2.0 or social networking) refers to Internet-based and mobile-based tools that allow individuals to communicate, share ideas, send personal messages, and images. Web 1.0 is the "read-only Web." Consumers are allowed to read information created by the provider of the online information. Web 2.0 allows users to create information, send posts and share audio, graphics, text, and video online [4].

Social media are computer-mediated communication tools that enable users to share and consume content through varied modalities such as text, image, and video [5]. Recently, the use of social media has been extended to the healthcare field. Healthcare professionals now use SM as part of their daily activities. Social networking sites allow users to share ideas, activities, events, and interests. The majority of those who use social networking sites use them to form self-aggregated interest groups for fundraising, awareness, marketing, and general support.

SM sites may include wikis, blogs, and social networks

- *Wikis*: These are easy-to-publish websites. They can be quickly and easily edited by multiple users. Wiki" is a Hawaiian term meaning "quick." Wikipedia happens to be the most commonly used wiki in the medical community as healthcare professionals use Wikipedia to find medical information. However, Wikipedia sometimes contains factual errors that lacks depth compared to traditionally edited, peer-reviewed information sources.

- *Blogs:* These are the oldest, most established, and evaluated form of social media. They provide the opportunity to publish large amounts of information in a variety of media (text, video, and audio) in an open forum. Blogs have been used by healthcare workers for peer-to-peer communication. Medical blogs generally target one of two different audiences: patients or providers. Microblogs provide dynamic and concise form of information exchange through social media.

- *Social Media:* Social media platforms such as Facebook allow individuals to post photos and messages and share them with friends, relatives, and acquaintances all over the world. Media sharing sites comprise social media tools that are optimized for viewing and sharing. They are great resources for education, community building, marketing, and research. They have become encyclopedic resources.

Today, many social media tools, including social networking sites, blogs, microblogs, wikis, media-sharing sites, are influential in our everyday life and are available for healthcare professionals (HCPs).

Social media in healthcare has introduced the term Social Health, which can be described by the following 6 Ps'[6].

1 *Personalization*: Healthcare is becoming more personalized, both in terms of access and treatment.

2 *Participatory:* Internet has introduced the terms of online patient communities and ePatients, introducing participatory medicine.

3 *Preventative:* Preventative medicine represents the need to not just cure, but to encourage behavior change that would lead to a healthier lifestyle, which in turn could prevent an illness.

4 *Peer-to-Peer/Patients*: Patients are at the heart of everything that Social Health stands for. Patients are now helping themselves and seeking other people who have the same illness.

5 *Portability:* It refers to having access to someone's personal health data.

6 *Passion:* Usually, it is about some personal experience that have fueled the passions of individuals and groups to do what they do.

21.3 POPULAR SOCIAL MEDIA

Social media sites serve different purposes which may include blogs, social networks, video- and photo-sharing sites, wikis, or a myriad of other media. These uses can be grouped by purpose as [7].

- Social networking (Facebook, Instagram, Twitter, Snapchat)
- Professional networking (LinkedIn)
- Media sharing (YouTube, Flickr)
- Content production (blogs [Tumblr, Blogger] and microblogs [Twitter, Instagram])
- Knowledge/information aggregation (Wikipedia)
- Virtual reality and gaming environments (Second Life)

Social media tools are available for healthcare professionals, including social networking platforms, blogs, microblogs, wikis, media-sharing sites, and virtual reality. Social media is consumer-generated media that covers a variety of new sources of online information, created, and used by consumers with the intent on sharing information with others. It employs mobile and web-based technologies to create, share, discuss, and modify consumer-generated content. Consumers are most likely to leverage their power in social media to be more demanding of marketers [8]. Social networks have become an important healthcare resource. The five most popular social media platforms are described here [9,10].

- *Facebook:* This is the most popular social media in the US and the rest of the world. It has the largest user base of any social media platform, with 2 billion active monthly users. It was launched on February 2004 by Mark Zuckerberg as a Harvard social networking site, expanding to other universities and eventually to every one. Facebook can sensitize individuals (consumers) about many products and services. A company can use Facebook to communicate their core values to a wide range of customers. Marketing strategists have found Facebook to be useful because it covers a range of personal and organizational interests. Facebook groups can use social media for healthcare professionals and patients to interact. Facebook Advertising costs extra, and this is how Facebook makes money. Facebook is uncommonly used for medical education.

- *Twitter:* Twitter was launched on July 2006 to provide a microblogging service. Twitter provides a real-time, Web-based service which enables users to post brief messages for other users and to comment on other user posts. Tweets are extracted from Twitter. A tweet is a small message of no more than 140 characters that users create in order to communicate thoughts. Microblogging is a newer blog option made popular by Twitter. Many Twitter posts (or "tweets") focus on the minutiae of everyday life. Twitter has been used at medical conferences to enhance speaker presentations by posting real-time comments and feedback from the audience.

- *LinkedIn*: This a networking website for the business community. It is a professional network that provides a platform for professionals to participate in networking with each other. By setting up an account on LinkedIn one can link with professional individuals of similar interests. LinkedIn remains the most popular social networking site for organizations to recruit new employees. It allows people to create professional profiles, post resumes, and communicate with other professionals. LinkedIn is where companies see their largest audiences. Many regard LinkedIn as a strictly professional networking site and would never post personal information there.

- *YouTube*: YouTube has established itself as social media. It was launched in May 2005. This is a video sharing platform where many people can discover, watch, and share user-generated videos. It is a website of participatory culture. It has become the most successful Internet website providing a short video sharing service since its establishment in early 2005. Since YouTube is a Google property, its required to have a Google account to prior to signing up for a YouTube account. YouTube may serve as home to aspiring filmmakers who might not have industry connections. YouTube can be both a blessing and a curse for some companies.
- *MySpace*: This social networking site bases its existence on advertisers who are paying for page views. It has a lot that users could do. There are MySpace sites in United Kingdom, Ireland, and Australia.
- *Instagram:* This is an image-based social media platform with more than 700 million active monthly users. The design is centered on a visual mobile experience. Instagram allows a simple and creative way to capture, edit, and share photos, videos and messages with friends and family.

Other social media include Reddit, Pinterest, Flickr, Snapchat, WeChat, and Vine Camera. A number of healthcare professional networking sites exist. These include Sermo, Asklepios, Doctors' Hangout, Ozmosis, Doc2Doc, ASHP Connect, and PharmQD. Social media provide healthcare professionals with tools to share information, promote health behaviors, educate, and to interact with patients, caregivers, students, and colleagues.

21.4 APPLICATIONS

Healthcare organizations are using social media for many purposes. Social media tools can be used by healthcare professionals to enhance professional networking and education, organizational promotion, patient care, patient education, public health, medical care, research, and education. Figure 21.2 illustrates what one can derive from healthcare social media [11]. Someone has noted that [12]:

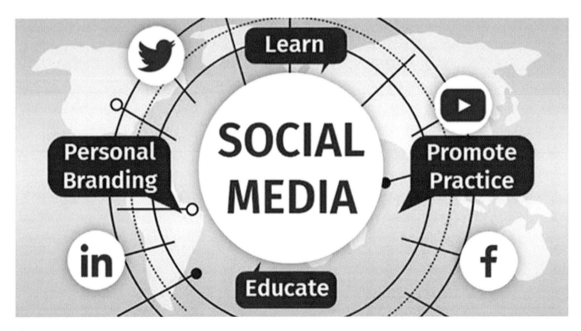

Figure 21.2   What one can derive from healthcare social media [11].

SOCIAL MEDIA + HEALTHCARE = SUCCESS

The application of social media in healthcare continues to expand. Examples of social media applications in healthcare include [13,14]:

- *Professional Networking:* Social media sites can benefit physicians and pharmacists as they participate in online communities, network professionally to listen to experts, and communicate with colleagues regarding patient issues. Sermo is a physician-only social networking, where physicians all over US gather to discuss treatment options and to query peers for expert advice. Doximity is a newer physician-only social networking community that offers text and images and provides peer-to-peer interaction. Physician- Sermo, Ozmosis, Medscape, PatientsLikeMe, and Inspire are social media specifically dedicated to healthcare. Other social networking sites are available for medical and for pharmacists.

- *Health Education:* Communication opportunities are being provided by social media. Recently, medical educators have begun to use social media tools to deliver educational content directly to learners, and enhance clinical students' understanding of communication, professionalism, and ethics. They are also widely used in pharmacy academic programs. Professors can establish Twitter handles so that pharmacy students can participate in class discussions anonymously. Twitter enhances the clinical decision-making skills of nursing students in critical care situations. The hashtag #MedTwitter is an online community on twitter for medical students, residents or attendings to discuss different topics specific to the field of medicine. Media sharing sites such as YouTube can also be used in the classroom to stimulate discussion, to illustrate a point, or to reinforce a concept. Social media enables patient education and the surgeon-patient engagement to occur remotely. It is increasingly utilized by patients to educate themselves. It can help patients to have access to healthcare information and educational resources, find hospital and physicians most capable of treating their condition. The main problem with health information found on social media, is that its mostly posted by unknown authors that lack quality and reliability. The incorporation of social media into clinical education has met with mixed acceptance. Social media–based education has a major advantage: it can reach and teach greater numbers of individuals than traditional forms of education. It has a major challenge: with the large number of participants in social media, the quality of the education is hard to determine.

- *Patient Care:* Although patients are central to healthcare delivery, their input has not been largely considered by healthcare providers. Things are changing as patient-centered healthcare has emerged. Using social media for direct patient care is gradually being accepted by healthcare professionals. Physicians have started to use social media, including Twitter and Facebook, to interact and communicate with people online for the purpose of providing education and health monitoring. Patient-centered healthcare is part of a shift in focus which has drawn increasing interest in recent years [15]. However, some feel it is ethically problematic to interact with patients on social networks for professional reasons.

- *Avoiding HIPAA Violations:* In 1996, US Congress enacted the Healthcare Insurance Portability and Accountability Act (HIPAA) to provide patients more control over their healthcare records. HIPPA is designed to reduce healthcare fraud and provide health insurance to individuals.

HIPAA compliance is one of the biggest challenges of social media in healthcare. One way to avoid HIPPA violations is to prominently post policies and procedures on all social media platforms. Healthcare providers need to obtain consent from patients to post their photos on social media sites.

Other applications of social media in healthcare include radiology, oncology, pharmacy, and crisis communications.

Mobile social media has emerged as the combination of social networking and mobile technologies. It is mediated by mobile devices such as smartphones, tablets, or laptop computers [16]. The use of mobile social media for healthcare purposes is growing. With this growth come new opportunities for deploying new services for healthcare. Big data is driving the development in biomedical and healthcare informatics because big data has unlimited potential for storing, processing, and analyzing meical data. Factors influencing social media and healthcare big data is shown in Figure 21.3 [17]

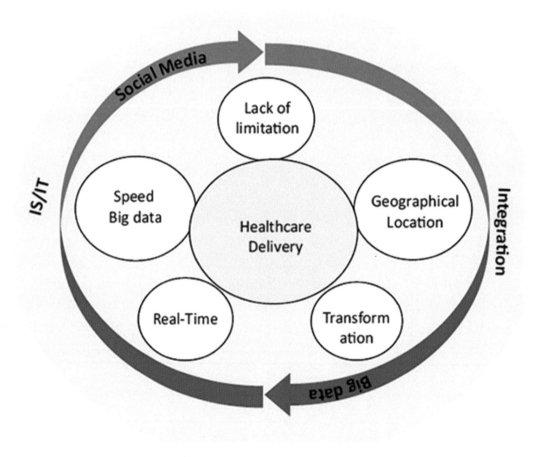

Figure 21.3 Factors influencing social media and healthcare big data [17].

21.5 BENEFITS

Social media is a popular platform used by healthcare providers (HCPs) to communicate with their patients. Using social media can connect individuals around the globe who share the same health conditions. Social media enable HCPs to market their services and gain a competitive advantage over other providers [18]. Advocates of the use of social media in healthcare makes a good argument that the SM tools allow for personalization, presentation, and participation.

In 2010, the American Medical Association (AMA) released official guidelines to guide physicians in their ethical use of social media. In 2011, the National Council of State Boards of Nursing (NCSBN) issued similar guidelines for nurses. Hospitals can communicate and educate their patients using social media platforms such as Facebook and Twitter. SM can facilitate disease surveillance, mass communication, health education, knowledge translation, and collaboration among healthcare providers [19]. The use of SM allows doctors in the same area to be in constant touch with each other.

Patients use social media to find healthcare resources. They use it to look for information, gather real-time research, find support, and make healthcare decisions. Other benefits are presented as follows [20].

- *Quick Spreading of Medical Information:* By their very nature, social media can spread information quickly to diverse groups of people, faster than ever before. SM enables high-speed and large-scale reach for information sharing and distribution. More users can become more informed about topics they are interested. Social media is a means of ensuring the public is aware of the latest issues, guidelines, and advisories. It can be used to direct followers to credible sources of current information. It is a useful tool for showcasing achievements.

- *Access to Information:* The convenience of accessing information is a major advantage of using SM for health-related purposes. The power of social media to share information is incredible. People with serious illness use social media to seek advice from others with similar health conditions. Social networks provide a meeting place for patients to share experiences and learn from each other. People can post information about new technologies, techniques, and treatments online.

- *Networking:* Social media is a great tool for networking with others globally. Social media allows everyone to share whatever they want to, with little or no restrictions. For example, Facebook allows people to remain in touch, regardless of distance. Professionals can use social media as a marketing platform to drive business to any industry and increase awareness about products offered. *Universities and colleges use social media to attract and retain students. Social media sites help employers fill positions and job-seekers find jobs.*

- *Your Patients Are Online:* Across the United States, there are more than 250 million people on Facebook. Over 99 percent of hospitals have an active Facebook page. Approximately two billion people worldwide use social media. Physicians can reach their patients where they already are with a well targeted healthcare social media marketing strategy. Using social media allows the patients to have two-way communication with other patients and healthcare providers. You can easily find out how they are feeling, discuss ongoing care with them, provide updates, encourage them to use the medications, share success stories, sharing tips for staying healthy, and ask them to reach out to your office to book their appointment. Since social media can provide healthcare professionals with a wealth of information about a patient, it can be used in a positive way to aid clinical care and disseminate health related information.

- *Senior Citizens Can Socialize:* Social media is no longer optional, even to the elderly people. Social media is a great platform for senior citizens to reconnect with society, socialize with their peers, stay in tune with younger generations, stay in touch with their loved ones (i.e., grandkids), and learn more about new technology. Connecting with people through social media has proven to have health benefits and constitute a privilege to stay connected to the outside world.

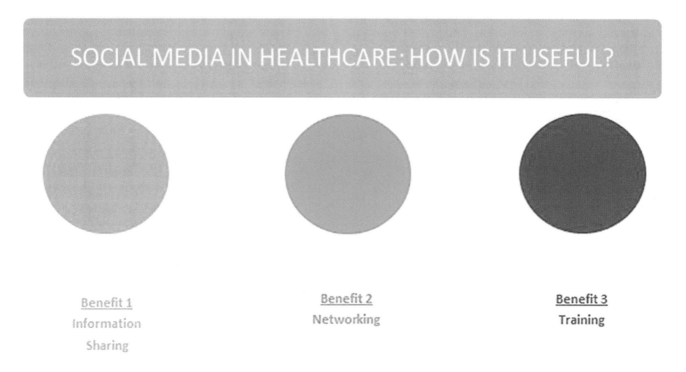

Figure 14.4 Some benefits of healthcare social media.

Figure 14.4 shows some of the benefits of healthcare social media. They are being used by nurses, doctors, and other healthcare professional on a daily basis. Healthcare organizations, including hospitals, health systems, and pharmacy are using social media for many purposes. Typical uses include interacting with patients online, education, marketing, promotions of products and services, and fund-raising.

21.6 CHALLENGES

There are always both pros and cons associated with using social media in a healthcare organization. In spite of the benefits, challenges persist in the world of social media in healthcare. Several questions in terms of governance, ethics, professionalism, privacy, and confidentiality remain unanswered. Another issue is whether a health care provider should be held liable for health-related recommendations provided through social media. Other challenges include the following [21-25]:

- *Information Overload:* Information overload occurs when one is trying to process too much information. It is being bombarded with too much information all at the same time. The amount of information that is available on social media platforms is staggering. The abundance of health information available on SM can backfire and prevent people from acquiring the information needed. Consumers can be overloaded and overwhelmed by the amount of online health information. Unfortunately, one cannot completely trust the sources of the information available on SM .

- *Misinformation:* This appears in the form of untrue statements or rumors. These can easily be debunked. For example, misinformation about COVID-19 symptoms and treatment was falsely attributed to Standford on social media. Citing information from credible sources or turning to government health officials is the best way to counter this type of misinformation.

- *Patient Privacy:* An important issue is the degree of privacy and security available in the medium. Confidentiality is a basic patient right which must be respected . Direct conversations with patients may inadvertently expose patient health information and violate HIPAA regulations. Violating HIPAA privacy policies can result in stiff penalties. Although most healthcare professionals use social media in a safe and ethical manner, some physicians violate privacy and confidentiality regulations. They may violate a patient's personal boundary by making inappropriate use of their information on social media. Misuse of social media could threaten the trust needed for a strong patient–physician relationship. Interaction with their patients on social media may be violating the patient's privacy even if patients initiate the online communication. The patient's consent is a critical issue to consider when using social media. Protected health information (e.g., names, social security numbers, date of birth, diagnoses, and photos) must be protected when dealing with medical problems.

- *Ethical Considerations:* Social media pose many risks for healthcare organizations that could potentially affect the confidentiality, safety, and security of patient information. Posting content that can damage the reputation of providers, students, and the healthcare institution is risky. Healthcare organizations should develop institutional policies that encompass discrimination, harassment, leaking of confidential information, and other ethical issues. Some user utilize SM to promote false information. It is difficult for social media platforms to mitigate cyberbullying, which is the use of technology to harass someone else.

- *Legal Issues:* The widespread use of social media has introduced new legal problems. Doctors and nurses have an ethical and legal responsibility to maintain their patients' confidentiality. Breaching confidentiality endangers the public's trust in the medical profession. Healthcare social media accounts are subject to strict rules and regulations. New legal questions are arising from some providers' use of social media to transcend geographic barriers in delivering care. Traditionally, doctors are licensed state by state so that a doctor in Texas would need to be licensed in Florida to serve patients there. Social networks might not recognize borders or geographic boundaries.

- *Social Stigma:* The fear of the unknown seems to be a major barrier against the adoption of social media in healthcare. This is due to the conservative nature of healthcare professionals. There is a growing movement of physicians who look down on social media. Some pharmacists have been reluctant in adopting social media. There continues to be conflict between the values of healthcare providers and those of social media. The main challenges that prevent physicians from adopting social media are: maintaining confidentiality, lack of active participation, finding time, lack of trust, workplace acceptance and support, and information anarchy. With the popularity of physician-only social media outlets like Sermo and Doximity, things may change in favor of social media.

- *Social Media Addiction:* This is a real phenomenon. People increasingly spend their time on social media sites such as Facebook, Twitter,and Instagram. Any addiction to these outlets are potentially harmful, since it saps one's energy from other activities such as work and offline relationships. Social media can also cause stress, lead to comparison and other negative emotions. One can also get eyestrain from staring at screens for too long.

- *Cost:* Doctors may want to try new technologies until they find them to be a financial burden. Doctors in small practices typically do not have the time, money, or other incentives to make the changes.
- *Lack of trust:* Physicians do not readily trust other people on social media when sharing medical information related to medical knowledge and practice. Social media is open to everyone and users credentials are not always assessable to check for creditability. Consequently, there is a lack of trust to accept what has been shared on social media. Anonymity is a major barrier to developing a trusted relationship on social media.

All things considered, the advantages of using SM in healthcare outweigh the disadvantages.

21.7 GLOBAL SOCIAL MEDIA IN HEALTHCARE

Social media is an easy way to connect with people locally and globally on a personal or professional basis. It is the fastest advertising and tracking marketing medium available. It is a liberating tool for millions of people throughout the world. Billions of people around the world use social media to interact and communicate with one another. There are significant discrepancies among nations in terms of their access to the Internet and use of social media in healthcare. Those countries with the most widespread access were United Kingdom, Australia and the USA. Although legal norms governing privacy and confidentiality in different nations may differ, one could argue that ethical norms should not.

Here we consider healthcare related social media policy in different countries around the world.

- *United States:* The growing use of social media tools such as Facebook, YouTube, and Twitter has led to a social media revolution. In the US, over 80% of Internet users are using social media sites. Patient's information is protected by the Health Insurance Portability and Accountability Act (HIPAA) and cannot be shared on social media. Sharing such information is considered a breach of patient privacy rules. Nearly all medical schools in US have a Facebook presence and have policies clearly stating the balance between what is forbidden or appropriate on social media, in order to help students navigate their online interactions.
- *Canada:* Consumers everywhere are using social media to position themselves at the center of care. Social media seems to be unevenly used in Canadian healthcare. Concerns with social media use by hospitals in Canada include data security, privacy, and compliance issues with applicable regulations. Challenges noted have been categorized into three areas: reputation, productivity, and privacy. In Canada, the Personal Information Protection and Electronic Documents Act (PIPEDA) dictates data privacy and how electronic documents containing personal health information can be transmitted [26].
- *India:* Hospitals across India are turning to social media as a means of distributing their message, educating their patients, and marketing their services. The government of India developed a Facebook Messenger chatbot, which can answer questions, direct citizens to the right resources, and counter misinformation [27].

- *Australia:* The Australian Nursing and Midwifery Federation (ANMF) published an online networking guidelines for nurses, which will help them to understand their professional responsibilities and adhere to high ethical standards while using social media [28].
- *Taiwan:* In Taiwan, a well-known emergency physician blogger created a public group to ask his colleagues how they could improve patient wait times in the emergency room. The group grew and received so much attention that the Minister of Health himself (and his staff) joined the group and commented directly. This caused the minister to make visits to emergency departments in ten different cities and promised to improve funding and reduce wait times in emergency departments [29].
- *Saudi Arabia:* This country has the highest number of active twitter users in the world. The majority of HCPs are in agreement with the utility of social media in the provision of health services. Social media can represent a useful tool by which physicians may advertise their services and disseminate general health information [30].

21.8 CONCLUSION

The healthcare industry lags behind many other industries in adopting social media as part of their practice. Social media tools are now becoming a presence in healthcare and transforming it in the process. They introduce a new dimension to healthcare, employing a platform used by the public, patients, and health professionals to communicate about health issues with the intent of improving health outcomes. It is no longer a matter of whether a healthcare organization should utilize social media to communicate with patients, but rather how and with what platforms. Although healthcare social media is still evolving, it has made a profound impact on the healthcare industry. Social media has gone beyond a tool for sharing photos and messages to fostering serious discussion on health and business. It have infiltrated our lives, personally and professionally. They are rapidly transforming the nature of healthcare interaction.

Healthcare social media provides new prospects and new avenues for research. Educational institutions should teach professional behavior and conduct of healthcare students' use of social media. There are great opportunities and advantages for social media to improve healthcare. More work is yet to be done in understanding the impact of social media on patient-professional relationship. Healthcare social media is here to stay as a game changer. More information about it can be found in the books in [31-34].

REFERENCES

[1] L. Campbell, "Social media use by physicians: A qualitative study of the new frontier of medicine," *Master's Thesis*, University of Washington, 2015.

[2] M. L. Antheunis, K. Tates, and T. E. Nieboer, "Patients' and health professionals' use of social media in health care: Motives, barriers and expectations," *Patient Education and Counseling*, vol. 92, 2013, pp. 426-431.

[3] J. A. H. Kareem et al., "Social media and consumer awareness toward manufactured food," *Cogent Business & Management*, vol. 2016.

[4] J. Sarasohn-Kahn, "The wisdom of patients: Health care meets online social media," April 2008, https://www.chcf.org/publication/the-wisdom-of-patients-health-care-meets-online-social-media/

[5] M. N. O. Sadiku, M. Tembely, and S.M. Musa, "Social media for beginners," *International Journal of Advanced Research in Computer Science and Software Engineering*, vol. 8, no. 3, March 2018, pp. 24-26.

[6] I. Apostolakis et al., "Use of social media by healthcare professionals in Greece: An exploratory study," *International Journal of Electronic Healthcare*, vol. 7, no. 2, 2012, pp. 105-124.

[7] C. L. Ventola, "Social media and health care professionals: Benefits, risks, and best practices," *P&T*, vol. 39, no. 7, July 2014, pp. 491-499.

[8] C. Kohli, R. Surib, and A. Kapoor, "Will social media kill branding?" *Business Horizons*, 2015, vol. 58, pp. 35-44.

[9] G. Merchant, "Unravelling the social network: theory and research," *Learning, Media and Technology*, vol. 37, no. 1, 2012, pp. 4-19.

[10] M. N. O. Sadiku, A. A. Omotoso, and S. M. Musa, "Social networking," *International Journal of Trend in Scientific Research and Development*, vol. 3, no. 3, Mar-Apr. 2019, pp. 126-128.

[11] "Should I be on social media as a healthcare professional?" https://www.pcronline.com/About-PCR/social-media-healthcare-professionals/Should-I-be-on-social-media-as-a-healthcare-professional

[12] "Social media for healthcare," November 2015, https://www.mpowermed.com/ever-wonder-how-social-media-can-help-your-practice/the-technicians-of-healthcare-1-1/

[13] M. N. O. Sadiku, N. K. Ampah, and S. M. Musa, "Social media in healthcare," *International Journal of Trend in Scientific Research and Development*, vol. 2, no. 5, June/July 2018, pp. 665-668.

[14] "Social media: A review and tutorial of applications in medicine and health care," *Journal of Medical Internet Research*, vol. 16, no. 2, Feb. 2014.

[15] R. Rozenblum and D. W Bates, "Patient-centred healthcare, social media and the Internet: The perfect storm? " *BMJ Quality and Safety*, vol. 22, no. 3, 2013, pp. 183–186.

[16] M. N. O. Sadiku, P. O. Adebo, and S.M. Musa, "Mobile social media," *International Journal of Advanced Research in Computer Science and Software Engineering*, vol. 8, no. 3, March 2018, pp. 8-10.

[17] S. Mgudlwa and T. Iyamu, "Integration of social media with heathcare big data for improved service delivery," *South African Journal of Information Management*, vol. 20, no. 1, 2018.

[18] M. S. Alhaddad, "The use of social media among Saudi residents for medicines related information," *Saudi Pharmaceutical Journal*, 2018.

[19] E. Hagg, V. S. Dahinten, and L. M. Currie, "The emerging use of social media for health-related purposes in low and middle-income countries: A scoping review," *International Journal of Medical Informatics*, vol. 115, 2018, pp. 92-105.

[20] D. Snipelisky, "Social media in medicine: A podium without boundaries," *Journal of the American College of Cardiology*, vol. 65, no. 22, 2015, pp. 2459-2460.

[21] "Top benefits of social media in the healthcare industry," https://www.businesswire.com/news/home/20180705005245/en/Top-Benefits-Social-Media-Healthcare-Industry-Infiniti

[22] M. N. O. Sadiku, A. E. Shadare, and S. M. Musa, "Information overload: Causes and cures," *Journal of Multidisciplinary Engineering Science and Technology*, vol. 3, no. 4, April 2016, pp. 4540-4542.

[23] K. M. Lambert, P. Barry, and G. Stokes, "Risk management and legal issues with the use of social media in the healthcare setting," *Journal of Healthcare Risk Management*, vol. 31, no. 4, 2012, pp. 41-47.

[24] S. J. Mansfield et al., "Social media and the medical profession," *MJA*, vol. 194, no. 12, 20 June 2011, pp. 642–644.

[25] S. Panahi, J. Watson, and H. Partridge, "Social media and physicians: Exploring the benefits and challenges," *Health Informatics Journal*, vol. 22, no. 2, 2016, pp. 99-112.

[26] K. Read and D. Giustini, "Social media for health care managers: Creating a workshop in collaboration with the UBC Centre for Health Care Management," *JCHLA / JABSC*, vol. 32, 2011, pp. 157-163.

[27] S. P. Singh et al., "Effect of social media in health care: Uses, risks, and barriers," *World Journal of Pharmacy and Pharmaceutical Sciences*, vol. 5, no. 7, 2016,pp. 282-303.

[28] J. Hao and B. Gao, "Advantages and disadvantages for nurses of using social media," *Journal of Primary Health Care and General Practice*, vol. 1, no.1, 2017.

[29] F. J. Grajales III et al., Social media: A review and tutorial of applications in medicine and health care," *Journal of Medical Internet Research*, vol. 16, no. 2, 2014.

[30] F. " Alshakhs and T. Alanzi, The evolving role of social media in health-care delivery: Measuring the perception of health-care professionals in Eastern Saudi Arabia," *Journal of Multidisciplinary Healthcare*, vol. 11, 2018, pp. 473–479.

[31] R. Nelson, I. Joos, and D. M. Wolf, *Social Media for Nurses: Educating Practitioners and Patients in a Networked World*. New York: Springer, 2013.

[32] C. B. Thielst, *Social Media in Healthcare: Connect, Communicate and Collaborate*. Health Administration Press, 2nd edition, 2013.

[33] Mayo Clinic Center for Social Media, *Bringing the Social Media Revolution to Health Care*. Mayo Foundation for Medical Education & Research, 2012.

[34] G. W. Lawson, *Healthcare Social Media: Transformation 3.0*. CreateSpace Independent Publishing Platform, 2015.

CHAPTER 22

HEALTHCARE GAMIFICATION

"Gamification is the use of game elements and game thinking in non-game environments to increase engagement and improve better targeting." - Mehreen Siddiqua

22.1 INTRODUCTION

Rapid advances in digital technologies are constantly unveiling new ways for us to interact with the world. Due to these technologies, the healthcare industry has undergone major transformation. One of the trends sweeping the healthcare industry is gamification. Numerous social and technological trends support the use of gamified products in the healthcare industry.

The games industry is one of the most lucrative industries due to the billion dollar sales of digital games. The global game marketplace includes video game console hardware and software and online, mobile, and PC games. Games are designed systematically, thoughtfully, and artistically for the purpose of creating fun and enjoyment. Although games and gamification have a lot in common, they are not exactly the same [1,2].

Gamification (or game-based approach) is basically adapting game-design elements (fun, play, transparency, reward, incentive, competition, and challenge) and game-thinking to non-game services and applications. It focuses on applying game mechanics to non-game purposes such as business and healthcare, other than their expected entertainment use. It is the most exciting and promising area in gaming. It improves player/user motivation, enhances engagement, and changes behavior. Recently, gamification has raised a lot of popular interest both in industry and academia. Understanding how gamification applies to the healthcare industry is essential.

The healthcare sector has witnessed a rapid adoption of gamification. Healthcare professionals have used gamification in self-management of chronic diseases and common mental disorders. Health gamification practices, involving children and parents, lead to better quality of life, reduced risk of disease, and increase life expectancy. *Fitocracy* is a typical example of gamification app used for motivating user exercise behavior. *SuperBetter* is an app that offers rewards for achieving mental health goals. When applied to mobile health care, gamification has the potential of greatly facilitating patient self-management [3].

This chapter provides an introduction to gamification in healthcare. It begins by explaining what gamification is all about. It presents different components of gamification. It discusses some applications of gamification in healthcare. It highlights some benefits and challenges of healthcare gamification. It covers healthcare gamification around the world. The last section concludes with comments.

22.2 CONCEPT OF GAMIFICATION

Gamification is the process of applying the science and psychology of digital gaming (such video game elements) in a non-game environment. It is the craft of deriving all the fun in games and applying them to productive activities. Some regard it as a mass-market consumer software that takes inspiration from video games. It involves taking something that already exists and integrating game mechanics into it to motivate participation and increase engagement [4]. For example, it is being employed to enhance user engagement by adding playfulness and fun to existing information systems.

Gamification (or game-based techniques) does not involve playing games, but it is simply absorbs the fun game-like elements (attractive interfaces, medals, progress bars, leader boards, etc.) in a game into real-world applications. It is the process of applying game-thinking to solve problems and engage individuals. It works by making technology more engaging, informing, and educating. Gamification has positive influence on individuals. When you gamify high-value interactions with customers, you boost sales, enhance stronger collaboration, deeper loyalty, and customer satisfaction.

The history of gaming goes back to ancient times when games constituted the oldest forms of social interaction. The word "gamification" was coined in 2002 by Nick Pelling, a British inventor, but it did not gain popularity until 2010. The idea of gamification came from the fact that the gaming industry was the first to master human-focused design and now we are learning from games. Gamification is not a new concept, but it is deeply rooted in marketing endeavors, such as points cards, grades, and degrees, and workplace productivity [5]. The main goal of gamification is to motivate individuals to change behaviors, develop skills, or foster creativity. Typical examples of target behavior can be donating money, buying a product or sharing ideas with a friend. Companies that are using gamification include Cisco, Microsoft, eBay, American Express, Samsung, Foursquare, Dell, and Siemens.

Gamifying healthcare has recently become important due to the following reasons [6]. First, as the healthcare industry is increasingly becoming expensive, wellness care has become more critical. Second, the great success of Pokémon GO demonstrated how willingly people will play games simply for the fun of earning points. Third, the proliferation of mobile devices creates natural platforms for gaming. Integrating gamification techniques into mobile applications may influence their usability.

22.3 COMPONENTS OF GAMIFICATION

Gamification is essentially a set of rules from the world of games (video games in particular) that aim at applying gaming elements to a non-game experience. It is a multidisciplinary technique covering a wide range of domains including game study, human-computer interaction, and psychology. Looking at the components (or core drives) of gamification will help us understand what a gamified system actually consists of.
- *Games*: Figure 22.1 shows various uses of games. The basic idea behind a game is to reward or punish the player with some reinforcements. Positive reinforcement tends to be more effective in producing results than negative reinforcements. Most games also provide motivations like

points, badges, rewards, or levels. Digital games involve programming computers to play games. They have become the fastest growing section of the entertainment industry. The educators, military, government, and healthcare providers use digital games. Games used for serious purposes or "serious games" are used by the military. Good game mechanics keep people engaged, motivated, and always desiring more. Today, games are not just for fun anymore; everything from dating to manufacturing has been gamified. Gamification mechanics produce four outcomes in patients: challenge, entertainment, social dynamics, and escapism [7,8].

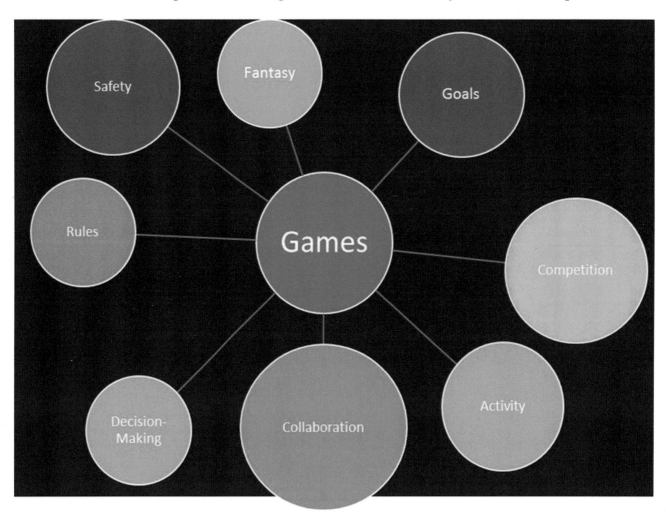

Figure 22.1   Different uses of games.

- *Gamification Elements*: These include [9]:
    - (a) Awards: A particular award is given to the player on the completion of a behavior.
    - (b) Point-based reward system: The players obtain a reward in the form of points on the completion of a certain behavior.
    - (c) Badges: These represent certain achievements of the player. They are common extrinsic rewards employed in gamification efforts.
    - (d) Levels: The users have a level that increases as they reach a certain number of points.
    - (e) Quests: The tasks the player has to complete are presented as a quest.
    - (f) Voting: Players can vote on another player's behavior.

(g) Ranking: A ranking with a list of the top players is presented to all players to increase competitiveness.

(h) Betting: Players bet on a certain event, such as an estimation, for example. The winner of the bet is rewarded.

• *Game mechanics:* Gamification model are based on games mechanics such as rewarding system, customization, and leader-boards. Game mechanics help break down large tasks into small, achievable goals and reward achievement. The game mechanics represent the modes of interacting with games. These consist of rules, roles, and stories [10].

Fun is the secret ingredient that makes the gamification a truly unique experience. It is a consequence of brain adaptation to pattern recognition. Like games, gamification includes goals, challenges, competition, and collaboration.

22.4 APPLICATIONS

Gamification is the application of elements of video games, game-thinking, and game-mechanics to help solve everyday real-life problems. It is an umbrella term for using video game elements in non-gaming platforms with the goal of improving user experience and engagement. It can be used almost everywhere; thanks to smartphones, tablets, and computers. It has been widely applied in different areas such as education, business, marketing, workplace, healthcare, edutainment, information studies, human–computer interaction, financial services, transportation, engineering, computer science, manufacturing, medicine, cybersecurity, and military [11,12]. Figure 22.2 illustrates some of these areas of applications of gamification [13].

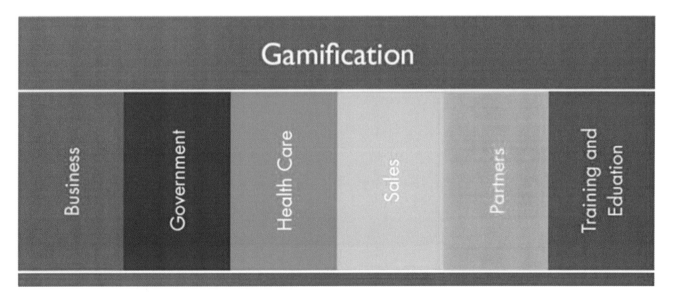

Figure 22.2   Different ways gamification can be used [13].

Gamified applications are designed for a variety of healthcare topics such as chronic disease management and rehabilitation, mental health, eHealth, mHealth, medication adherence, medical education, nutrition, weight control, fitness, wellness and different diseases (i.e., diabetes, Alzheimers, cardiovascular disease). Some of these applications of healthcare gamification are shown in Figure 22.3. Gamification naturally complements existing digital tools including electronic health records (EHRs), cutting-edge robotics, social media, and big data analytics. Key gamification market players include Fitbit,, Ayogo Health, Microsoft, Bunchball, EveryMove, Akili Interactive Labs, JawBone, Mango Health, and Nike.

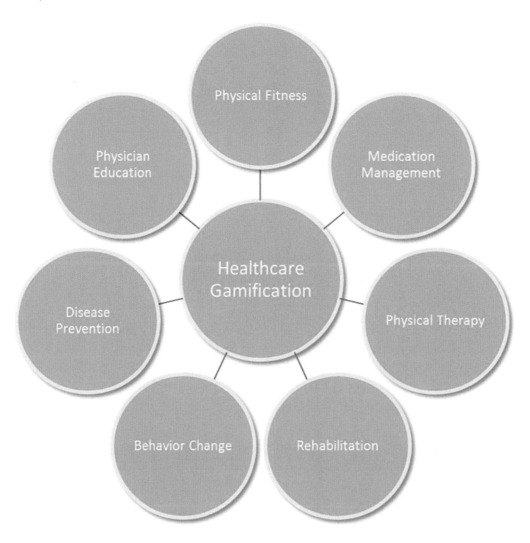

Figure 22.3   Different applications of healthcare gamification.

Some of the applications of gamification in healthcare include the following [14-16].
* *Physical Fitness:* Chronic disease management and physical fitness are the most popular applications of gamification in healthcare. Physical fitness encompasses both fitness and exercise for people who do not have to be necessarily ill and supports people who want to have a healthier lifestyle. Wellness can become fun via social media. Gamification of fitness and exercise is very popular. Gamification seeks to restructure a typically boring activity into something enjoyable and engaging. As the healthcare industry becomes more expensive, wellness care has become more critical. Nike is a good example of a sports manufacturer offering apps

and engaging with their customers online. Some companies such as BP, IBM, and Bank of America give their employees Fitbit devices to track their health habits.

- *Medication Management:* Patients often do not follow their physician's instructions. Busy lifestyles make people forget to take their medication. Not taking medicines on time is a widespread problem with patients. For example, strict adherence to a medication regimen is a crucial factor in patients with epilepsy to remain seizure free for years.[17]. Gamification is essentially a tool for motivation, helping patients commit and stick to activities they want to do. Thus, gamification seems to be a valuable technique to motivate people to adhere to medication regimens. A smartphone application was developed by *Mango Health* to motivate patients to take their medications at the right time. The use of tailored games can raise patients' willingness to manage their condition and increase their medical adherence. *Play-It Health* is an adherence platform that helps patients adhere to all key components of their disease management. *Medisafe is* a medication reminder app with more than 5 million users.

- *Physical Therapy:* Applying gamification in physical therapy is motivated by characteristics such as attractiveness, motivation, and engagement. It has potential to increase participants' motivation and engagement in therapy. Physical therapists use gaming technologies to motivate their patients to exercise. Gamification is offered at a low cost, which means it can positively impact patients with serious injuries. It helps motivate patients to do their exercises when not being supervised by a physical therapist. Increasing the efficacy of physical therapy will certainly result in increased patient satisfaction.

- *Rehabilitation:* Traditional rehabilitation treatments involve different types of visual and physical coordination tasks, many of which are 'paper and pen' based. It is quite monotonous and boring. Gamified therapies can help make rehabilitation more fun and divert attention from pain. It is important to help people stick with their treatment. The *Reflexion Health VERA* (Virtual Exercise Rehabilitation Assistant) is a tele-rehabilitation system that allows patients to perform physiotherapy at home in a monitored environment. The objective is to use technology to make rehabilitation fun and engaging.

- *Behavior Change:* Gamification is already being used widely to encourage healthy behaviors, as well as helping change maladaptive behavior. It can be used to influence patient behavior. Business, education, and healthcare all use gamification to affect some desired behaviors. Physicians often face difficulty in helping their patients change their health behaviors, such as cessation of smoking, losing weight, poor food choices, etc. . Combining behavioral economics and gamification holds promise for achieving behavior change. While gamification can be used to affect the behavior of learners, its actual effects are greatly dependent on characteristics of the learners and the context in which the gamification is implemented. Gamification programs are unlikely to engage people at higher risk (of what??) who could benefit most from changing their behavior. Embedding behavioral insights into gamification could represent a significant opportunity to improve health and wellbeing [18]. Game designers strongly believe that gamification is strong enough to help us make behavior changes. Motivating people to make lifelong health changes is challenging. Patients need to adopt the recommended behavioral change to achieve success. Smartphones can serve as a conduit to behavior change, as game applications can be downloaded which could alter patient's health behavior. Mobile phones have been shown to be effective platforms for delivering health interventions.

- *Disease Prevention:* The healthcare industry is heading toward a focus on prevention. Prevention of diseases like diabetes or cardiovascular disease is an area where gamification can show promise. Games can include a wellness plan that encourages patients to exercise regularly and eating a well-balanced diet to help prevent those diseases.

- *Physician Education:* Education is perhaps the most successful and well-known area of application for gamification. Traditional education has been found to be ineffective in motivating and engaging many students. Gamification is being increasingly used in medical education, as it has the ability to make learning fun, memorable, and more effective. It facilitates better learning experience and environment, increases recall and retention, provides instant feedback, engages and entertains learners, and drives strong behavioral change. Medical students should cease seeing their education as a challenge to overcome. Gamification in medical education is a viable alternative to some of the existing educational delivery methods. The goal of education gamification is not to replace regular lectures but to be a supplemental tool for students in learning concepts. Gamification simply means improving the learning that occurs as an experience. It unifies educators and engages learners through an effective, systematic approach [19,20]. Over the years, medical education games, mobile applications, and virtual patient simulations for medical education have been developed. Gamification can act as a catalyst for collaborative learning, where teams of learners can work together towards a shared goal.. Whether medical schools incorporate gamification in their curriculum remains to be seen. The concept of "serious games" was introduced by Abt in 1970; they are games that have an explicit and carefully thought-out educational purpose [21,22]. The main reason for using games for healthcare is their ability to motivate. Figure 22.4 shows how serious games are related to other kids of games [23].

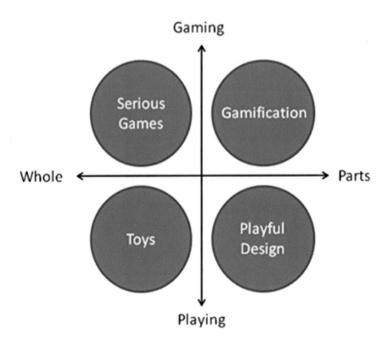

Figure 22.4   Gamification between game and play, whole and parts [22].

Other applications of healthcare gamification include surgery, obesity, health insurance, active ageing, stress reduction, diabetes, and cardiovascular disease. Physicians are having success with using online video games as their primary learning tool Overall, gamification offers benefits to all members of the healthcare community.

22.5 BENEFITS

Gamification has shown promise in the healthcare setting. It has provided the healthcare industry several benefits by engaging patients and tracking overall improvement. Gamification works well for enhancing brand awareness, boosting employee performance, accelerating learning. It benefits the patients by helping them manage chronic health conditions, take their medications at the right time, endure through physical rehabilitation easier, and improve emotional health. Gamification improves health literacy for patients, students and doctors. Healthcare professionals, game designers, behavioral scientists, investors, and governments can be united in using game-play to foster creative, collaborative, and healthy populations. Other benefits include the following.

- *Customer Engagement:* The major benefit of gamification in healthcare is ensuring users' regular engagement, known as "stickiness." Video gaming is a form of entertainment that engages participants emotionally and mentally. Gamification is designed to improve multiple aspects of engagement including fun and enjoyment, and create a sense of mastery. It can get people more engaged and responsible for their health-related decisions. Anyone with a smartphone can download various game applications that can encourage them to foster a healthier lifestyle. Players of these games can win rewards (may be cash) if they hit their health goals.
- *Weight loss:* Several weight loss programs have tried many different methods to help their clients succeed. Gamification has provided a cost effective option that is able to track their weight loss progress and meet their individual goals.
- *Social-Sharing:* Developing positive social relationships and promoting a feeling of integration are the key social benefits of gamification. Gamification has a great potential for improving communication and mutual encouragement among users by means of social-sharing. For an example, on the Nike app you can create a challenge to run 50 miles in 1 month and share it with friends who also have the app, where you can track everyone's progress throughout the month. While you run with your smartphone it would automatically track how many miles you run.
- *Competition:* There are the obvious links of gamification to competition. Humans are wired to be competitive, to win, and to enjoy rewards. Gamification aids in cognitive development since it stimulates the brain and helps in competition because its social by design. Gamifying your goals encourages communal participation and healthy competition in the workplace, classroom, among companies, etc. For example, competition in the classroom context may result in material rewards or simply winning.

22.6 CHALLENGES

As a new trend, gamification has many advocates and critics alike. Like any other emerging concept, gamification is suffering from growing pains. There are concerns and limitations to consider when applying gamification. Some worry that gamification may trivialize the learning experience. Others doubt whether it works.

While we can benefit from the applications of gamification, not every learning activity can be gamified [24]. The same gamification mechanism can be motivating to some students while disliked by others [25]. Sometimes gamification can encourage unintended behaviors. Some critics will argue that social gaming is detrimental to progress and it is ineffective for improving patient engagement in the long run. The role of practitioners (or the "digital practitioner") in the era of gamification has not been clearly established. Identifying gamification involves high level of subjectivity and contextuality. When gamification is not properly implemented, it runs the risk of making learning become a game where people participate only to have fun rather than to improve their skills. There are a lack of standards. Other challenges include the following [26]:

- *Engaging Participation*: A major challenge for all healthcare-related gamification schemes is engaging participation, particularly among high-risk patients. Organizations that plan to use a gamification strategy must understand the target audience's behavior and motivation and decide how success will be measured. People who struggle with health issues such as obesity, diabetes, or cancer, may feel undue pressure to lose weight or change their diet.

- *Protecting Privacy:* Healthcare gamification faces the added challenge of protecting patient privacy. Health providers must abide by the Health Insurance Portability and Accountability Act (HIPAA), which requires them to conceal personal health information.

- *Legal Restrictions:* Rigorous regulatory processes are important for safe applications of gamification to healthcare. Multiple legal restrictions (such as virtual currencies, data privacy laws, and data protection) may apply to gamification. Gamification features in some local cultures may require incentives that include ideals of reciprocity, face-saving, and social obligation. Healthcare providers that intend to provide games to their customers must ensure that they are not violating federal patient privacy regulations.

- *Lack of Education*: Gamification may be flawed and misleading for those unfamiliar with gaming. Poor or insufficient clinical reasoning can have serious consequences. Gamification may be difficult to implement effectively. Failure to successfully implement gamification will bring costs in morale and productivity. It may produce adverse and unanticipated consequences.

Some of challenges of gamifications are depicted in Figure 22.5. These issues prevent researchers from applying gamification in healthcare to its full potential [27].

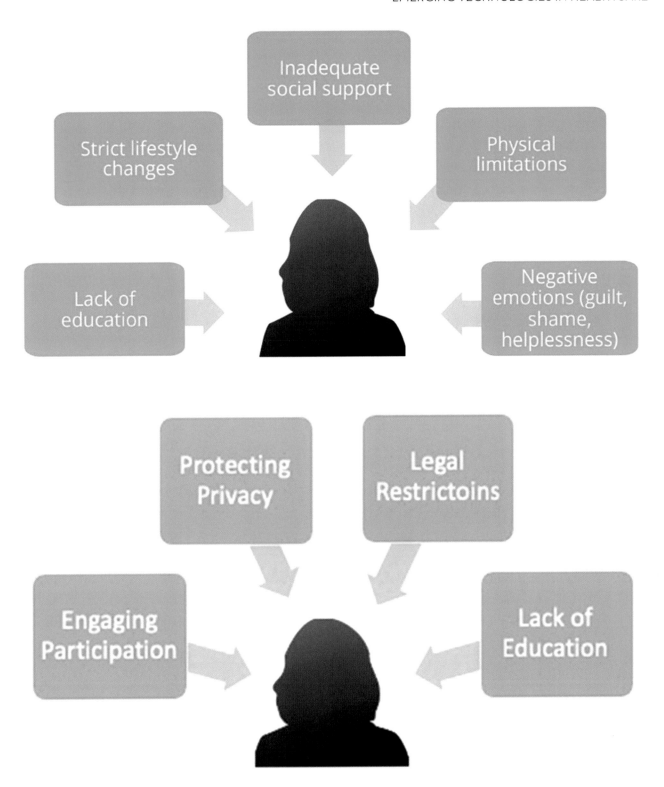

Figure 22.5 Some challenges facing healthcare gamification.

22.7 GLOBAL HEALTHCARE GAMIFICATION

The use of smartphones has increased rapidly in developed and developing countries. Accompanying this rapid increase in smartphones, is an expansion in applications targeting health-related behaviors as well as a remarkable increase in gaming. The healthcare sector has only recently been introduced to the concept of gamification and is still at a relatively early stage of product adoption. Many global players are already chasing the huge market potential for healthcare gamification products. Gamification strategies include goal setting, providing feedback on performance, reinforcement, self-monitoring of behavior, and comparing progress. Game-play tends to focus control, and capture the minds of many around the world and different age groups. People enjoy playing games and winning.

Healthcare gamification industry is highly competitive. The use of healthcare gamification worldwide is presented as follows:

- *United States:* Healthcare costs are skyrocketing in the US, but gamification leverages behavioral principles to instill personal responsibility. Wide adoption of gamification in healthcare will make great strides in making our therapeutic experiences significantly better. Popular culture, social media, and smartphones have fed into the desire to play and win. Gamification is typically employed in wellness, disease prevention, medication adherence, and medical education. The Health Insurance Portability and Accountability Act (HIPAA) security and privacy rules establish the standards for protection of health information in the US.

- *Canada:* Testing gamification principles within provincial health improvement campaigns has been successful. Use of gamification in this context worked well. A Canadian company, GestureTek Health, has developed applications specific to health, disability, and rehabilitation.

- *United Kingdom:* Every month, software developers, clinicians, behavioral scientists, and investors get together at the Google Campus in London to discuss new strategies to influence health behaviors. The main purpose of these networking events is to develop digital games that have been created for specific health conditions. For example, Bant, a mobile app was developed to target improving the frequency of glucose monitoring of adolescents with diabetes [28]. The UK National Health Service (NHS) uses a rigorous approach to ensure health apps for all ages that incorporates gamification comply with trusted sources of information and to identify apps that may potentially cause harm.

- *South Africa:* This nation has witnessed a robust growth pertaining to increasing need for healthcare services to meet the demand and reducing the high cost of services. It has a sophisticated healthcare system, where gamification in healthcare has reached a popular level. Health care companies and banking industries in South Africa are increasingly adopting gamification in their operations. Some forms of gamification have been applied in health-related programs in South Africa such as Multiply's Active Dayz™ and Discovery's Active rewards. Some of these programs encourage exercise which can help prevent heart disease by decreasing blood pressure, improving blood circulation, increasing fat loss, and building muscle mass [29].

- *Saudi Arabia:.* It is one of the top countries for prevalence of diabetes, particularly Type 1 diabetes. Diabetes is an illness that requires time and effort to self-manage. Apps from US and Europe and are out of reach to many Saudi patients because of language barriers. *Sukr* is a gamified self-management system for Arab diabetic patients. It is an application that uses gamification to help users self-manage their condition [30].

22.8 CONCLUSION

Gamification is the new concept of applying game-design thinking to non-game, real-world applications. As a new concept, its key theoretical understandings are still unfolding. It involves using game-based mechanics, game dynamics, and game-thinking to engage people, change behavior, motivate action, and solve problems.

Gamification of healthcare is a promising endeavor. It is a powerful weapon for effective learning, marketing, and behavioral change. It can facilitate innovative learning and promote de-stress activities. It has flourished in the corporate world and is gradually driving popular interest in the healthcare community as reflected in the growing number of papers published. It is a concept that needs to be part of every professional's tool box.

The healthcare industry will increasingly leverage gamification to engage customers and drive them toward healthier outcomes. Software developers will continue "gamifying" applications for healthcare in droves. Gamification is yet to attain the mainstream of any academic discipline. It is here to stay. More information about gamification can be found in the books in [24, 31-36].

REFERENCES

[1] M. N. O. Sadiku, S.M. Musa, and R. Nelatury, "Digital games," *International Journal of Research and Allied Sciences*, vol. 1, no. 10, Dec. 2016, pp. 1,2.

[2] B. Kim, "The popularity of gamification in the mobile and social era," *Understanding Gamification*, chapter 1 or *Library Technology Report*, vol. 51, no. 2, February-March 2015, pp. 1-10.

[3] A. S. Miller, J. A. Cafazzo, and E. Seto, "A game plan: Gamification design principles in mHealth applications for chronic disease management," *Health Informatics Journal*, vol. 22, no. 2, 2016, pp. 184–193

[4] J. Dale Prince, "Gamification," *Journal of Electronic Resources in Medical Libraries*, vol.10, no. 3, 2013, pp. 162-169.

[5] K. Seaborn and D. I. Fels, "Gamification in theory and action: A survey," *International Journal of Human-Computer Studies*, vol. 74, 2015, pp. 14–31.

[6] J. Schepke, "What's your healthcare gamification strategy?" May 2018, https://www.beckershospitalreview.com/healthcare-information-technology/what-s-your-healthcare-gamification-strategy.html

[7] D. Keefe, Gamification in Healthcare – Let's Play!," March 2016, https://hcldr.wordpress.com/2016/03/19/gamification-in-healthcare-lets-play/

[8] W. Hammedi, T. Leclerq, and A. C.R. Van Riel, "The use of gamification mechanics to increase employee and user engagement in participative healthcare services: A study of two cases," *Journal of Service Management*, vol. 28, no. 4, August 2017, pp. 640-661.

[9] O. Pedreira et al., "Gamification in software engineering – A systematic mapping," *Information and Software Technology*, vol. 57, 2015, pp. 157–168.

[10] A. Martens and W. Mueller," Gamification - A structured analysis," *Proceedings of IEEE 16th International Conference on Advanced Learning Technologies*, 2016, pp. 138-142.

[11] "Gamification," *Wikipedia*, the free encyclopedia https://en.wikipedia.org/wiki/Gamification

[12] Y. Chen, "Examining the use of user-centered design in gamification: A Delphi study," *Doctoral Dissertation*, Purdue University, 2015.

[13] "Gamification 101: An introduction to game dynamics," https://www.bunchball.com/gamification101

[14/] R. J. Law, "Networked integration required for healthcare gamification to succeed," May 2012, https://pharmaphorum.com/views-and-analysis/networked_integration_required_for_healthcare_gamification_to_succeed/

[15] "The top 15 examples of gamification in healthcare," July 2017, https://medicalfuturist.com/top-examples-of-gamification-in-healthcare/

[16] L. Sardi, A. José, and L. Fernández-Alemán, "A systematic review of gamification in e-Health," *Journal of Biomedical Informatics,* vol. 71, July 2017, pp. 31-48.

[17] M. I. A. Rahim and R. H. Thomas, "Gamification of medication adherence in epilepsy," *Seizure,* vol. 52, November 2017, pp. 11-14.

[18] M. S. Patel, S. Chang, and K. G. Volpp, "Improving health care by gamifying it," May 2019, https://hbr.org/2019/05/improving-health-care-by-gamifying-it

[19] C. I. Muntean, " Raising engagement in e-learning through gamification," *Proceedings of the 6th International Conference on Virtual Learning* (ICVL), 2011, pp. 323 -329.

[20] D. J. Fisher, J. Beedle, and S. E. Rouse, "Gamification: A study of business teacher educators' knowledge of, attitude toward, and experiences with the gamification of activities in the classroom," *The Journal of Research in Business Education*, vol. 56, no. 1, January 2014, pp. 1-16.

[21] S. Singhal, J. Hough, and D. Cripps, "Twelve tips for incorporating gamification into medical education," https://www.mededpublish.org/manuscripts/2678

[22] S. V. Gentry et al., "Serious Gaming and Gamification interventions for health professional education," *Journal of Medical Internet Research*, vol. 21, no. 3, March 2019.

[23] R. A. C. Marques., "Using gamification for reducing infections in hospitals," Master's Thesis, April 2016

[24] K. M. Kapp, *The Gamification of Learning and Instruction: Game-based Methods and Strategies for Training and Education*. San Francisco, CA: John Wiley & Sons, 2012.

[25] L. Hakulinen and T. Auvinen, "The effect of gamification on students with different achievement goal orientations," *Proceedings of International Conference on Teaching and Learning in Computing and Engineering*, 2014, pp. 9-16.

[26] "Gamification (as you know it) is wrong," October 2014, https://www.pcpcc.org/sites/default/files/Michael%20Fergusson%20Slides.pdf

[27] M. R Floryan, L. M. Ritterband, and P. I. Chow, "Principles of gamification for Internet interventions," *Translational Behavioral Medicine*, vol. 9, no. 6, December 2019, pp. 1131–1138.

[28] D. King et al., "'Gamification': Influencing health behaviours with games," *Journal of the Royal Society of Medicine*, vol. 106, no. 3, March 2013, pp. 76 –78.

[29] T. Devar and M. Hattingh, "Gamification in healthcare: Motivating South Africans to exercise," *Nature Public Health Emergency Collection*, March 2020, pp.108–119.

[30] A. A. Al-Marshedi, . G. B. Wills, and A. Ranchhod, "Gamification to improve adherence to diabeteic treatment in Saudi Arabia," *International Conference on Information Society, London, United Kingdom.* November 2014.

[31] T. Reiners and L. C. Wood (eds.), *Gamification in Education and Business.* Springer, 2015.

[32] G. Zichermann and J. Linder, *The Gamification Revolution: How Leaders Leverage Game Mechanics to Crush the Competition.* McGraw-Hill Education, 2013.

[33] S. Stieglitz et al. (eds.), *Gamification: Using Game Elements in Serious Contexts.* Springer, 2017.

[34] D. Novák et al., *Handbook of Research on Holistic Perspectives in Gamification for Clinical Practice.* IGI Global, 2015.

[35] M. Herger, *Gamification in Healthcare & Fitness (Enterprise Gamification).* CreateSpace Independent Publishing Platform, 2015.

[36] G. Wigmore, *Gamification of healthcare.* Medical Xpres, 2016.

CHAPTER 23

FUTURE OF HEALTHCARE TECHNOLOGIES

"If we don't know where we are going, we won't know when we don't get there." — Yogi Berra.

23.1 INTRODUCTION

Technology is a tool that usually helps improve efficiency and effectiveness. Technologies that are designed for the treatment and care of patients have been profound and have caused the healthcare industry to be constantly evolving. They have enabled better quality research, treatment, and access to healthcare. Technology-focused companies such as Google, Amazon, and Apple are beginning to make significant impact on the existing market [1]. The ongoing COVID-19 pandemic has further propelled the importance of emerging technologies in disease management and prevention.

Nothing is more important than our health and healthcare system. Health is crucial to human, social, and economic development. We all interact with the healthcare system one way or another. The cost of healthcare affects individuals, families, and employers as well as local, state, and federal budgets. The present healthcare system consists of disconnected components -- health plans, hospital systems, pharmaceutical companies, medical device manufacturers. The system is not designed to handle the current surge of chronic diseases nationwide. The system continues to evolve in an everchanging landscape. Changing the system is an uphill task. In order for the health systems to remain successful and flexible, healthcare systems need a clear goal about adopting new technologies and a strategic plan that will help them get there. Health systems have more opportunity to leverage data and technology to deliver the best care to all patients. Healthcare industry has been a fertile ground for technology applications and research over the years. Decision making technologies have developed and applied in healthcare delivery [2].

This chapter discusses the future of technology in healthcare. It begins by looking at the trends in healthcare technologies. It covers the future of technology in healthcare. It describes the future of global healthcare technology. It highlights some challenges facing future healthcare technology. The last section concludes with comments.

23.2 TRENDS IN HEALTHCARE TECHNOLOGIES

By trends, we mean a chain of data about progress in the past, present, and future, which can be measured or estimated. It is well known that healthcare is a bit behind other industries when it comes to adopting technology. Becoming familiar with emerging healthcare technologies puts future healthcare leaders in a winning position when they are planning for the future. Emerging technologies expand the options for where patients are seen. Doctors will be less tethered to the hospital and able to perform more procedures in the office, making care more convenient and accessible. Some of the trends in healthcare can be summarized as follows [3].

- The Affordable Care Act
- Automated procedures and services
- Telehealth and remote patient monitoring
- Digital transformation and interoperability
- Cloud growth is inevitable
- RFID implants for recreational purposes
- Artificial intelligence is controlling the world
- Nearly all procedures will be done by AI and robots
- Virtual reality (VR) is changing the lives of patients and physicians alike
- Price transparency initiatives are changing care delivery models
- Prescription drug prices are skyrocketing
- Improving patient experience, engagement, and satisfaction
- Consumerization of healthcare payments
- Physicians are becoming data-driven
- Healthcare organizations are struggling to attract the needed talent
- Pharmacy costs and pricing continue to generate debate
- Patients will take a more active role in managing their healthcare
- The hospital of the future puts patients first
- Care will happen anywhere and everywhere
- Need for a healthcare reform
- Stem cells, nanobots, and other scientific breakthroughs
- Digitization of the consumer experience
- The use of telecare and E-healthcare will mean shorter waiting times for patients
- 3D printing will be used to produce medicine, eliminating the need for pharmacies
- The future of pharma will be 3D-printed drugs
- Telemedicine will be used as an appropriate alternative for the first post-operation visit in adolescents.

23.3 FUTURE OF TECHNOLOGY IN HEALTHCARE

The healthcare sector is seeking for ways to treat patients virtually, predict, and prevent diseases, increase hospitals' efficiency, as well as to address privacy and security issues. From telemedicine to 3D printing, healthcare is starting to look a lot like the tech industry. The future of healthcare is shaping up with advances in healthcare technologies, such as telehealth, artificial intelligence, robotics, cloud computing, 3D-printing, and nanotechnology. Future technologies in healthcare include the following [4,5].

- *Telehealth:* This is the provision of health-related services using telecom technologies. It is the ability to engage in healthcare quickly and seamlessly through technology like smartphones, laptops, and streaming services. It allows remote advice, care, education, monitoring, and treatment assessment. Reliance on telehealth and the technology to maintain it will grow. Telehealth services benefit both the patient and the medical physicians. They allow patients to make virtual appointments from the comfort of their homes. Patients also take advantage of the availability of telehealth services to manage and monitor chronic illnesses. Telehealth allows doctors to see more patients efficiently and giving office staff more time to process paperwork. More healthcare systems, doctors, and medical staff are providing telehealth services.

- *Artificial Intelligence:* AI focuses on how computers learn from data and mimic human thought processes. It has affected healthcare in a big way. It has the potential to redesign healthcare completely. The AI algorithm has outperformed all human radiologists on pre-selected data sets to identify breast cancer. It revolutionizes drug development. AI algorithms are able to mine medical records. In the coming years, the adoption of robotics, machine learning, and artificial intelligence in healthcare will become a part of the "new norm." AI-powered systems will be widely used in personalized medicine. Autonomous AI will begin to replace human doctors. As patient trust increase, AI will become more reliable and widely adopted. The computing power of AI will drastically reduce the time scientists spend analyzing data.

- *Robotics:* This is one of the most exciting and fastest growing fields of healthcare, with developments ranging from robot companions through surgical robots. In healthcare, robots can help alleviate loneliness, treat mental health issues or even help children with chronic illness. Robots can allow paralyzed patients to move around. Robotic surgical operations will continue across the healthcare system, especially in spine, cardiology, and oncology. Robot health assistants can be used to help keep an eye on the health of people in a household. Figure 23.1 shows a robot as a doctor [6].

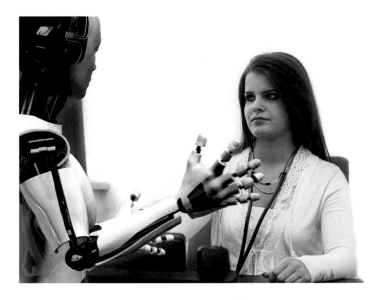

Figure 23.1 Robot as a doctor [6].

- *Internet of Things:* The Internet is becoming the media for healthcare delivery. IoT is disrupting the notion of who and what can be monitored and managed—and from where, and for how long. The future of eldercare and at-home healthcare, in particular, will leverage the gathering wave of IoT. The convergence of IoT and telemedicine has brought about a variety of wearable devices. Figure 23.2 shows how IoT is used in healthcare for varying purposes [7]. The Internet of Medical Things (IoMT) covers a variety of smart devices: ECG, EKG monitors, smart beds, connected inhaler, etc.

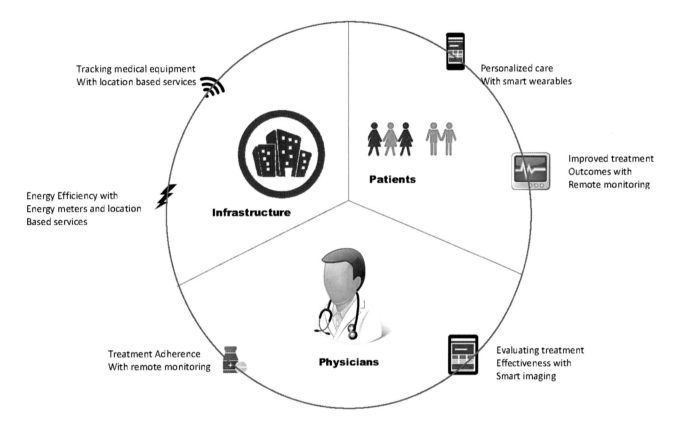

Figure 23.2 IoT is used in healthcare for varying purposes [7].

- *3D-printing:* This has emerged as a disruptive technology in healthcare. It is being leveraged to create personalized medical devices and provide training to future medical professionals. 3D printers are beginning to infiltrate homes and enter the mainstream. It has created a new generation of at-home and do-it-yourself manufacturers and children are starting to adopt it. The technology has enormous potential for the healthcare industry and will significantly change its future. It can bring wonders in all aspects of healthcare. The pharmaceutical industry is also benefiting from this technology. Figure 23.3 displays some medical applications of 3D printing technology [8].

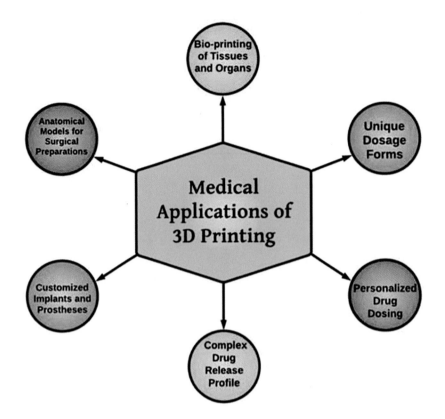

Figure 23.3 Medical applications of 3D printing technology [8].

- *Nanotechnology:* This is perhaps the most advanced and promising solution for healthcare. It is a relatively new interdisciplinary field that studies materials at the nanoscale (about 1 to 100 nanometers). We are living at the dawn of the age of nanomedicine. For example, nanotechnology can be used to treat as well as diagnose. It also has the potential to transform current chemotherapy treatments. As nanotechnology evolves, we will see more practical examples in medicine. Nanodevices are expected to improve the drug delivery system.

- *Cloud Computing:* Cloud computing is a promising technology that has the potential to transform the healthcare. It has many benefits like flexibility, cost and energy savings, resource sharing, and fast deployment [9]. The cloud provides unprecedented scaling, data integration, and access advantages. Easy access to and sharing of data is an essential foundation for building a healthcare system. Cloud computing will allow physicians to have access to complete information on a patient's electronic health record, prescriptions, test results, imaging, etc. Concerns about interoperability, security, legal compliance, and potential downtime when dealing with the most sensitive personal data can all be addressed. Global collaboration depends on cloud computing.

- *Cybersecurity:* As a result of the increasing use personal data, cybersecurity has emerged to be important more than ever before due to healthcare providers and healthcare systems being entrusted with personal information. Cybersecurity is also a new priority as ransomware attackers hit hospitals and health systems. Cybercriminals will continue to discover and exploit new attacks and manage to stay one step ahead of cybersecurity. The game changer for cybersecurity could be next-generation technologies.

These technologies have the potential to make an enormous impact on patients, their families, and caregivers. Their applications are poised to grow rapidly in the near future. Other emerging technologies in healthcare include precision medicine, personalized medicine, genome sequencing, virtual/augmented reality, health wearables, business intelligence, and blockchain. These are the key enablers of technology advances in healthcare.

23.4 GLOBAL HEATHCARE TRENDS

Healthcare systems globally have experienced intensive changes, reforms, developments, and improvement over the past three decades. Across the globe, there are significant disparities in how money is spent on health on a nation level. Unfortunately, the global healthcare system still relies heavily on manual processes, obsolete technologies, and in-person interactions. It has caused the global healthcare system not to be prepared for the COVID-19 crisis. A significant number of caregivers around the world have considered quitting their jobs due to work-related stress. However, every crisis makes way for new opportunities. As governments worldwide start to ease the lockdowns, it is expedient to start analyzing how to make the future healthcare system more resilient to potential emergencies.

Anticipating the future of healthcare demand is not an insignificant exercise. The future is a complex mix of predictable trends, unpredictable dislocations, and interactions between them. Healthcare is changing rapidly and so is the industry's need for technologies which helps foster up solutions. The future of healthcare and healthcare technology is rapidly evolving. We now consider the future of healthcare technologies in the following nations:

- *United States:* The United States healthcare system is larger than the gross domestic product of all but five other nations. One out of every six dollars of the nation's annual production of goods and services is spent on healthcare. Several problems come from such a large, expensive, and ever-growing healthcare system [10]. During the past several years, hospitals in the US have witnessed a decline in inpatient volumes, while outpatient volumes to grow. Health care systems in the United States are creating virtual hospitals through extensive use of telehealth technology. The coronavirus pandemic has unveiled our vulnerabilities, transformative opportunities, resourcefulness, and empathy.
- *Turkey*: Increasing demand of healthcare and limited resources have led to reorganization and improvement of healthcare systems in Turkey, where healthcare is cheap and safety regulations of patients are not well applied. Turkey cannot use technology intense treatments due to high cost of importing medical devices. Promoting the decentralization of healthcare governance to increase competitions of healthcare is a challenge for the future to improve efficiency [11].
- *South Africa:* Many governments in sub-Saharan Africa desire to establish public–private partnerships (PPPs) for the financing and operation of new healthcare facilities and services. The Lesotho PPP is an ambitious attempt to outsource new healthcare facilities. The deal was initiated by the Government of Lesotho and the International Finance Corporation, an arm of the World Bank. The experience of the Lesotho PPP is mixed. New facilities were constructed and delivered to time. The quality of clinical services provided has been high. However, there is no evidence that these outcomes resulted from the deal itself [12].

- *Iran:* National governments are mainly responsible for protecting and promoting health in their respective countries. Increasing healthcare cost due to uncontrolled increase in using new technologies in healthcare is one of the most important threats facing healthcare system in Iran. The technological trends affecting healthcare system in Iran include demographic transition, epidemiologic transition, increasing bio-environmental pollution, increasing slums, increasing private sector partnership in health care delivery, moving toward knowledge-based society, increasing use of high technologies in health system, and development of traditional and alternative medicine [13].

- *United Kingdom:* In the United Kingdom, there is ample evidence to suggest that women are disproportionately impacted by austerity cuts. The workforce metrics for the two largest segments of the health care workforce, doctors and nurses, indicate a growing divide and marked misalignment in growth rates over the past decade. Since nursing is a major part of the solution to building a better future in health care, future policy options should consider scaling up the participation of nurses in designing future policy [14].

- *Canada:* While healthcare has advanced, the funding and delivery of healthcare in Canada have basically remain the same. The delivery of healthcare occurs mainly on a face-to-face basis and is funded on the basis of volume. There are three major developments that hold the potential to revolutionize the delivery of medicine and health care in Canada: (1) virtual care, the use of electronic means to reduce face-to-face interaction; (2) big health data, the ability to analyze large volumes of different types of data from a variety of sources; (3) technological developments such as robotics, 3D printing, virtual and augmented reality, nanotechnology, and the Internet of things [15].

- *China:* A recent research shows that China is leading the way in adoption of digital health technology. Digital technologies, such as telehealth and artificial intelligence, have the potential to alleviate China's overstretched healthcare professionals and help provide better care. However, global health technology innovators see China facing many barriers such as an ageing population, a medical and digital infrastructure that is vastly different from other countries, unique regulatory demands, and a lack of affordability of existing solutions that are needed in rural or impoverished regions. For technologies that are still in a nascent stage in healthcare, the situation is complex because regulations need further development [16].

As these trends unfold, healthcare is likely to experience revolutionary changes.

23.5 FUTURE OF GLOBAL HEALTHCARE TECHNOLOGY

Technologies are evolving at a rapid pace all over the world. They are regarded to be the driving force behind improvements in healthcare. After decades as a technological laggard, the healthcare industry has entered the digital age. Global advances in technology have changed the way consumers manage their own healthcare and interact with medical providers. These advances have laid the foundation for a core component of the next revolution: data-driven healthcare. The data-driven healthcare creates the possibility of turning every health care environment into a data-driven learning environment.

In the fast-paced area of global healthcare, it is hard to find moments to reflect on the events of the past, the challenges of the present, and the hopes for the future. Although we cannot foresee exactly what the future of healthcare will be in the next ten or twenty years, there are a handful of advances in healthcare that we can expect. The future of global healthcare will likely be driven by digital transformation, enabled by artificial intelligence, and the integration of newly emerging technologies.

To some degree, predictions of the healthcare environment can be made. In his <u>lecture</u>, Dr. Merson shared his top six predictions for the future of global healthcare [17].

(1) *The rise of chronic and non-communicable diseases (NCDs):* NCDs will be the <u>predominant</u> cause of death worldwide. Chronic diseases include heart disease, cancer, and diabetes.

(2) *Continued growth of infectious diseases:* infectious diseases will play a role in the future of global health, such as HIV and Tuberculosis.

(3) Climate change influencing health: Climate change is one of the most significant long-term risk to human health and biodiversity.

(4) *Refugee migration:* With refugee movement comes malnutrition, decrease vaccinations, decreased disease surveillance and lack of psychosocial support.

(5) *Health technology:* Patients are receiving greater access to and quality of healthcare through technology

(6) *Increased longevity:* With health technologies developing more rapidly each day, life expectancies have been on the rise.

Researchers have predicted that more than half of the world's adult population will be overweight or obese by 2030.

In planning for the future, stakeholders can navigate uncertainties by factoring in past and current drivers, which include a growing and aging population, rising prevalence of chronic diseases, complex healthcare technology, rising health care costs, changing patient demographics, evolving consumer expectations, workforce shortages, and the expansion of health care systems in developing markets. Healthcare systems should work toward a future in which there is a shift away from treatment, to prevention and early intervention [18].

The future healthcare system must address the issues of access, affordability, comprehensiveness, and relevance for the users. It must start by imaging what that future looks like and make the decision today for a dual transformation to move to that future [19].

23.6 CHALLENGES

While the technologies mentioned earlier promise a new world of healthcare, there are some significant challenges to their implementation. The challenges faced by the global healthcare system in recent years have been increased in population and urbanization, behavioral changes, rise in chronic diseases, traumatic injuries, infectious diseases, regulation, patient choice, specific regional conflicts and healthcare delivery security. The healthcare systems around the world have faced multiple challenges [20]. Some of them are listed below:

- *Consumer Demand or Patient-centricity*: Patient/consumer choice is at the forefront of the debate on the future direction of healthcare. Patient wellness is the heart of healthcare. Today, patients are well informed about their health and therefore play a more active role in their own healthcare, fueling the drive towards personalized medicine. People around the world are now living longer than in previous generations. Currently, consumers bear more cost for their care. There is a need to increase the quality of patient care at a lower cost to address our country's health disparities and inequities. Customers are becoming ever more tech-savvy and demanding. Consumers have been used to transformations that have occurred in other sectors, such as e-commerce and mobility. These consumers will demand that healthcare follow suit. The consumer will determine when, where, and with whom he or she engages for care or to sustain well-being. Consumers have grown used to wearable devices that track their health and fitness. The center of gravity in this new system will be patients, not the acute-care hospital. This is central to market liberalism and democracy because its focus is on property rights, individual freedom, competition, and the emphasis on self-interest as the driver of human behavior [21]. Figure 23.4 illustrates the shift toward patient-centric care [22].

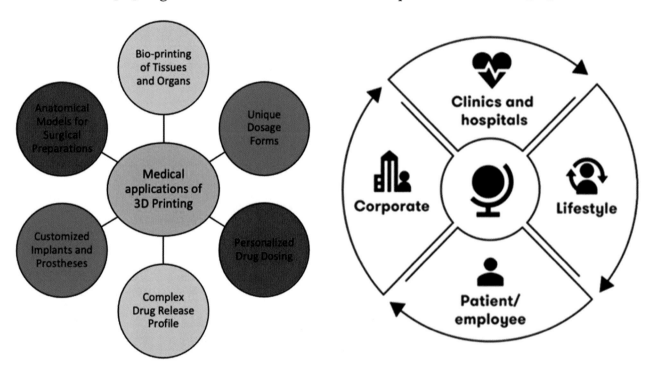

Figure 23.4 The shift toward patient-centric care [22].

- *Healthcare Regulation:* Changes in the healthcare industry usually occur at the legislative level, but once enacted these changes have a direct impact on facility operations. The healthcare system itself is managed and regulated by dozens of federal and state agencies, including the Department of Health and Human Services, the Centers for Disease Control, the Center for Medicare and Medicaid Services, the Veterans Administration, the Food and Drug Administration, and the Agency for Healthcare Research and Quality. These regulators will set the standards for how business are transacted. The regulators of the future will influence policy while promoting consumer and public safety.
- *Workforce:* Human factors will remain one of the major limitations of technological breakthroughs. The entire healthcare workforce will evolve, mainly because technology will expand the capabilities of healthcare professionals. Figure 23.5 depicts the future of healthcare professionals

[23]. The cooperation between people and technology may result in amazing achievements. The healthcare industry lacks expertise, regulatory expertise, a targeted consumer base, and existing partnerships with other incumbents. There is also an increase in demand for primary care and the shortage of primary-care physicians. It is projected that in just over a decade we will face a shortage of more than 100,000 physicians. There will also be a need for engineers and designers working with 3D printers to print artificial bones, limbs, braces, etc. [24].

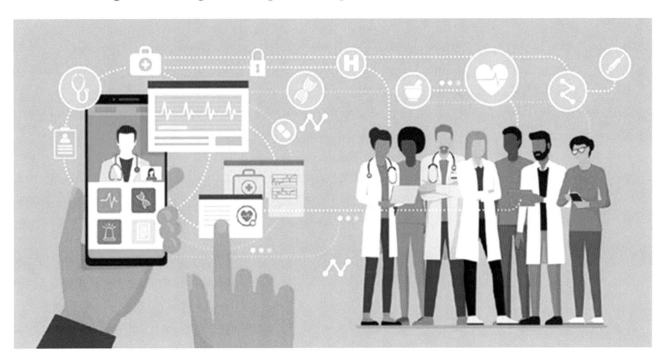

Figure 23.5 Future healthcare professionals [23].

- *Complexity:* There can be no doubt that the healthcare industry is a massive and complex business. The healthcare industry is the US's largest employer and takes more than 18% of the GDP [25]. With the rapid growth of online social networking for health, healthcare systems are increasing in complexity. Partly due to this complexity, clinical trials are expensive and time-consuming. Regulatory approval is crucial but challenging to obtain. Concerns about the contribution of healthcare materials to toxic waste and how it impacts the environment, health care has been growing for about two decades.
- *Risk:* Computer security is a growing field in computer science that focuses on protecting computer systems and electronic data against unauthorized access, hardware theft, data manipulation, and against common threats and attacks. Healthcare systems generate a mammoth amount of data that requires storage and protection of patient data. Innovation spurs growth and helps maintain a competitive advantage, but introduces risks. Classic approaches to hacking like ransomware and phishing schemes continue to pose serious threats to healthcare organizations. The challenges of data protection by healthcare providers is underlined by the risk of financial, legal and reputational damage in the wake of a data breach. It is for this reason that any chosen data protection system must guarantee safety against cyberattacks. Emerging technologies and

the threats of cybersecurity breaches require tight protection, strong detection and response tactics to protect patients and the health organizations [26].

Other challenges include costs, aging population, healthcare consumerism, health inequities, and cultural change. These challenges shape the future of healthcare.

23.7 CONCLUSION

Technological innovations are changing the face of the healthcare industry with each year passing. New technologies and innovations are being introduced within the industry, creating excitement among medical practitioners, researchers, and patients. Over the coming decades, health will be described holistically as an overall state of well-being encompassing mental, social, emotional, physical, and spiritual health. Care will be organized around patients and their familes, rather than around the institutions currently driving the existing healthcare system. The future of healthcare will be focused on optimal well-being, prevention, and early intervention rather than treatment. From time to time, we need to familiarize ourselves with the latest developments in emerging healthcare technologies in order to be able to control technologies and not the technologies controlling us. The future promises a continued utilization of technology and a greater focus on patient outcomes.

Although the future is hard to predict, we know for sure that the future of healthcare is bright for both patients and health care professionals. The future of healthcare will be shaped by forward-looking leaders' curiosity, compassion and courage, and their ability to develop connections with the people and communities they serve [27]. Technology will continue to transform and revolutionize the healthcare industry, and its adoption is somewhat unstoppable. There is still plenty of room for improvement in the applications of the current and emerging technologies. More information about the future of technology in healthcare can be found in the books in [19, 28-30] and related journals: *Future Healthcare Journal* and *Journal of Medical Systems,*

REFERENCES

[1] "Forces of change: The future of health," https://www2.deloitte.com/content/dam/insights/us/articles/5169_forces-of-change-future-of-health/DI_Forces-of-change_Future-of-health.pdf

[2] M. Hatcher and I. Heetebry, "Information technology in the future of health care," *Journal of Medical Systems,* Vol. 28, No. 6, December 2004, pp.673-688.

[3] M. Vatandoost, "The future of healthcare facilities: How technology and medical advances may shape hospitals of the future," December 2019, https://www.middleeastmedicalportal.com/the-future-of-healthcare-facilities-how-technology-and-medical-advances-may-shape-hospitals-of-the-future/

[4] "10 Ways technology is changing healthcare," January 2020, https://www.healthcareguys.com/2020/01/15/10-ways-technology-is-changing-healthcare/

[5] M. N. O. Sadiku, P. O. Adebo, A. Ajayi-Majebi, and S. M. Musa, "Future of Healthcare: A Primer," *International Journal of Trend in Research and Development,* vol. 8, No. 2, March-April 2021, pp. 177-181.

[6] A. Sakharkar, "A power user is more likely to accept a robot doctor, than a non-power user," May 2019, https://www.techexplorist.com/power-user-more-likely-accept-robot-doctor-non-power-user/23005/

[7] A. Yuksel, "Energy IQ: Three trends that will change the future of health care infrastructure," August 2019, https://www.cummins.com/news/2019/08/15/energy-iq-three-trends-will-change-future-health-care-infrastructure

[8] A. Ali, U. Ahmad, and J. Akhtar, "3D printing in pharmaceutical sector: An overview," January 2020, https://www.intechopen.com/books/pharmaceutical-formulation-design-recent-practices/3d-printing-in-pharmaceutical-sector-an-overview

[9] Y. Al-Issa, M. A. Ottom, and A. Tamrawi, "eHealth cloud security challenges: A survey," *Journal of Healthcare Engineering*, 2019.

[10] "Health care primer," https://www.concordcoalition.org/primer/health-care-primer

[11] I. Aslana, O. Çınar, and Ü. Özen, "Developing strategies for the future of healthcare in Turkey by benchmarking and SWOT analysis," *Procedia - Social and Behavioral Sciences*, vol. 150, 2014, pp. 230 – 240.

[12] M. Hellowell, "Are public–private partnerships the future of healthcare delivery in sub-Saharan Africa? Lessons from Lesotho," *BMJ Journal*, vol. 4, no. 2, 2019.

[13] F. Rajabi et al., "Future of health care delivery in Iran, opportunities and threats," *Iranian Journal of Public Health*, vol. 42, supple.1, 2013, pp. 23-30.

[14] A. M. Rafferty, "Nurses as change agents for a better future in health care: The politics of drift and dilution," *Health Economics, Policy and Law*, vol. 13, 2018, pp. 475–491.

[15] "The future of technology in health and health care: A primer," https://www.cma.ca/sites/default/files/pdf/health-advocacy/activity/2018-08-15-future-technology-health-care-e.pdf

[16] World Economic Forum, "How global tech can drive local healthcare innovation in China," June 2019, https://europeansting.com/2019/06/21/how-global-tech-can-drive-local-healthcare-innovation-in-china/

[17] "Six predictions for the future of health," November 2020, https://www.innovationsinhealthcare.org/six-predictions-for-the-future-of-health/

[18] "2020 US and global health care outlook: Laying a foundation for the future," https://www2.deloitte.com/us/en/pages/life-sciences-and-health-care/articles/global-health-care-sector-outlook.html

[19] H. O. Tontus and C. Chuah, *Future of Healthcare*. Newport, UK: Self-Published, H. Omer Tontus, 2019.

[20] H. Durrani, "Healthcare and healthcare systems: Inspiring progress and future prospects." *Mhealth*, vol. 2, no. 2, 2016.

[21] M. Fotaki, "Is patient choice the future of health care systems?" *International Journal of Health Policy and Management*, vol.1, no. 2, 2013, pp. 121–123.

[22] "Healthcare at the edge: A vision for a smart healthcare system," https://www.dxc.technology/healthcare/insights/146041-healthcare_at_the_edge_a_vision_for_a_smart_healthcare_system

[23] "Future healthcare technologies flat concept vector image," https://www.vectorstock.com/royalty-free-vector/future-healthcare-technologies-flat-concept-vector-24957643

[24] M. Kimberl, "Healthcare Jobs 2.0: The future of healthcare and tech," January 2019, https://www.td.org/insights/healthcare-jobs-20-the-future-of-healthcare-and-tech

[25] Stasha, "The state of healthcare industry – Statistics for 2021," January 2021, https://policyadvice. net/insurance/insights/healthcare-statistics/

[26] Y. Al-Issa, M. A. Ottom, and A. Tamrawi, "eHealth cloud security challenges: A survey," *Journal of Healthcare Engineering*, 2019.

[27] T.Jones and J. Besser, "The future of healthcare," March 2020, http://www.dukece.com/insights/ the-future-of-healthcare/

[28] D. M. Berwick, *Escape Fire: Designs for the Future of Health Care*. John Wiley & Sons, 2010.

[29] S. Gordon, J. Buchanan, and T. Bretherton, *Safety in Numbers: Nurse-to-Patient Ratios and the Future of Health Care*. Cornell University Press, 2006.

[30] B. Mesko, *The Guide to the Future of Medicine: Technology and The Human Touch*. Webicina Kft, 2014.

INDEX

24-7 availability, 139
3D Printing, 5, 238, 242, 245, 280
    In healthcare, 235
4D Printing, 244-246

A

Acceptance, 172
Accessibility, 34, 42
Additive manufacturing, 5, 237, 244
Affordability, 34, 57
Africa, 159, 193
Aging, 101
Alzheimer patient, 169
Ambient assisted living, 169
Ambient intelligence, 165-167, 171, 231
American Diabetes Association (ADA), 101
American Medical Association (AMA), 256
Anatomical models, 239
Artificial intelligence, 3, 94, 106, 110, 111, 123, 134,
    227, 279
    In healthcare, 99
Augmented reality, 200, 204, 208, 210
    Benefits of, 208
    Challenges of, 209
Australia, 194, 260

B

Battery life, 22
Behavior change, 268
Behavior analysis, 217
Big data, 79, 90
    Benefits of, 87
    Challenges of, 88, 89
    Characteristics of, 81
    In healthcare, 66, 80
Big data analytics, 82
Big data ethics, 83, 84, 88
Biomedical research, 86
Bitcoin, 176, 178
Blockchain, 7, 172, 183
    Features of, 178

Properties of, 177
Types of,178
Blockchain 2.0, 179
Blockchain 3.0, 179
Blog, 251
Body sensor network, 55
Business intelligence, 213, 215, 217
    Clinical type, 216

C

Canada, 103, 193, 259, 283
Cancer, 100, 137
    Breast type of, 100
    Colorectal type, 129
    Therapy of, 190
Cancer treatment, 54
Cardiology, 19
Cardiovascular care, 86
Cardiovascular disease, 192
Care, 147
    Delivery of, 157
Care robots, 147
Change, 105
Charles Hall, 237
Chatbots, 133, 134, 140
China, 103, 160, 181, 283
Chronic diseases, 9, 117
Clinical data, 126
Clinical decision, 115
Clinical decision support, 126, 129
Clinical psychology, 205
Clinical trials, 180
Cloud Computing, 6, 281
    In healthcare, 66
Collaboration, 89
Communicable diseases, 138, 193
Competition, 270
Complexity, 35, 105, 221, 286
Computer-aided coding, 127
Computer emotion, 99
Computer Science, 3, 95

Computer vision, 99
Confidence, 171
Confidentiality, 35
Connectivity, 21, 51, 57
Convenience, 21, 34
Copyright, 243
Cost advantages, 161
Cost-effectiveness, 150
Cost saving, 183
Costs, 59, 73, 88, 104, 259
    Of care, 149
COVID-19, 258, 277, 282
Customer engagement, 270
Cybersecurity, 227, 281
Cybersickness, 209

D

Data, 130
Data accuracy, 22, 180
Data management, 214
Data mining, 99, 217
Data overload, 59
Data ownership, 184
Data security, 57, 58, 139
Data standards, 221

Limitations of, 162
Medical uses of, 157
Drug anti-counterfeiting, 54
Drug delivery, 191, 195
Drug development, 180, 195
Drug management, 52

E

Education, 206, 207, 241
    Lack of, 271
Effective care, 51
Efficiency, 104
Egypt, 219
Ehealth, see Electronic health
Elderly care, 19, 85, 137, 147, 159, 171
Elderly independent living, 54
Electronic health, 39, 40, 43, 46
    Benefits of, 44
    Challenges, 44
Electronic health record (EHR), 9, 21, 85, 101, 116, 126, 129, 227
    Analysis of, 217
Electronic medical record (EMR), 84
Emergency, 159
Emerging healthcare technologies, 12
Emerging technologies, 2, 8, 11, 72

Data visualization, 208
Data warehousing, 213, 214
Databases, 178
Decision support systems, 217
Deep learning, 98
Democratization of technology, 244
Dentistry, 101, 205, 240
Diabetes care, 101
Diabetes monitoring, 44
Diabetics, 20
Diagnosis, 208
Digital divide, 45
Digital hospital, 54
Digital revolution, 224, 232
Digital wellness, 232
Digitalization, 15, 224, 232, 233
Disease diagnosis, 100
Disease management, 43, 100
Disease prediction, 115
Disease prevention, 269
Distraction, 22
Do-it-yourself manufacturing, 241
Doctors, 9, 39, 48, 52, 55-57, 64, 68, 71, 74, 75, 95, 100, 102, 105, 110, 117, 137, 142, 256, 257, 278
Donor shortage, 242
Drones, 154-157

Employee satisfaction, 21
Encryption, 178
Energy, 59
Environment, 167, 200
Estonia, 181
Ethereum, 176, 178
Ethics, 88, 117, 150, 172, 196, 243, 258
    Risks of, 105
European Commission's Information Society Technologies
    Advisory Group (ISTAG), 170
European Union, 148, 193, 230
Excessive information, 22
Experience, 73
Expert systems, 96, 110
Extreme learning machine, 113

F

Facebook, 250, 252
Fear(s), 105, 118, 139
Federal Aviation Administration (FAA), 155, 157, 160, 244
Fitness, 19
Food and Drug Administration (FDA), 285
Forecasting, 104

Fourth industrial revolution, 166, 225
France, 103
Fraud, 117
    Detection of, 181
Fraud reduction, 85
Fun, 266
Funds, 221
Future Internet, 48
Future of technology, 277
Fuzzy logic, 97

G

Games, 264, 265
    Digital type of, 265
Games industry, 263
Gamification, 264-274
    Benefits of, 270
    Challenges of, 270, 71
    Elements of, 265
    Mechanics of, 265, 266
Gamifying healthcare, 264
Garbage-in-garbage-out, 130
Genomic medicine, 115
German government, 225, 229
Global blockchain healthcare, 181
Global healthcare, 283
Global healthcare chatbots, 159
Global healthcare gamification, 272
Global healthcare industry, 128
Global healthcare robotics, 147
Global healthcare system, 284
Global positioning systems (GPS), 156
Global virtual reality, 208
Glucose monitoring, 54

H

Hacking, 163
Head-mounted display, 203
Health, 15, 175
Health/healthcare gamification, 263, 271, 273
Health-IoT, 50
Health Insurance Portability and Accountability Act
    (HIPAA), 45, 254, 258, 271, 273
Healthcare, 7, 48, 62, 91, 133, 170, 175, 213, 216, 224,
    238, 241, 255, 277, 282, 283
Healthcare 1.0, 231
Healthcare 2.0, 231
Healthcare 3.0, 231
Healthcare 4.0, 224, 226-228, 232
Healthcare 5.0, 230-232
Healthcare business intelligence, 218, 219
Healthcare consultant, 137

Healthcare delivery,117
Healthcare industry, 6, 8, 15, 34, 52, 62, 79, 208, 214, 214,
    218, 221, 224, 235, 241, 244 257, 260, 263, 264,
    270, 274, 277, 286
Healthcare practitioners, 170
Healthcare professionals, 27, 39, 43, 91, 118, 140, 150, 218,
    249, 251, 253, 258, 263, 270
    Shortage of, 105
Healthcare providers, 6, 244, 255
Healthcare robots, 148-150
Healthcare social media, 260
Healthcare technologies, 1, 2, 65, 277, 282
    Benefits of, 10
    Challenges of, 11
Hospital 4.0, 228, 229
Hospitals, 217, 221, 241, 244
    Administration of, 137
Human errors, 88

I

IBM Watson, 182
Illness, 85
Imaging, 191
Implants, 240
Inclusivity, 42
India, 103, 160, 194, 230, 259
Industrial robots, 144
Industry 4.0, 225, 226, 228
Information and communication technologies (ICT), 25,
    26, 36, 69, 75
Information infrastructure, 203
Information overload, 45, 257
Infrastructure, 58
Inkjet, 237
Instagram, 250, 253
Integration, 89, 171, 220
Integrity, 183
Intellectual property, 89
Intelligence, 88
Internet, 49, 51, 56, 249
Internet medical things (IoMT), 49, 52, 53, 226, 280
Internet of services (IoS), 226
Internet of things (IoT), 6, 48, 52, 56, 57, 59, 280
Interoperability, 58, 182, 221
IoT healthcare, 6, 49, 66
Iran, 282
Irreversibility of records, 178

J

Japan, 148, 194, 230
John McGarty, 95
Just-in-time manufacturing, 241

K

Karel Capek, 143
Knowledge, 221
Korea, 148

L

Languages, 122
Legal issues, 258
LinkedIn, 250, 252
Litcoin, 176
Location-as-a-service, 57

M

Machine accuracy, 117
Machine learning, 66, 97, 110, 111, 118, 123, 135
    Challenges of, 117
    Classification of, 112
    Healthcare applications of,
Made-in-China, 229
Malpractice, 35
Mammography, 44
Manufacturing jobs, 243
Manufacturing of medicine, 238
Materials, 243
Media sharing
Medical data management, 179
Medical device, 242
Medical device manufacturing, 227
Medical health, 126
Medical imaging, 101
Medical professionals, 9, 88
Medical research, 102
Medication adherence, 72, 181
Medication errors, 9, 72, 85, 220
Medicine, 72
Mental health, 137, 205
Mhealth, see Mobile health
Microwave, 3
Misinformation, 258
Mixed reality, 204
Mobile health, 28, 39, 40, 43, 102
Benefits, 44
Challenges, 44
Mobile phones, 3, 28, 39, 40, 85, 102
Mobile social media, 255
Mobile technology, 3
Mode of transportation, 161
Monitoring, 22, 52, 57, see also Remote monitoring
    Of patients, 9, 85, 86
Monitoring system, 18
Morphology, 124

Myspace, 253

N

Nanomaterials, 189
Nanomedicine, 6, 67, 187, 188, 191, 193, 196
    Applications of, 190
    Benefits of, 194
    Challenges of, 195
Nanoparticles, 188
Nanorobots, 192
Nanoscience, 189
Nanotechnology, 6, 187, 189, 193, 196
Narrowband IoT (NBIoT), 50
National Aeronautics and Space Administration
    (NASA), 160
National Council of State Boards of Nursing
    (NCSBN), 256
National Health Service (NHS), 273
Natural language processing, 96, 122, 123-128, 134, 135
    In healthcare, 125, 135
    Global use of, 128
Netherlands, 219
Neural networks, 96
Neuroscience, 101
Nick Pelling, 264
Nike, 268
Noise, 89
Non-communicative diseases, 138, 193, 230
Nurses, 39, 48, 52, 55, 57, 88, 105, 139, 143, 158, 256, 257
Nursing, 146

O

Oncology, 115
Online analytical processing (OLAP), 217
One-size-fits-all medicine, 85
Online booking, 33
Opportunities, 73

P

Pakistan, 161
Pain reduction, 206
Passion, 251
Pathology, 115
Pathology detection, 68
Patient analysis, 217
Patient-centered care, 183
Patient experience, 206
Patient monitoring, 53, 68, 231
Patient reminders, 137
Patients, 75, 95, 137-140, 142, 158, 217, 251, 256, 268, 273,
    278, 284
    Care of, 104, 129, 149, 220, 254

Safety of, 127
Peer-to-peer network, 178
Personalization, 251
Personalized care, 139, 241
Personalized healthcare/medicine, 9, 115, 227
Pharmaceutical industry, 69
Pharmacists, 146, 158
Pharmacology, 239
Pharmacy, 116, 205
Phonetics, 124
Physical education, 269
Physicians, 87, 117, 139
Pinterest, 250
Portability, 21
Pragmatics, 125
Precision medicine, 85
Prediction, 220
Presentation, 214
Prior authorization, 127
Privacy, 35, 58, 74, 88, 105, 117, 139, 162, 171, 196
    Of patients, 258
Productivity, 171
Protection of data, 220
Poverty related diseases, 193
Psychiatry, 86
Public health, 84

Q

Quality, 56

R

Radiology, 100, 115, 125
Rapid prototyping, 237, 242
Readmission, 115, 117
Record management, 74
Reduced costs, 139
Regenerative medicine, 8
Regulation, 184, 243
    Compliance of, 231
    Of healthcare, 285
    Lack of, 23, 196
Rehabilitation, 146, 170
Reliability, 172
Remote monitoring, 9, 54, 74, see also Monitoring
Repeatability, 149
Reproductivity, 118
Research and development (R&D), 241
Richard Feymann, 189
Risks, 89, 286
Robotic nurses, 146
Robotic surgery, 55
Robotics, 3, 142, 143, 206, 279

Robots, 3, 4, 96, 142, 143, 150
    Applications of,144
    Different types of, 144
    Healthcare types, 148
    Medical type of, 96
Rural health/healthcare, 34, 157

S

Safety, 22, 149, 162, 172
Saudi Arabia, 260, 273
Security, 22, 74, 105, 149, 171
Self-care, 22
Semantics, 125
Sensors, 17, 18, 85, 96, 168, 203
Singapore, 161
Smart environment, 171
Smart everything, 51
Smart devices, 51, 64
Smart heath records, 116
Smart healthcare, 63
Smart home healthcare, 68
Smart hospitals, 69, 170, 228
Smart medication, 72
Smart technology, 54
Smartphones, 268
Social-sharing, 270
Social compatibility, 172
Social health, 251
Social media, 7, 8, 249-251, 256, 260
    Addiction of, 259
Social networking, 252
Social stigma, 258
Society 5.0, 230, 231
South Africa, 273, 282
Space shuttle, 33
Speech recognition, 127
Speed, 243
Sports medicine, 21
Standardization, 89
    Lack of, 184
Standards, 58
Sterolithography, 237
Stroke, 33
Supply chain analysis, 217
Surgery, 137, 206, 208
Syntax, 125

T

Taiwan, 260
Technologies, 1, 2, 49, 277, 283
Tele-education, 33
Teleaudiology, 32

Telecardiology, 33
Telecare, 29
Teleconsultation, 29, 43
Teledentistry, 32
Teledermatology, 30
Teleeverything, 10, 28, 29.33
Telehealth, 29, 74, 279
Telemedicine, 10, 25-28, 34, 35, 74, 86, 101, 133
    Types of, 27
Telementoring, 32
Telemonitoring, 29
Telenephrology, 32
Teleneuropsychology, 32
Telenursing, 32
Teleobstetrics, 32
Teleoncology, 32
Teleophthalmology, 31
Telepharmacy, 31
Telepathology, 31
Telepediatrics, 32
Telepresence, 146
Telepsychiatry, 30
Teleradiology, 30
Telerehabilitation, 30
Telesurgery, 31
Teletrauma care, 32
Testability, 43
Thailand, 230
Thailand 4.0, 230
Theft, 22
Third industrial revolution, 235
Tracking, 52, 57
Traditional healthcare/medicine, 62, 191, 246
Traditional manufacturing, 246
Training, 206, 207, 241
Transformation, 263
Transparency, 178
Trust, 139, 171
    Lack of, 259
Tuberculosis, 192

Tunisia, 181
Turkey, 282
Twitter, 250, 252

U

United Kingdom, 103, 181, 273, 283
United States, 160, 181, 193, 219, 229, 259, 273, 282
Universal access, 183
Unmanned aerial vehicles (UAV), 154, 155, see also
    Drones
User interface, 203

V

Virtual assistants, 102
Virtual environment, 200, 201
Virtual reality, 5, 200, 201, 204, 210
    Benefits of, 208
    Challenges, 209
Visualization, 88

W

Wearable biosensors, 20
Wearable devices, 19, 55
Wearable healthcare technology, 17, 23
    Applications of, 18
Wearable technologies, 3, 17, 23, 69, 168
Wearables, 15, 22
Weight loss, 270
Wiki, 251
Wikipedia, 251
Wireless body area network (WBAN), 20
Wireless sensor networks (WSN), 59, 168
Wireless technology, 2, 65
Workforce, 58, 74
World Health Organization (WHO)

Y

YouTube, 250, 253

Printed in the United States
by Baker & Taylor Publisher Services